# Handbook of
# Pediatric Radiology

# HANDBOOKS IN RADIOLOGY SERIES

## Other Volumes in Series

*Handbook of Chest Radiology,* Second Edition
**STUART A. GROSKIN, M.D.**

*Handbook of Gastrointestinal and Genitourinary Radiology*
**STEPHEN R. ELL, M.D., Ph.D.**

*Handbook of Head and Neck Imaging,* Second Edition
**H. RIC HARNSBERGER, M.D.**

*Handbook of Interventional Radiology and Angiography,* Second Edition
**MYRON WOJTOWYCZ, M.D.**

*Handbook of Neuroradiology: Brain and Skull,* Second Edition
**ANNE G. OSBORN, M.D. AND KAREN A. TONG, M.D.**

*Handbook of Nuclear Medicine,* Second Edition
**FREDERICK L. DATZ, M.D.**

*Handbook of Skeletal Radiology,* Second Edition
**B.J. MANASTER, M.D., Ph.D.**

*Handbook of Syndromes and Metabolic Disorders: Radiologic and Clinical Manifestations*
**HOOSHANG TAYBI, M.D.**

# Handbook of Pediatric Radiology

**Vesna Martich Kriss, M.D.**
Associate Professor
Section Chief, Pediatric Radiology
Departments of Radiology and Pediatrics
University of Kentucky Medical Center
University of Kentucky Children's Hospital
Lexington, Kentucky

with 170 *illustrations*

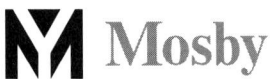 Mosby

St. Louis   Baltimore   Boston   Carlsbad   Chicago   Minneapolis   New York   Philadelphia   Portland
London   Milan   Sydney   Tokyo   Toronto

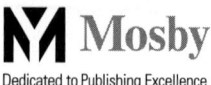
Mosby
Dedicated to Publishing Excellence

A Times Mirror
Company

*Managing Editor:* Elizabeth Corra
*Associate Developmental Editor:* Marla Sussman
*Project Manager:* Linda Clarke
*Associate Production Editor:* Theresa M. Petosa
*Senior Composition Specialist:* Kevin D. Dodds
*Designer:* Carolyn O'Brien
*Manufacturing Manager:* William A. Winneberger, Jr.

Copyright © 1998 by Mosby, Inc.

All rights reserved. No part of this publication may be reproduced, stored in a retrieval system, or transmitted, in any form or by any means, electronic, mechanical, photocopying, recording, or otherwise, without written permission of the publisher.

Permission to photocopy or reproduce solely for internal or personal use is permitted for libraries or other users registered with the Copyright Clearance Center, provided that the base fee of $4.00 per chapter plus $.10 per page is paid directly to the Copyright Clearance Center, 222 Rosewood Drive, Danvers, MA 01923. This consent does not extend to other kinds of copying, such as copying for general distribution, for advertising or promotional purposes, for creating new collected works, or for resale.

Printed in the United States of America
Composition by Mosby Electronic Production, Philadelphia
Printing/binding by R.R. Donnelley & Sons, Inc.

Mosby, Inc.
11830 Westline Industrial Drive
St. Louis, Missouri 63146

**Library of Congress Cataloging in Publication Data**
Kriss, Vesna Martich.
    Handbook of pediatric radiology / Vesna Martich Kriss.
       p.   cm. — (Handbooks in radiology series)
    Includes bibliographical references and index.
    ISBN 0-8151-3749-4
      1. Pediatric radiology—Handbooks, manuals, etc.  I. Title.
  II. Series.
      [DNLM: 1. Pediatrics—methods—handbooks.  2. Radiology—methods—handbooks.
  WS 39 K92h 1998]
  RJ51.R3K75   1998
  618.92′00757—dc21
  DNLM/DLC
for Library of Congress                                                   97–29968
                                                                               CIP

98  99  00  01  02  /  9  8  7  6  5  4  3  2  1

To my parents, Jovo and Slobodanka, and grandparents, Stevo and Stana:
you faced adversity with courage and integrity
and taught me what is truly important in life.

And to my husband Timothy,
for his unwavering love and support.

# Foreword

The amount of clinical information demanded of residents and nonspecialized practitioners of medicine at the present time has resulted in so many textbooks that limitations of time and expense handicap members of these two groups in the selection of information sources. One response to this circumstance has been the development of "handbooks" oriented toward easy access to varying degrees of knowledge in specialized fields. This *Handbook of Pediatric Radiology* is designed by Dr. Kriss for quick study of pertinent facts concerning practical pediatric radiology topics, which are presented in six sections covering anatomic systems and a seventh devoted to trauma. All in all, 44 chapters (frequently subdivided) provide key concepts in the identification of normal and pathologic processes in common and some less common conditions. Imaging techniques are emphasized, especially in regions where infections or trauma are frequent; interpretation clues and differential diagnoses are included throughout. Helpful clues for both anatomic variants and physical variations are noted, and technical suggestions are occasionally provided. Each chapter includes carefully selected references from journals as well as textbooks.

In short, Dr. Kriss tells the reader where and how to look, and what to look for, when diagnostic imaging is considered for pediatric patients.

Frederic N. Silverman, M.D.

# Preface

The *Handbook of Pediatric Radiology* was written to be a quick outline guide for practicing physicians and as a study tool for residents and students learning the basics of pediatric radiology. This book was clearly not intended to be an all-inclusive work encompassing the entire field of pediatric radiology. Instead, I refer the reader to such outstanding texts as *Caffey's Pediatric X-Ray Diagnosis* (edited by Frederic Silverman and Jerald Kuhn), *Practical Pediatric Imaging* (edited by Donald Kirks), and *Radiology of Syndromes, Metabolic Disorders, and Skeletal Dysplasias* (by Hooshang Taybi and Ralph Lachman).

This handbook is designed to offer practical and useful comments concerning pediatric entities that are commonly encountered in daily practice. The book is divided into seven subsections that comprise the six organ systems (airway and chest, gastrointestinal, cardiac, genitourinary, musculoskeletal and neurologic) as well as a subsection on trauma. Each of the 44 chapters begins with "key concepts" that summarize the most common or important points of the chapter. Embryologic and developmental descriptions are also provided. Within each disease description is a listing of etiology, demographics, treatment, and prognosis, if possible. More unusual and rare diseases are still mentioned, albeit briefly. The main focus of the handbook, however, remains imaging findings and radiographic approach to pediatric diseases. Suggested readings are also provided at the end of each chapter for those who wish to further explore specific topics.

Vesna Martich Kriss, M.D.

# Acknowledgments

Such a project would not have been possible without the help and inspiration of many people. My sincere thanks to my proofreaders: Diane Babcock, Brad Betz, Carol Cottrill, Nirmala Desai, Elizabeth Jackson, Neil Johnson, Bernadette Koch, Lori Shook, and Janet Strife. Their insightful comments were greatly appreciated and certainly improved the manuscript. My thanks also to the illustrator, Melissa Garland, who developed the superb figures and illustrations seen throughout the book. Special thanks to Kim Dupin, my secretary, who helped in the cross-checking of some 500 references. My gratitude also to the editors at Mosby–Year Book. Elizabeth Corra, Marla Sussman, and Theresa Petosa were organized, helpful, efficient, and quite simply a pleasure to work with.

Personal thanks to the many mentors I have been so fortunate to have encountered in my academic career. From John Fennessy, who gave me my start in radiology, to Andrew Poznanski and the staff at Children's Memorial Hospital (Chicago), who first introduced me to the wonders of pediatric radiology. To Janet Strife and the staff at Children's Hospital Medical Center (Cincinnati), who gave me a world of knowledge and the confidence to use it. And finally, to Andrew Fried, who continues to teach me how to be a successful academic radiologist with grace and integrity.

I also must thank the many clinicians at the University of Kentucky Children's Hospital. It is a privilege and honor to work closely with these outstanding physicians. Their expertise and professionalism are to be commended. Contributing to the care of Kentucky's children continues to be one of the most rewarding aspects of my work.

And lastly, thanks to the countless radiology residents, clinical housestaff, and students for whom this book is written. Your continuing interest, curiosity, and enthusiasm is what makes our job fun.

# Contents

Foreword, vii

Preface, ix

Acknowledgments, xi

I  Airway and Chest, 1

    1  Airway, 2

    2  Neonatal Chest, 16

    3  Pneumonia, 29

    4  Pulmonary Circulation, 38

    5  Congenital Lung Lesions, 44

    6  Chronic Lung Disorders, 50

    7  Mediastinal Masses, 58

II  Gastrointestinal System, 71

    8  Neonatal Abdomen: Bowel Obstruction and Masses, 72

    9  Abnormalities of the Foregut (Esophagus and Stomach), 87

    10  Abnormalities of the Midgut (Small Bowel), 97

    11  Abnormalities of the Hindgut (Large Bowel), 109

    12  Acute Abdomen, 117

13 Hepatobiliary System, 126

14 Pancreas and Spleen, 137

## III Cardiac and Great Vessels, 147

15 Congenital Heart Disease: Radiographic Approach, 148

16 Congenital Heart Disease—Acyanotic, 156

17 Congenital Heart Disease—Cyanotic, 165

18 Surgical Repair of Congenital Heart Disease, 172

19 Situs Abnormalities, 177

20 Congenital Abnormalities of the Aortic Arch, 181

## IV Genitourinary System, 193

21 Congenital Renal Abnormalities, 194

22 Lower Urinary (Bladder and Urethra) Development and Disorders, 206

23 Urinary Tract Infection, 216

24 Acquired Renal Disease, 223

25 Renal Masses, 230

26 Genital Development and Disorders, 235

## V Trauma, 245

27 Musculoskeletal Trauma, 246

28 Nonaccidental Trauma (Child Abuse), 258

29 Abdominal Trauma, 266

## VI  Musculoskeletal System, 273

- 30  Musculoskeletal Infection, 274
- 31  Lesions of Bone—Benign and Malignant, 282
- 32  Axial Skeleton: Spine and Skull, 293
- 33  Hip and Knee, 301
- 34  The Foot, 314
- 35  Bony Abnormalities in Metabolic, Endocrine, and Hematopoietic Disorders, 321
- 36  Skeletal Dysplasias, 332

## VII  Neurologic System: Head and Neck, 341

- 37  Congenital Brain Malformations, 342
- 38  Neonatal Head, 354
- 39  Central Nervous System Infections, 364
- 40  Brain Neoplasms, 370
- 41  Metabolic Brain Disorders, 378
- 42  Head and Neck Lesions, 386
- 43  Spine, 395
- 44  Orbital Lesions, 404

Index, 412

# SECTION I
Airway and Chest

# 1
# Airway

### Key Concepts

1. Smaller size of the infant airway renders it highly susceptible to edema from infectious (viral) or reactive airway disease and can lead to significant air trapping of the lungs.
2. Normal expiratory film can demonstrate physiologic "shouldering" of the subglottic region versus pathologic "steepling" of the airway, seen with tracheobronchitis or croup.
3. Edematous enlargement of the epiglottis is an emergency (epiglottitis) and can radiographically manifest as the "thumbprint sign."
4. Airway masses in the pediatric population are almost always benign lesions, most commonly hemangiomas.
5. Infantile inspiratory stridor is most commonly caused by laryngomalacia, an abnormality due to soft, flaccid laryngeal tissues. Ninety percent of cases will resolve within 2 years.

A. Anatomy.
   1. Normal anatomy: Evaluation should be performed on nonrotated, inspiratory film.
      a. Lateral film (Fig. 1-1, *A*).
         *1.* Identify:
            *a.* Nasopharyngeal airway/adenoids.
            *b.* Soft palate, uvula.
            *c.* Oral airway, tongue.
            *d.* Epiglottis/aryepiglottic folds.
            *e.* Piriform sinuses.
            *f.* Retropharyngeal soft tissues.
      b. Anteroposterior (AP) film (Fig. 1-1, *B*).
         *1.* Identify:
            *a.* Subglottic region (at level of piriform sinuses).
            *b.* Smooth, symmetric, and parallel tracheal walls.
   2. Normal radiographic variants.
      a. Be aware of expiratory radiograph, which can be misleading.
         *1.* Normal expiratory lateral radiograph shows "buckling" or sharp anterior angulation of airway just above thoracic inlet (Fig. 1-2, *A*). This appearance often mimics retropharyngeal widening (normal prevertebral or retropharyngeal space is about one vertebral body length).
         *2.* Normal expiratory AP radiograph (Fig. 1-2, *B*) demonstrates shouldering at subglottic region (closure of vocal cords) versus pathologic steepling (Fig. 1-3; see discussion of croup).
      b. Obtaining adequate inspiratory radiograph from uncooperative pediatric patient can be difficult. In situations when adequate radiographs can not be obtained despite repeated attempts, airway fluoroscopy (with videotape of procedure) can be attempted to evaluate structures of airway.
B. Physiology.
   1. Most important factor: size. Narrower pediatric airway diameter (as compared with adults) is more readily compromised by infectious or inflammatory narrowing, internal lesions, or external compression.
   2. Result: the smaller the child, the more likely airway pathology will be symptomatic.
C. Pathology.
   1. Infectious or inflammatory.
      a. Viral croup (acute tracheolaryngobronchitis).
         *1.* Most common cause of upper airway obstruction (stridor) in children.
         *2.* Occurs between 3 months and 5 years, mostly in children less than 2 years of age.

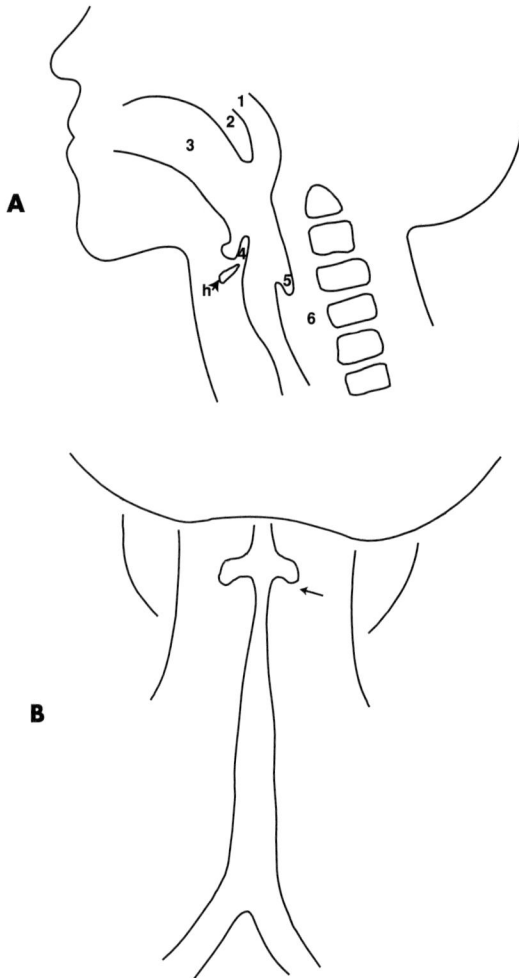

**Fig. 1-1** **A,** Lateral view of airway (inspiratory). Following structures are labeled: nasopharyngeal airway *(1)*, soft palate, uvula *(2)*, oral airway *(3)*, epiglottis *(4)*, piriform sinus *(5)*, retropharyngeal soft tissues *(6)*, hyoid bone *(h)*. **B,** AP view of airway (inspiratory). Subglottic region is seen at level of piriform sinuses *(arrow)*.

    3. Barky cough with inspiratory stridor; retractions may be present on physical examination.
    4. Subglottic edema is present; significantly reduces tracheal lumen diameter.
    5. Etiology is viral.
    6. Treatment.

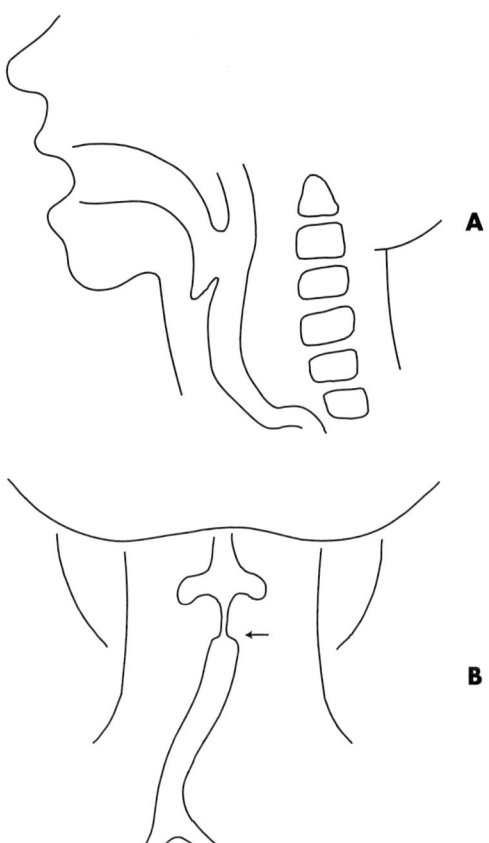

**Fig. 1-2 A,** Lateral view of airway (expiratory). Buckling is present in airway at lower cervical level just above thoracic inlet, mimicking retropharyngeal widening; **B,** AP view of airway (expiratory). Normal shouldering is seen in subglottic region *(arrow)*.

      *a.* Self-limiting viral etiology: supportive, symptomatic treatment only is needed.
      *b.* In rare cases, patients need to be hospitalized and even intubated due to potential for respiratory arrest.

**Imaging** Symmetric subglottic narrowing (steeple sign, Fig. 1-3) with distension or "ballooning" of hypopharynx on lateral radiograph of airway.

  b. Membranous croup (bacterial tracheitis).

**6** Handbook of Pediatric Radiology

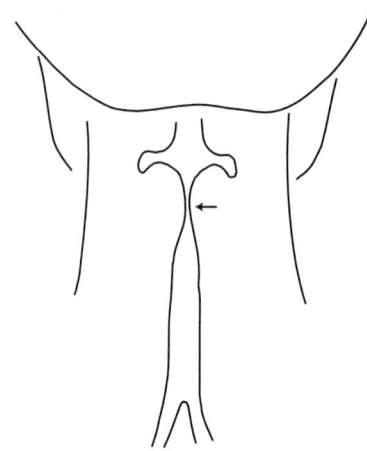

**Fig. 1-3** AP view of airway. Subglottic narrowing *(arrow)* or steepling, as seen with viral croup.

1. Emergency: necrotizing inflammation of airway can produce adherent mucopurulent membranes that can obstruct airway if they detach.
2. Etiology is bacterial, often in conjunction with viral infection.
3. Tends to be seen in older children (unlike viral croup, usually seen in infants and younger children).
4. Treatment.
   a. Emergent bronchoscopy.
   b. Performed to strip membranes from tracheal walls.

> **Imaging** Looks like croup with subglottic narrowing (steepling) on neck radiograph. However, check airway closely for irregular tracheal walls or visible soft-tissue strands along wall of trachea.

c. Epiglottitis.
   1. Emergency: edematous enlargement of epiglottits and aryepiglottic folds, which can close off airway.
   2. Etiology is *Haemophilus influenzae* (recently much lower incidence of this emergent entity owing to widespread *H. influenzae* immunizations).
   3. Presents with fever, sore throat, dysphagia, drooling, and anxiety.
   4. Usually seen in children 3 to 6 years of age.
   5. Subglottic narrowing (croup) may coexist.

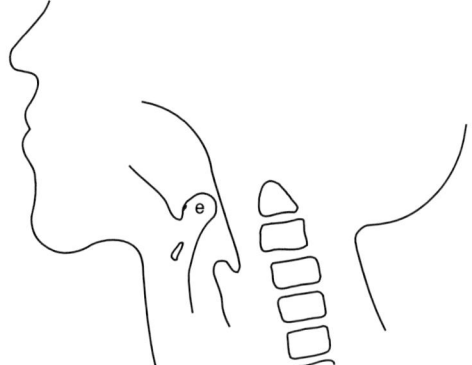

**Fig. 1-4** Epiglottitis. Marked enlargement of epiglottis *(e)*, known as thumbprint sign.

   6. Treatment.
      a. Elective intubation (by experienced person) to secure the airway.
      b. Antibiotics.

> **Imaging** Lateral neck radiograph demonstrates marked enlargement of epiglottis (thumbprint sign) and aryepiglottic folds (Fig. 1-4). Often see ballooning of hypopharynx owing to obstructive nature of enlarged epiglottis and aryepiglottic folds.

   d. Retropharyngeal abscess.
      1. Early childhood, usually related to suppurative lymphadenopathy from infections of ears, nose, sinuses, and throat. Can be a complication of penetrating neck injury.
      2. Presents with fever, sore throat, and often signs of airway compromise because of airway compression (shortness of breath, stridor, drooling).
      3. Treatment.
         a. Surgical drainage of retropharyngeal abscess.
         b. Recently, however, some physicians have advocated more conservative approach, using antibiotics only.
      4. Differential of prevertebral or retropharyngeal mass.
         a. Normal variant (expiratory film).
         b. Cystic hygroma.
         c. Hemangioma.
         d. Neuroblastoma.

e. Retropharyngeal goiter.
f. Lymphoma.
g. Rhabdomyosarcoma.
h. Esophageal foreign body.
i. Trauma.
   1) Hematoma from cervical spine injury.
   2) Traumatic diverticulum.

**Imaging** Lateral neck radiograph shows widening of prevertebral or retropharyngeal tissues with anterior displacement of airway. Piriform sinuses are usually missing (compressed by retropharyngeal pathology). Can sometimes see retropharyngeal gas within abscess. Contrast-enhanced computed tomography (CT) can define retropharyngeal abscess (low-density collection with mass effect upon airway).

e. Mononucleosis.
   1. Usually seen in older children or adolescents, rare in children less than 3 years of age.
   2. Etiology is Epstein-Barr virus.
   3. Highly infectious; often presents with fever, pharyngitis with dysphagia, generalized adenopathy and splenomegaly.
   4. Self-limiting; supportive, symptomatic treatment only.

**Imaging** Tonsils and adenoids may be massively enlarged, although usually without compromise to airway.

2. Airway masses.
   a. Airway masses in pediatric population are almost always benign lesions. However, tumors such as rhabdomyosarcoma and lymphoma of head and neck can involve airway (see Chapter 42).
   b. Papillomas.
      1. Most common laryngeal tumor in children.
      2. Etiology is papillomavirus, probably acquired from mother during delivery (may be history of maternal condylomata acuminata or genital warts).
      3. Lesions are characteristically found along anterior part of larynx (true or false cord) and extend into subglottic area, but can occur anywhere along respiratory tract.
      4. Presents with stridor, wheezing, or hoarseness.
      5. Transbronchial spread of laryngeal papillomatosis into lung; lesions can cavitate, worrisome complication.
      6. Treatment involves removal of papillomas, via laser therapy, if possible; however, lesions can recur.

> **Imaging** Neck radiograph can show multiple lobulated, eccentric, soft-tissue masses within airway, usually near glottic or subglottic area.

    c. Hemangiomas.
        *1.* Most common mass in infancy to cause airway obstruction.
        *2.* Most appear by 3 years of age; found more commonly in females than in males.
        *3.* Associated cutaneous hemangiomas ("strawberry") (50%).
        *4.* Presents with cough, inspiratory stridor and hoarseness if lesion actually involves true cords.
        *5.* Treatment.
            *a.* Often spontaneously regress with time.
            *b.* Laser therapy can remove symptomatic lesions.

> **Imaging** Radiograph of neck can show soft-tissue mass causing persistent, eccentric deformation of airway.

    d. Airway obstruction by foreign body.
        *1.* Usually toddlers, developmentally delayed patients.
        *2.* Presents with stridor, wheezing, cough, pneumonia.
        *3.* Aspirated foreign body usually lodges in bronchi (in right bronchi more commonly than in left).
        *4.* Type.
            *a.* Nonradioopaque (peanuts, hot dogs, candy, etc.).
            *b.* Radioopaque (coins, bone, eggshell, etc.).
        *5.* Complications.
            *a.* Esophageal foreign body can narrow airway.
            *b.* Long-term esophageal foreign body can also erode through esophageal wall, causing tracheoesophageal fistula or abscess.
        *6.* Treatment.
            *a.* If foreign body is in bronchi:
                *1)* Bronchoscopy to diagnose and remove foreign body.
            *b.* If foreign body is in esophagus:
                *1)* Some physicians have advocated removal using balloon-tipped catheter under fluoroscopic guidance. Procedure is risky owing to possible aspiration of esophageal foreign body, as it is being removed.
                *2)* Endoscopic removal.

> **Imaging** Look for asymmetric aeration of lungs on chest radiograph. If foreign body totally obstructs airway, atelectasis
>
> *Continued*

> *Continued from previous page*
> will ensue. Partial or "ball-valve" foreign body will permit air to enter lungs, but not to leave. As a result, affected side will be more lucent, as persistent air trapping occurs. In addition, decubitus films can also demonstrate persistent air trapping (better seen in older children). "Down" or dependent side should normally become less lucent than "up" side. If not, air trapping is suspected. Airway fluoroscopy has also been helpful: with forced expiration, the mediastinum moves to non–air-trapping side.

   e. Juvenile angiofibroma.
      1. Benign but highly vascular lesion in posterior nasal cavity.
      2. Found almost exclusively in adolescent males.
      3. Presents with epistaxis, nasal obstruction.
      4. Treatment.
         a. Angiography for embolization.
         b. Subsequent surgery if needed following embolization.

> **Imaging** Facial radiograph can demonstrate anterior bowing of posterior maxillary wall, which may have bony erosion. Nasal septum displacement can occur with mass in nasopharyngeal airway. Contrast-enhanced CT demonstrates enhancing soft-tissue mass in posterior nasopharynx.

   f. Malignant primary lesions of airway (rare).
      1. Bronchial carcinoid (neuroectodermal tumor).
      2. Adenocystic carcinoma (cylindroma).
      3. Mucoepidermoid (mucin producing).
      4. Granular cell myoblastoma (schwannoma).
3. Congenital or developmental.
   a. Choanal atresia.
      1. Most common congenital abnormality of nose (1:5000).
      2. Found more commonly in females than in males; more likely to be unilateral.
      3. Usually caused by focal choanal obstruction, which is bony or membranous (90%). Choanal narrowing can also be caused by maxillary hypoplasia or turbinate hyperplasia.
      4. Associated with craniofacial abnormalities (Treacher Collins syndrome).
      5. Respiratory distress at birth, especially with feeds.
      6. Diagnosis suspected clinically when unable to pass nasogastric (NG) tube.

**Imaging** CT scan shows medial bowing of lateral walls of nasal cavity with bony or membranous bridge seen in posterior nasal cavity. Bridge occludes or narrows nasopharyngeal passage (intranasal administration of decongestants to decrease secretions can help eliminate false-positive results by better visualizing bony or membranous bridge).

   b. Tracheal agenesis or atresia.
      1. During differentiation of primitive foregut (which eventually forms larynx, trachea, and esophagus), aberrant ventral deviation of tracheoesophageal septum can occur (at about the twenty-first to twenty-fifth day of gestation causing tracheal agenesis [Fig. 1-5]).
      2. Types (Fig. 1-6).
         a. Type I (absence of proximal trachea).
         b. Type II.
            1) Absence of trachea to level of carina.
            2) Most common.
         c. Type III (both bronchi arise directly from esophagus).
      3. Immediate respiratory distress, but no audible cry.
      4. Treatment.
         a. Aeration is maintained via esophageal intubation.
         b. No long-term treatment for this lethal abnormality.

**Imaging** Chest radiograph shows bilateral atelectasis of lungs, resembling severe surfactant deficiency disorder (SDD).

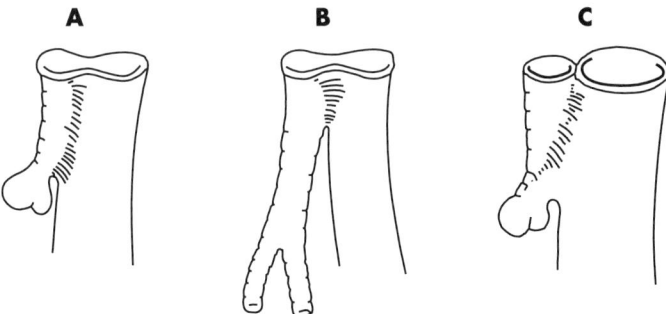

**Fig. 1-5** Tracheoesophageal septum. Normal formation. **A,** Developing foregut with lateral esophageal groove, beginning to separate into dorsal (digestive) and ventral (respiratory) portions. **B,** Near complete separation of normal developing trachea and esophagus. **C,** Aberrant lateral esophageal groove can "cut off" ventral tracheal portion causing tracheal agenesis.

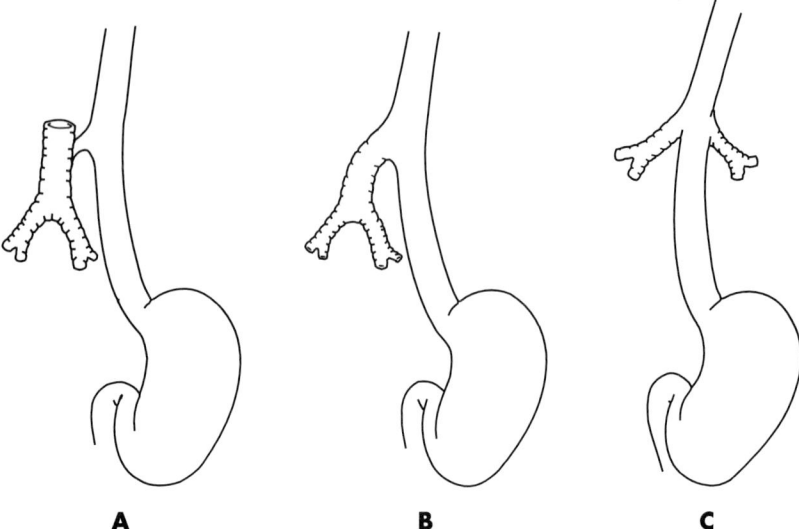

**Fig. 1-6** Types of tracheal agenesis.

    c. Tracheal bronchus ("pig bronchus").
        1. Tracheal bronchus is normal anatomy for pig, hence nickname.
        2. Right upper lobe (RUL) bronchus arises directly from trachea; difficulty in clearing secretions from RUL because of this anomalous bronchus.
        3. Usually asymptomatic, but can have recurrent RUL atelectasis and pneumonias.
        4. Associated with Down syndrome.
        5. Bronchoscopy confirms diagnosis with direct suction of RUL, performed to relieve obstruction or secretions.
        6. Surgical removal of RUL anomalous bronchus can be done in severely symptomatic patients.

> **Imaging** Chest radiograph demonstrates persistent RUL opacity, usually with volume loss.

    d. Esophageal bronchus.
        1. Extra lung bud from foregut is cause of anomalous bronchus.
        2. Anomalous esophageal bronchus connects to lower lobes of lungs and usually has systemic arterial supply.
        3. Found more commonly in females than in males (2:1).
        4. Presents with chronic, persistent pulmonary infections.
        5. Treatment is surgical resection of aberrant bronchus.

> **Imaging** Chest radiograph shows persistent lobar opacity (usually in the lower lobes). Occasionally, anomalous esophageal bronchus is seen during upper gastrointestinal (UGI) examination.

  e. Laryngomalacia.
    1. Infantile inspiratory stridor, worse when supine.
    2. Etiology is due to soft, flaccid laryngeal tissues that readily infold, leading to collapse and obstruction of airway upon expiration.
    3. Ninety percent of cases resolve within 2 years as airway matures and firms up.

> **Imaging** No abnormality is seen, except possibly marked collapse of airway upon expiration only. Persistent airway narrowing is not present.

  f. Tracheomalacia.
    1. Majority present before 1 year of age (90%).
    2. Narrowing of tracheal lumen with rigid and nondistensible tracheal walls, resulting in inhibited airflow.
    3. Primary (intrinsic) tracheomalacia.
        a. Caused by complete cartilaginous rings.
        b. Weak supporting cartilage.
            1) Larsen syndrome.
            2) Relapsing polychondritis.
    4. Secondary (extrinsic) tracheomalacia.
        a. Long-standing vascular compression.
            1) Vascular rings.
                a) Double aortic arch.
                b) Right arch with anomalous left subclavian.
                c) Pulmonary sling.
                d) Anomalous innominate artery compression.
                    (1) Innominate artery passes anterior to and can compress trachea, causing apnea, stridor, and cough.
                    (2) This entity is usually asymptomatic. Possibly related to more distal location of innominate artery, as it branches from aortic arch (see Fig. 20-7).
            2) Can lead to localized tracheal stenosis or tracheomalacia, even after vascular insult has been removed.
            3) Often associated with complete tracheal rings or severe tracheomalacia.

b. Granulation tissue or scarring from prior intubation or tracheal injury.
   c. Tracheoesophageal fistula.
   d. Mass (such as bronchogenic cyst).
5. Treatment of tracheomalacia.
   a. If possible, relieve obstruction causing airway compromise.
      1) Repair vascular ring.
      2) Remove tracheal granulation tissue.
      3) Reposition innominate artery more anterior to trachea, using aortopexy procedure (aorta is sutured to sternum).
   b. In some cases, tracheostomy is needed to bypass obstruction.
   c. Occasionally, nothing can be done to relieve obstruction (complete tracheal rings).

**Imaging** Persistent narrowing of air column can be seen on neck or chest radiograph. Airway fluoroscopy may also demonstrate lack of airway distension. Bronchoscopy can confirm significance of compression. Magnetic resonance imaging (MRI) is particularly helpful for imaging potential vascular rings or external airway compression.

   g. Macroglossia.
      1. Large tongue can cause airway obstruction.
      2. Often seen with congenital syndromes.
         a. Down syndrome.
         b. Beckwith-Wiedemann syndrome.
         c. Mucopolysaccharidoses (Hurler syndrome).
         d. Pierre Robin syndrome (small mandible with proportionally large tongue).
      3. Tracheostomy can be done in severe cases of airway obstruction; often tonsilloadenoidectomy is helpful.

**Imaging** Neck radiograph may show large tongue compressing vallecula; can cause significant airway compression, particularly in supine position.

**SUGGESTED READINGS**

Barkovich AJ: Congenital nasal masses. *AJNR* 1991; 12:105-116.
Benjamin B: Tracheomalacia in infants and children. *Ann Otol Rhinol Laryngol* 1984; 93:438-442.
Capitanio M, Kirkpatrick JA: Upper respiratory obstruction in infants and children. *Radiol Clin North Am* 1986; 6:265-277.

Esclamado RM, Richardson MA: Laryngotracheal foreign bodies in children. *Am J Dis Child* 1987; 141:259-262.

Greenholz SK, Karrer FM, Lilly JR: Contemporary surgery of tracheomalacia. *J Pediatr Surg* 1986; 21:511-514.

Han BK, Dunbar JS, Striker TW: Membranous laryngotracheobronchitis (membranous croup). *AJR* 1979; 133:53-58.

Manson D, Babyn P, Filler R, Holowka S: Three dimensional imaging of the pediatric trachea in congenital tracheal stenosis. *Pediatr Radiol* 1994; 24:175-178.

Oh KS, Newman B, Bowen A: Pediatric airway disorders: Practical approaches to imaging evaluation. *Curr Probl Diagn Radiol* 1989; 18:199-231.

Rothrock SG, Pignatiello GA, Howard RM: Radiologic diagnosis of epiglottitis. *Ann Emerg Med* 1990; 19:978-982.

Sato Y, Dunbar JS: Abnormalities of the pharynx and prevertebral soft tissues in infectious mononucleosis. *AJR* 1980; 134:149-152.

Simoneaux SF, Bank ER, Webber JB, Parks WJ: MR imaging of the pediatric airway. *Radiographics* 1995; 15:287-300.

Slovis TL, Renfro B, Watts FB: Choanal atresia: Precise CT evaluation. *Radiology* 1985; 155:345-348.

Strife JL, Baumael AS, Dunbar JS: Tracheal compression by the innominate artery in infancy and childhood. *Radiology* 1981; 139:73-75.

Strife JL: Upper airway obstruction in infants and children. *Radiol Clin North Am* 1988; 26: 2-12.

# 2
# Neonatal Chest

---

### Key Concepts

1. Surfactant deficiency disorder (SDD) occurs predominantly in premature infants. Hallmark radiographic findings include: small lung volumes, air bronchograms, and granular appearance of lungs.
2. When "white" or increasing opacity of the neonatal lung is present, general differential possibilities include:
    a. Atelectasis (SDD, mucus plugs, aberrent endotracheal [ET] tube placement).
    b. Fluid (pulmonary edema, hemorrhage, pleural effusion).
    c. Neonatal pneumonia (aspiration).
    d. Mass (sequestration, fluid-filled cystic adenomatoid malformation [CAM], herniated abdominal contents).
3. Air leak (pneumothorax, pneumomediastinum) can be subtle. Look for increasing lucency of the hemithorax or along the cardiac border.
4. Respiratory distress in the newborn can be broken down into two main categories: medically versus surgically treated conditions.

A. Medically treated conditions.
   1. Transient tachypnea of newborn (TTN).
      a. Full-term infants, often following cesarean section or infants of diabetic mothers.
      b. Symptomatic within first 2 to 4 hours of life, with grunting and/or tachypnea.
      c. Caused by retained fetal lung fluid (edema or pleural fluid); found more commonly in right than in left lung.
      d. Treatment is supportive only, as this condition usually resolves within 24 to 48 hours.

   **Imaging** Chest radiograph reveals normal lung volumes with increased pulmonary markings; often fluid can be seen within minor fissure.

   2. SDD (see box on p. 18).
      a. Previously known as hyaline membrane disease (HMD) or respiratory distress syndrome (RDS).
      b. Over 95% are premature infants, males more often than females.
      c. Lack of surfactant production (by immature Type II alveolar cells) in neonate results in increased alveolar surface tension, leading to increased alveolar atelectasis.
      d. Mild, uncomplicated cases can resolve in 48 to 72 hours, as normal physiologic surfactant production is initiated.
      e. Prevention.
         *1.* If possible, administer prenatal agents that can hasten lung maturity.
         *2.* Corticosteroids and thyroid releasing hormone.
      f. Treatment.
         *1.* Positive pressure ventilation.
         *2.* Tracheal surfactant administration.
      g. Complications of SDD.
         *1.* Generally result from ventilatory therapy used.
         *2.* "Air leak" problems.
            *a.* Pulmonary interstitial emphysema (PIE).
            *b.* Pneumothorax.
            *c.* Pneumomediastinum.
         *3.* Chronic lung changes (BPD).
      h. Abnormal surfactant production (surfactant B deficiency).
         *1.* First recognized inborn error of surfactant metabolism (inability to make surfactant protein B, one of four crucial surfactant proteins).
         *2.* Thought to be autosomal recessive.

## Classification of SDD: Changes with New Therapies over Last Three Decades

1. Original Northway classification (1967).*
   - Stage I: 2 to 3 days, HMD.
   - Stage II: 4 to 10 days (coarse reticular markings).
   - Stage III: 10 to 20 days (combination of atelectasis and emphysematous changes, pulmonary interstitial emphysema [PIE] often present).
   - Stage IV: greater than 20 days, bullae enlargement with cystic lung changes, or bronchopulmonary dysplasia (BPD).
2. Modified classification.†
   - 1 to 5 days.
     - SDD, or "evolving" SDD.
     - Outcome: Infant either becomes "normal" or will have chronic lung changes (ranging from mild to severe). However, need to wait at least 21 days prior to administering chronic lung "label."
   - 6 to 20 days.
     - Pulmonary insufficiency of the premature (PIP) also known as "hazy lungs of prematurity" (related to mild residual atelectasis and "hypoplastic" lungs of the premature).
     - Majority of infants with PIP will have normal lungs as they grow and mature. (Remember to always look out for appearance of air leak [PIE or pneumothorax] in ventilated infants.)
     - During this time, some infants develop increased pulmonary markings and/or early air trapping, findings that can signal impending chronic change. This appearance has been called "Leaky lung syndrome" (LLS), condition that is probably precursor to chronic lung changes, and is presumed caused by capillary damage from oxygen therapy and ventilatory support.
   - Greater than 21 days.
     - Last stage is chronic lung, defined as persistently abnormal chest x-ray in infant more than 21 days old.
     - Clinical definition of chronic lung change is similar: oxygen requirement in infant greater than 1 month of age.
     - Previous term of BPD is reserved for those infants who develop classic "bubbly" lung appearance with diffuse air trapping of lungs.

*Data from Northway WH, Rosen RC, Porter DY. Pulmonary disease following respiratory therapy of hyaline membrane disease: Bronchopulmonary dysplasia. *N Engl J Med* 1967; 276:357-368.
†Data from Swischuk LE, John SD: Immature lung problems: Can our nomenclature be more specific? *AJR* 1996; 166:917-918.

3. Fatal respiratory disease; some physicians have suggested lung transplantation as possible treatment.
4. Presents like regular SDD, except occurs in full-term infants who temporarily improve with surfactant administration. However, progressive hypoxic respiratory failure occurs.
5. Alveolar proteinosis is present.

**Imaging** Chest radiograph shows classic triad of SDD: hypoventilated lungs, "granular" lungs, and air bronchograms. Ranges from mild to severe changes (complete "white out" of lungs).

3. PIE.
    a. Rupture of terminal airways or alveoli.
    b. Air dissects along bronchovascular sheaths to lung periphery.
    c. More common in "micro" premature infants.
        1. Have larger interstitial space.
        2. Due to decreased alveolar volume in immature lungs.
    d. Treatment.
        1. Reduce ventilatory pressures, allowing interstitial air to resorb on its own.
        2. Use high-frequency ventilation.
        3. Can try selective intubation away from affected side or place infant decubitus with affected side down. This allows affected side to collapse, and may hasten resorption of PIE.

**Imaging** Chest radiograph demonstrates bubbly lungs (linear lucent bubbles of air trapped in interstitium, radiating out from hilar regions). Lungs often appear hyperaerated, changing little with expiration.

4. Air leak (pneumothorax and pneumomediastinum).
    a. Can be spontaneous finding; usually complication of mechanical ventilation. Can see PIE prior to actual pneumothorax; therefore, PIE can act as warning of impending further air leak.
    b. Cross-table lateral film helpful in elucidation of anterior pneumothorax.
    c. Pneumomediastinum.
        1. Uplifted thymus.
        2. Lucency around cardiothymic silhouette.
    d. Treatment.
        1. Pneumothorax.
            a. Nitrogen "wash out."
                1) Administer 100% oxygen, causing absorption of nitrogen.

2) Contraindications.
    a) Premature infants, because of risk of retinopathy of prematurity (ROP).
    b) Positive pressure ventilation.
   b. "Needling chest" or chest tube placement to remove air leak.
   c. Remember, most of air will be anterior in supine child; therefore, anterior location of chest tube is advantageous. Occasionally, in minimally symptomatic child, air is resorbed on its own, without intervention.
2. Pneumomediastinum.
   a. Usually no intervention.
   b. Watch for potential pneumothorax.

> **Imaging** Can be subtle finding. On chest radiograph, look for increasing lucency of hemithorax as compared with other side. Can also have flattening or inversion of diaphragm and mediastinal shift, with increasing tension of pneumothorax. Costophrenic angles can also appear more lucent and deep.

5. BPD.
   a. Results from prolonged $O_2$ therapy and positive pressure ventilation; factors such as air leaks and lung infections can accentuate development of BPD.
   b. Previously, 35% of ventilator-dependent SDD developed BPD. However, classic "cystic BPD" is less common today, because mainstay of treatment is surfactant administration not just positive pressure ventilation. Use of oscillating ventilators and lung-maturing agents administered prenatally have also reduced and changed appearance of chronic lung from prematurity.
   c. Treatment.
      1. Supportive treatment only as needed (oxygen therapy).
      2. Some physicians advocate course of steroid therapy to reduce initial severity of BPD.
      3. Lung alveoli are still capable of formation and growth after birth (up to about 8 years of age); therefore, infant with BPD and/or oxygen dependence will improve with time.

> **Imaging** Originally described as persistently hyperaerated lungs with cystic bubbly change and chronic fibrotic markings on chest radiograph. Today, with improving therapies, true bubbly BPD is not commonly seen. Instead, lungs demonstrate mild air trapping with varying degrees of

increased pulmonary markings (presumed chronic fibrotic change).

6. Wilson-Mikity syndrome.
   a. Unknown etiology; initially described in infants prior to modern ventilatory therapy. Some physicians have suggested infectious etiology.
   b. No initial symptoms; respiratory difficulties develop in first few weeks and months of life.
   c. Treatment.
      1. Like BPD, no definitive treatment except for supportive.
      2. Again, antenatal lung growth often results in improvement of condition with time.

**Imaging** Can resemble BPD with radiographic findings of air trapping, coarse reticular markings, and cystic lung changes. However, unlike BPD, these infants did not undergo oxygen or ventilatory support.

7. Neonatal aspiration (meconium).
   a. Usually full-term or postmature infants.
   b. Intrauterine fetal distress can result in early release of meconium.
   c. Aspiration can vary from only amniotic fluid (mild lung changes) to aspiration of thick, tenacious meconium, which can cause severe chemical pneumonitis.
   d. Can be associated with pneumothorax.
   e. Treatment.
      1. Can be prevented with early suctioning of aspirate at birth (perineal suction) if possible. Nothing but supportive care in milder cases.
      2. Aspiration of meconium with resulting severe pneumonitis can be life threatening; ventilatory support with extracorporeal membrane oxygenation (ECMO) has been used in these infants. ECMO provides ventilatory and perfusion support to rest lungs, allowing them to heal.

**Imaging** Chest radiograph demonstrates hyperaeration of lungs (due to air trapping caused by thick, tenacious meconium) with varying degrees of reticular, often nodular infiltrate. Pneumothorax may be present.

8. Neonatal pneumonia.
   a. Often associated with maternal early rupture of membranes.
   b. Infection can occur in utero, during passage through vagina, or shortly after birth.

c. Afebrile, can have marked respiratory distress; often few if any clinical signs.
d. Usually bacterial source.
 1. Group B *Streptococcus*.
 2. *Escherichia coli*.
e. *Ureaplasma urealyticum*.
 1. Considered when lungs display "precocious chronic change" (similar appearance to chronic lung change in infant during first 2 weeks of life).
 2. Associated with subsequent chronic lung changes.
 3. Treat with erythromycin (often empiric treatment, because of long time period for laboratory diagnosis and rapidity of lung damage from this organism).
f. Treatment is appropriate antibiotic and supportive therapy.

**Imaging** Findings on chest radiograph vary, but can be commonly seen as coarse, patchy infiltrates. Can mimic SDD or edema (reticular pattern); can appear like precocious chronic change.

9. Pulmonary hemorrhage.
  a. Usually secondary to severe hypoxia or capillary damage, as can be seen in SDD, meconium aspiration, patent ductus arteriosus (PDA), or neonatal pneumonia.
  b. Can manifest clinically as blood within ET tube.
  c. Treatment.
   1. Introduction of epinephrine, via ET tube, to induce vascular constriction.
   2. Positive end expiratory pressure (PEEP) attempts to "tamponade" hemorrhage.

**Imaging** Chest radiograph usually demonstrates normal lung volumes with air space disease and air bronchograms. Can have homogeneously opaque lungs with massive hemorrhage.

10. Pulmonary edema.
  a. Can be related to congenital heart disease (most commonly PDA).
  b. Other etiologies include iatrogenic fluid overload or capillary damage (LLS).
  c. Treat cause of edema.
   1. Indomethacin to close open ductus arteriosus.
   2. Diuresis for fluid overload.

> **Imaging** Chest radiograph shows increased perihilar markings, often losing sharp cardiothymic silhouette. Look for cardiac enlargement and elevation of left mainstem bronchus (due to enlarging left atrium).

11. Chylothorax.
    a. Due to traumatic tear of thoracic duct during delivery.
    b. General anatomic rule: If chylothorax is right-sided, tear is below T7. If chylothorax is left-sided, damage occurred in thoracic duct above T7.
    c. Initial treatment is thoracentesis; if chylothorax persists, then chest tube is placed.

> **Imaging** Chest radiograph can demonstrate varying degrees of pleural effusion, ranging up to opaque lung, with contralateral mediastinal shift in more severe cases.

12. Persistent pulmonary hypertension of the newborn (PPHN).
    a. Also known as persistent fetal circulation.
    b. As lungs first expand, pulmonary vascular resistance drops. However, high pulmonary pressures can persist, and prevent pulmonary blood flow from perfusing lungs.
    c. Usually transient condition; if persistent, can be life threatening.
    d. Treatment.
        *1.* Usually supportive, until pulmonary pressures drop.
        *2.* ECMO has been used in severe cases.
        *3.* Other therapies have included vasodilators (nitric oxide), artificially raising systemic pressures (via pharmocologic pressors) above pulmonary pressures, to induce perfusion of lungs.

> **Imaging** Chest radiograph shows normal or near-normal lungs (can occasionally see mild decreased pulmonary flow). The key to diagnosis is presence of near-normal chest film, yet poor clinical picture.

13. Pulmonary hypoplasia (agenesis).
    a. Usually right-sided; can have isolated agenesis in right upper lobe (RUL) and/or right middle lobe (RML).
    b. Could be related to external compression.
        *1.* Diaphragmatic hernia.
        *2.* Oligohydramnios from renal agenesis or infantile polycystic kidneys.
    c. Associated with scimitar syndrome.
        *1.* Right lung hypoplasia.

2. Abnormal venous return or partial anomalous pulmonary venous return (PAPVR).
    d. If hypoplasia is severe (particularly in cases of diaphragmatic hernia), it is fatal. However, hypoplastic lung is commonly asymptomatic, and is often an incidental finding. However, if PAPVR is present, it needs to be surgically repaired.

> **Imaging** Opacification of hemithorax (usually right), with mediastinal shift to affected side, can be seen on chest radiographs. Associated pulmonary artery is usually small and hypoplastic as well. Look for "scimitar": curvilinear density at medial base of lung (corresponds with PAPVR).

14. Lymphangiectasia.
    a. Rare; can be seen in infants with generalized lymphangiectasia, or associated with congenital heart disease (CHD), particularly Noonan syndrome.
    b. Symptoms include: respiratory distress and cyanosis.
    c. Etiology.
        1. May be due to early arrest of embryonic pulmonary lymphatic development with persistence of dilated, obstructed channels.
        2. When CHD is present, impaired lymphatic drainage may be due to increased pulmonary venous pressure. Chylothorax may be present.
    d. No treatment; early death.

> **Imaging** Chest radiograph reveals reticulonodular infiltrate with "congested" appearance; often with hyperaeration and pleural effusions.

15. Restrictive lung.
    a. Chest movement is restricted by external factors.
    b. Etiology.
        1. Neuromuscular etiology.
            a. Severe asphyxia with neurologic impairment.
            b. Paralyzing agents such as pancuronium bromide (Pavulon).
        2. Asphyxiating thoracic dystrophy or congenitally small thorax.
            a. Jeune syndrome.
            b. Thanatophoric dwarf.
            c. Ellis-van Creveld syndrome.

> **Imaging** Chest radiograph demonstrates bell-shaped thorax with subsequent low lung volumes. In case of asphyxiating

thoracic dystrophy, short malformed ribs are present, resulting in abnormally narrow chest. Abnormal spine and ribs usually result in severe scoliosis, and flail chest can disrupt respiration.

B. Surgically treated conditions.
   1. Diaphragmatic hernia.
      a. Intrauterine herniation of abdominal contents (usually bowel loops) into chest, via diaphragmatic defect.
      b. Bochdalek is most common (left, posterior).
      c. Because of mass effect of abdominal contents in chest, pulmonary hypoplasia is concern.
      d. Morgagni hernia.
         1. Right-sided; often with liver herniation.
         2. Associated with group B *Streptococcus* infection.
      e. Treatment.
         1. Surgical correction with bowel returned to abdomen and closure of diaphragmatic defect.
         2. Unfortunately, morbidity and mortality is related to amount of compressive pulmonary hypoplasia that exists.

**Imaging** Chest radiograph can show cystlike lucencies in hemithorax with gasless, often scaphoid abdomen. Significant mediastinal shift is usually present, away from affected side. Pneumothorax is common complication.

   2. CAM.
      a. Congenital hamartomatous lesion, characterized by proliferation of terminal respiratory bronchioles with no alveolar communication. After birth, air trapping in malformed tissue results in characteristic cystic appearance.
      b. Comprises 25% of all congenital lung lesions and 95% of congenital cystic pulmonary lesions.
      c. Usually presents in neonate with respiratory distress. Ten percent present after first year of life, often with recurrent pneumonias.
      d. Can initially appear as unilateral fluid-filled cysts that gradually fill with air; can mimic diaphragmatic hernia.
      e. Types: (Fig. 2-1).
         1. Type 1.
            a. Several dominant cysts (greater than 2 cm) with multiple smaller cysts.
            b. Most common, best prognosis.
         2. Type II.
            a. Numerous, uniform small cysts (less than 1 to 2 cm).

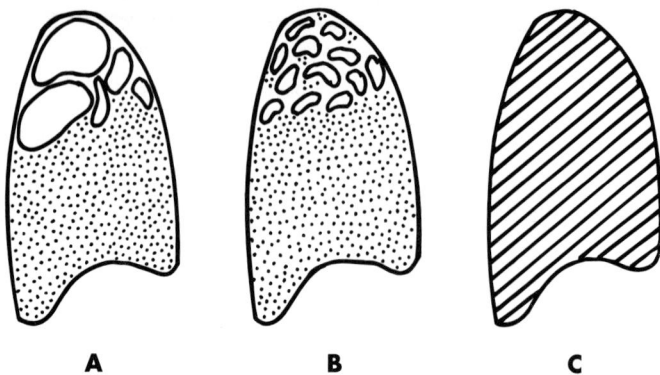

**Fig. 2-1** CAM types. **A,** Type 1; **B,** type 2; **C,** type 3.

       *b.* Associated with other congenital abnormalities (such as pulmonary sequestration, CHD, and hydrops).
   3. Type III.
       *a.* Solid mass (many tiny cysts).
       *b.* Often associated with anasarca and hydrops.
       *c.* Least common, worst prognosis.

> **Imaging** Chest radiograph can initially have solid (opaque) appearance, due to fluid filling cysts. As lungs aerate and fluid is resorbed, air fills lesion, giving it characteristic lucent (cystic) appearance. Size of aerated cysts determines type (see previous discussion). Look for mediastinal shift; can be significant and can cause compressive pulmonary hypoplasia.

3. Pulmonary sequestration.
   a. Nonfunctioning pulmonary tissue.
      *1.* Without bronchial connection.
      *2.* With abnormal vasculature.
   b. Usually located in lower lobes; found more commonly in left than in right.
   c. Two types.
      *1.* Extralobar (distinct pleural covering).
         *a.* Systemic arterial supply with systemic venous drainage (left-to-right shunt).
         *b.* Etiology is abnormal budding of foregut.
      *2.* Intralobar (within visceral pleura).
         *a.* Systemic arterial supply with pulmonary venous drainage.

b. Possibly acquired etiology as intralobar sequestration is usually discovered in older children with repeated infections.

**Imaging** Persistent opacity, usually in lower lobes, is seen on chest radiograph. Computed tomography, magnetic resonance imaging, or angiography may demonstrate systemic arterial supply (from aorta).

4. Congenital lobar emphysema.
   a. Usually found in left upper, right upper, or right middle lung (LUL, RUL, or RML).
   b. Etiology is unknown, but may be related to underdeveloped bronchial cartilage, which can cause "ball-valve" air trapping of adjacent lung lobe.
   c. Involved lobe can be opaque early on in life, secondary to fluid accumulation; gradually fluid will clear.
   d. Surgical resection is performed in symptomatic patients.

**Imaging** Progresssive overdistension of lung lobe, resulting in air trapping; lucent appearance on chest radiograph. Significant mediastinal shift is often present.

5. Congenital lung cysts.
   a. Quite rare; 95% of cystic pulmonary lesions are CAM.
   b. Usually present with recurrent infections; difficult to distinguish from postinfectious pneumatoceles.
   c. Congenital lung cysts, particularly in apices, have been associated with Down syndrome.

**Imaging** Cystic, thin-walled lesions are seen on chest radiograph; can be found anywhere in lungs.

## SUGGESTED READINGS

Clark EA, Siegle RL, Gong AK: Findings on chest radiographs after prophylactic pulmonary surfactant treatment of premature infants. *AJR* 1989; 153:799-802.

Cleveland RH: A radiologic update on medical diseases of the newborn chest. *Pediatr Radiol* 1995; 25:631-637.

Crouse DT, Odrezin GT, Cutter GR, Reese JM, Hamrick WB, Waites KB, Cassell GH: Radiographic changes associated with tracheal isolation of *ureaplasma urealyticum* from neonates. *Clin Infect Dis* 1993; 17(suppl 1):S122-130

Dinger J, Schwarze R, Rupprecht E: Radiological changes after therapeutic use of surfactant in infants with respiratory distress syndrome. *Pediatr Radiol* 1997; 27:26-31.

Edwards DK, Hilton SVW, Merrit TA, Hallman M, Mannino F, Boynton BR: Respiratory distress syndrome treated with human surfactant: Radiographic findings. *Radiology* 1985; 157:329-334.

Edwards DK, Jacob J, Gluck L: The immature lung: radiographic appearance, course and complications. *AJR* 1980; 135:659-666.

Hamvas A, Nogee LM, Colten HR: Lung transplant for treatment of infants with surfactant protein B deficiency. *J Pediatr* 1997; 130:231-239.

Heneghan MA, Sosulski R, Baguero JM: Persistent pulmonary abnormalities in newborns: The changing picture of bronchopulmonary dysplasia. *Pediatr Radiol* 1986; 16:1-6.

Herman TE, Nogee LM, McAlister WH, Dehner LP: Surfactant protein B deficiency: Radiographic manifestations. *Pediatr Radiol* 1993; 23:373-375.

Merten DF, Goetzman BW, Wennberg RP: Persistent fetal circulation: An evolving clinical and radiographic concept of pulmonary hypertension. *Pediatr Radiol* 1977; 6:74-80.

Northway WH, Rosan RC, Porter DY: Pulmonary disease following respiratory therapy of hyaline membrane disease: Bronchopulmonary dysplasia. *N Engl J Med* 1967; 276:357-368.

Panicek DM, Heitzman ER, Randall PA, Groskin SA, Chew FS, Lane EJ, Markarian B: The continuum of pulmonary developmental anomalies. *Radiographics* 1987; 7:747-772.

Sindel LJ, Blackburn WR, Brogden BG, Harris RO: Progressive pulmonary lymphangiectasia. *Pediatr Pulmonol* 1991; 10:57-62.

Swischuk LE, John SD: Immature lung problems: Can our nomenclature be more specific? *AJR* 1996; 166:917-918.

Swischuk LE, Shetty B, John SD: The lungs in immature infants: How important is surfactant therapy in preventing chronic lung problems? *Pediatr Radiol* 1996; 26:508-511.

Wood BP, Sinkin RA, Kendig JW, Notter RH, Shapiro DL: Exogenous lung surfactant: Effect on radiographic appearance in premature infants. *Radiology* 1987; 165:11-13.

# 3
# Pneumonia

---

**Key Concepts**

1. Viral infections (such as respiratory syncytial virus [RSV]) are the most common cause of respiratory infection in children.
2. Pneumococcal pneumonia (often radiographically manifesting as a "round" pneumonia) is the most common bacterial pneumonia in children.
3. Unexplained pleural effusion and hilar or mediastinal adenopathy are classic chest radiographic findings of tuberculosis in children.
4. Differential diagnosis for children with multiple pneumonias includes:
   a. Cystic fibrosis.
   b. Anatomic defect, such as tracheoesophageal fistula and cleft palate.
   c. Gastroesophageal reflux.
   d. Vascular ring.
   e. Impaired neurologic state.
   f. Immunodeficiency.
5. Human immunodeficiency virus (HIV) or acquired immunodeficiency syndrome (AIDS) usually occurs via transplacental spread in infants. This earlier presentation tends to be a more rapidly progressive course, with multiple episodes of pneumonia such as *Pneumocystis carinii* and lymphocytic interstititial pneumonitis (LIP).

A. Typical pneumonias.
   1. Bronchiolitis (viral airways disease).
      a. Viral infection of lower tracheobronchial tree.
      b. Viruses are most common etiologic agents causing pediatric respiratory infections (95% of pneumonias in preschoolers).
         *1.* RSV is most common.
         *2.* Adenovirus.
      c. Seasonal (November to February).
      d. Clinical presentation.
         *1.* Fever.
         *2.* Wheezing.
         *3.* Tachypnea and/or retractions.
      e. *Chlamydia* may mimic clinical and radiographic "bronchiolitis" in 4- to 7-week-old infant. Conjunctivitis may also be present.
      f. Children at greater risk for mortality or morbidity with RSV infection.
         *1.* Infants born premature with bronchopulmonary dysplasia.
         *2.* Children with congenital heart disease.
      g. Treatment.
         *1.* Bronchiolitis or viral airways disease is usually self-limiting and requires only supportive care.
         *2.* Occasionally air trapping is severe, and can lead to respiratory distress and subsequent intubation.

   **Imaging** Obstructive airway disease is seen on chest radiograph as air trapping (hyperaerated lungs with flattened diaphragms, best appreciated on lateral film) and increased perihilar markings (also called "perihilar infiltrates" or "peribronchial cuffing or edema"), due to increased secretions and edema of bronchial wall. When dealing with bronchiolitis, always evaluate trachea. Look for signs of viral upper airways disease or croup ("steepling" or subglottic edema).

   2. Bacterial pneumonia.
      a. Common organisms.
         *1.* Neonate.
            *a.* Group B *Streptococcus*.
            *b.* *Escherichia coli*.
            *c.* *Listeria*.
            *d.* Can be associated with persistent pulmonary hypertension of the newborn.
         *2.* Age 2 months to 5 years.

a. *Haemophilus influenzae* used to be most common pathogen in age group, but it is much less frequent today because of widespread immunizations.
   b. Today, pneumococcal is most common nonneonatal pneumonia.
  3. Older child or adolescent.
   a. *Mycoplasma.*
   b. *Pneumococcus.*
 b. Round pneumonia.
  1. Occurs as result of less well-developed collateral ventilation present in children.
  2. Collateral channels of lung (pores of Kohn and canals of Lambert) become fully developed by age 8. Prior to that time, there is poor collateral drift. Therefore, lung lobes (particularly right middle lobe) can easily become atelectatic (mucus-plugging). Similarly, pneumonia in lung segment has few avenues by which to spread; therefore, it tends to remain concentrated in one region, forming round pneumonia.
  3. Common locations include left lower lobe, behind heart, and right middle lobe.
  4. Can obtain repeat radiograph at resolution of symptoms if round opacity is suspicious for mass lesion.

**Imaging** Chest radiograph can show alveolar infiltrate in child with pneumonia in typical segmental or lobar distribution. Round pneumonias can have almost coin-like appearance in lung. These well-circumscribed and spherical lesions differ from more ill-defined adult pneumonia. Often concomitant viral airways disease is present as well. Older children can have more vague, ill-defined alveolar infiltrates (often caused by *Mycoplasmas*).

 3. Aspiration pneumonia.
  a. Causes.
   1. Neurologically or mentally impaired children.
   2. Tracheoesophageal (TE) fistula.
   3. Seizures.
   4. Hiatal hernia or gastroesophageal (GE) reflux.
  b. Infiltrate is usually located in dependent parts of lungs (classic sites for aspiration in supine position include right upper lung [RUL], right lower lung [RLL], and left lower lung [LLL] in young infants and posterior basilar lung in older child).

> **Imaging** Chest radiograph reveals vague, ill-defined, predominantly basilar opacity. Look for signs of previous aspiration (chronic pulmonary markings or scarring). In addition, look for signs of chronic illness or neurologic impairment, such as osteopenia of bones, C-shaped neuromuscular scoliosis, or dislocated hips.

4. Multiple pneumonias.
    a. Commonly encountered problem in pediatrics.
    b. Diagnostic differential.
        1. Anatomic defects.
            a. TE fistula.
            b. Tracheoesophageal cleft.
            c. Cleft palate.
        2. Neurologic abnormality.
            a. Swallowing dysfunction.
            b. Depressed cough or gag.
        3. GE reflux.
            a. Upper gastrointestinal (UGI) examination can evaluate reflux.
                1) Using intermittant fluoroscopy, one can document how extensive reflux is, and how many episodes are present.
                2) UGI examination can also estimate gastric emptying time (important when drug therapy to facilitate gastric emptying is considered).
            b. Nuclear medicine reflux study is more sensitive, yet has poor anatomic detail.
        4. Chronic foreign body.
            a. Look for asymmetrical inflation of lungs (affected side is air trapping and lucent; will not collapse on decubitus films).
            b. Less than 10% of foreign bodies are radiopaque.
            c. Peak age is 1 to 2 years of age; higher in mentally compromised children.
            d. Clinical signs.
                1) Choking episode.
                2) Stridor or cough.
                3) Recurrent pneumonia.
            e. Found more commonly in right lung than in left.
        5. Cystic fibrosis.
        6. Immunodeficiency.
            a. DiGeorge syndrome (absent thymus).

           b. Chronic granulomatous disease of childhood.
              1) Poor phagocytic activity.
              2) Predominantly seen in boys (X-linked).
              3) Characteristic gastric antral narrowing.
           c. Other types of hypogammaglobulinemia.
              1) Chédiak-Higashi syndrome.
              2) Wiskott-Aldrich syndrome.
           d. AIDS, HIV.
        7. Vascular ring (see Chapter 20).
           a. Look for presence of right arch.
           b. "Missing tracheal segment" sign.
              1) Portions of trachea are persistently not visualized.
              2) Due to external compression.
        8. Asthma and other allergic conditions.
     5. Bronchiolitis obliterans.
        a. Also known as Swyer-James syndrome.
        b. Sequelae of infectious insult (usually adenovirus), probably prior to age 8.
        c. Can involve single lobe only or entire lung.

  **Imaging** Unilateral hyperlucent lung with diminished perfusion and hypoplasia of pulmonary artery can be seen on chest radiograph. Air trapping of affected side is often present.

B. Unusual or opportunistic pneumonias.
   1. Tuberculosis (TB).
      a. Organism is *Mycobacterium tuberculosis*.
      b. Primary TB.
         *1.* Inhalational pulmonary parenchymal infection.
         *2.* Subsequently can spread to hilar and mediastinal lymph nodes; these nodal groups enlarge and may later calcify.
         *3.* Any unexplained hilar mediastinal adenopathy merits purified protein derivative (PPD) test for evaluation for possible TB.
         *4.* Pleural effusion.
      c. Can be seen in immunocompromised, especially AIDS patients; more common in adults.
      d. Reinfection or chronic TB is not commonly seen in children.

  **Imaging** Chest radiograph may demonstrate hilar adenopathy, pleural effusion, pneumonic infiltrate, granulomas, or any combination of these findings. Miliary pattern (tiny nodular opacities) can also be seen with hematogenous spread of TB. Hematogenous TB also can affect spine (Pott's disease), central nervous system (CNS), and kidneys.

2. *Staphylococcus aureus.*
   a. Usually produces only pneumonic infiltrate, but can lead to lung abscess, pneumatoceles, and sterile or infected pleural effusion (empyema).
   b. *Staphylococcus* and *Haemophilus* are common causes of pediatric empyema (pus in pleural space).
   c. Often need to perform drainage of any concomitant abscess or empyema.

   **Imaging** Segmental, lobar, or multilobar alveolar consolidation can be seen on chest radiograph. Look for pleural effusions or lung abscess (air-fluid level).

3. Varicella (chicken pox).
   a. Highly contagious, but usually self-limiting cutaneous disorder in children.
   b. In adolescent and adult, there is increased risk of developing varicella pneumonia, which can be quite severe, even life-threatening (particularly in pregnant women and immunocompromised patients).
   c. Acyclovir can be given to high-risk patients; varicella vaccine is now available.
   d. Abnormal pulmonary function tests are common after varicella pneumonia; indicative of secondary pulmonary fibrosis.

   **Imaging** Chest radiograph may initially show diffuse, patchy alveolar infiltrates that can be somewhat nodular. Following resolution of acute phase, diffuse pulmonary calcifications can appear within 2 years of original infection.

4. Epstein-Barr virus.
   a. Causes infectious mononucleosis.
   b. Usually seen in adolescents ("kissing disease").
   c. Has been implicated as etiology for African Burkitt lymphoma.

   **Imaging** Look for adenopathy (lingual or palatine tonsils and adenoids); best seen on lateral airway radiograph. Can rarely cause patchy pulmonary opacities.

5. Pertussis.
   a. Also known as whooping cough (distinctive cough usually limited to infants).
   b. Organism is *Bordetella pertussis.*
   c. Decreasing incidence, probably because of widespread immunizations.

> **Imaging** Classic chest radiographic finding is hyperaeration and "shaggy heart" due to perihilar and right middle lung or lingular infiltrates (similar finding as in adenovirus, RSV, and measles pneumonia).

6. Fungal.
   a. Histoplasmosis *(Histoplasma capsulatum)*.
      1. Endemic in central United States (Ohio River Valley).
      2. Several clinical forms.
         a. Mild course (only remnant is hilar mediastinal calcified lymph nodes. Scattered pulmonary parenchymal granulomas may also be present).
         b. Disseminated form (severe pneumonitis, particularly in immunocompromised patient).
      3. Can cause fibrosing mediastinitis.

> **Imaging** Similar imaging findings to TB, namely hilar mediastinal adenopathy (often calcified). Look for scattered granulomas (tiny nodules). Can see diffuse alveolar infiltrate with acute pneumonitis.

   b. Candidiasis.
      1. In immunocompromised patient, debilitated patient, premature infant, or AIDS patient.
      2. Organism is *Candida albicans*.
      3. Can also involve liver, spleen, kidneys, and CNS.

> **Imaging** No pathognomonic pattern. Usually scattered alveolar consolidation is present on chest radiograph. Adenopathy or cavitation is not usually present.

   c. *Aspergillus*.
      1. Saprophytic to mycetoma.
         a. Noninvasive; coexists with host, usually within preexisting pulmonary cavities.
         b. May be asymptomatic and incidental radiographic finding; can cause hemoptysis.
         c. Usually seen in upper lobes (sites of previous TB cavities).

> **Imaging** Well-defined opacity is present on chest radiograph, often within pulmonary cavity; "fungal ball" (mycetoma) is often mobile within cavity.

      2. Allergic bronchopulmonary aspergillosis.
         a. Associated with asthma, bronchiectasis.

    b. Increased eosinophils in blood.

> **Imaging** "Finger-in-glove" appearance on chest radiograph, usually in upper lobes (due to mucoid impaction).

   3. Invasive *Aspergillus*.
      a. Rapid progression with high mortality.
      b. Seen in immunocompromised patients.
      c. Prompt administration of appropriate antibiotics (amphotericin B) is crucial.

> **Imaging** Chest radiograph may initially have scattered, subtle nodular densities, which can rapidly progress to coalescing consolidation.

   d. Other fungal infections (less common).
      1. Actinomycosis.
         a. Rare in children.
         b. Frequently spreads to involve pleura and chest wall, with rib destruction and empyema.
      2. Mucormycosis.
         a. Extremely lethal and destructive fungal infection.
         b. Seen in compromised patients, diabetes, leukemia, or lymphoma.
      3. Blastomycosis.
         a. Nonspecific.
         b. Often have hilar or mediastinal adenopathy that can be quite extensive.
      4. Coccidioidomycosis.
         a. Endemic in southwestern United States.
         b. Pulmonary infiltrate with adenopathy (similar appearance to TB).
      5. Cryptococcus.
         a. "Infiltrating mass" with adenopathy.
         b. Cavitation and/or pleural effusion is uncommon.
7. AIDS.
   a. HIV.
   b. Transplacental spread in infants; earlier presentation tends to have more rapidly progressive course.
   c. Multiple episodes of pneumonia.
   d. *P. carinii* (usually seen in older children or adolescents).
   e. LIP tends to be seen in younger children (less than 5 years of age).
   f. Increased incidence of lymphoma or leukemia.

> **Imaging** Subtle, often insidious onset with basilar or hilar interstitial infiltrate seen on chest radiograph that can progress to consolidation. LIP is described as small nodular infiltrate, although biopsy is needed for definitive diagnosis.

## SUGGESTED READINGS

Cremin BJ: Tuberculosis: The resurgence of our most lethal infectious disease: A review. *Pediatr Radiol* 1995; 25:620-626.

Griscom NT: Pneumonia in children and some of its variants. *Radiology* 1988; 167:297-302.

Griscom NT, Wohl MEB, Kirkpatrick JA: Lower respiratory infections: How infants differ from adults. *Radiol Clin North Am* 1978; 26:367-387.

Haller JO, Cohen HL: Pediatric HIV infection: An imaging update. *Pediatr Radiol* 1995; 24:224-229.

Haller JO, Ginsberg KJ: Tuberculosis in children with immunodeficiency syndrome. *Pediatr Radiol* 1997; 27:186-188.

Haney PJ, Yale-Loehr AJ, Nussbaum AR, Gellad FE: Imaging of infants and children with AIDS. *AJR* 1989; 152:1033-1041.

Hardy KA, Schidlow DV, Zaeri N: Obliterative bronchiolitis in children. *Chest* 1988; 93:460-466.

Klein DL, Gamsu G: Thoracic manifestations of *Aspergillus*. *AJR* 1980; 134:543-547.

Kline MW, Lorin MI: Childhood tuberculosis. *Adv Pediatr Infect Dis* 1987; 2:135-160.

Radkowski MA, Prantzler JK, Beem MO: Chlamydia pneumonia in infants. *AJR* 1981; 137:703-707.

Sivit CJ, Miller CR, Rakusan TA, Ellaurie M, Kushner DC: Spectrum of chest radiographic abnormalities in children with AIDS and *Pneumocystis carinii* pneumonia. *Pediatr Radiol* 1995; 25:389-392.

Strouse PJ, Dessner DA, Watson WJ, Blane CE: Mycobacterium tuberculosis infection in the immunocompetent children. *Pediatr Radiol* 1996; 26:134-141.

Turner RB, Lande AE, Chase P, Hilton N, Weinberg D: Pneumonia in pediatric outpatients: Cause and clinical manifestations. *J Pediatr* 1987; 111:194-200.

Wahlgren H, Mortensson W, Eriksson M, Finkel Y, Forsgren M: Radiographic patterns and viral studies in childhood pneumonia at various ages. *Pediatr Radiol* 1995; 25:627-630.

Weller MH, Katzenstein AA: Radiologic findings in group B streptococcal sepsis. *Radiology* 1976; 118:385-389.

Wildin SR, Chonmaitree T, Swischuk LE: Roentgenologic features of common pediatric viral respiratory tract infections. *Am J Dis Child* 1988;142:43-46.

# 4
# Pulmonary Circulation

---

### Key Concepts

1. Three mechanisms for pulmonary edema are: increased hydrostatic pressure, decreased oncotic pressure, and capillary leak.
2. Unlike in adults, cardiogenic cause for pulmonary edema in children is uncommon.
3. Renal dysfunction is the most common cause of new onset of pulmonary edema in children.
4. Pulmonary emboli are rare in pediatric patients yet can be seen in children with predisposing conditions like trauma or hypercoagulable states.

A. Pulmonary edema.
   1. Arises from three mechanisms.
      a. Increased hydrostatic pressure.
         *1.* Cardiogenic edema.
         2. Fluid overload.
      b. Decreasing oncotic pressure.
         *1.* Hypoproteinemia.
         2. Liver disease.
      c. Capillary damage or leakage.
         *1.* Adult respiratory distress syndrome (ARDS).
         2. Inhalational insults.
         3. Drug reaction or overdose.
   2. Etiology of pulmonary edema.
      a. Renal dysfunction.
         *1.* Most common cause of "pulmonary edema of unknown etiology" in children.
         2. Glomerulonephritis, especially poststreptococcal.
         3. Nephrotic syndrome.
      b. Fluid overload (often iatrogenic).
         *1.* Patients with central venous catheters.
         2. Postoperative patients.
      c. Cardiogenic.
         *1.* Unusual in pediatric population.
         2. Congenital heart disease.
         3. Cardiomyopathy.
            *a.* Viral (often Coxsackievirus).
            *b.* Glycogen storage disease.
      d. Neurogenic.
         *1.* Head injury or stroke.
         2. Any central nervous system event that results in increased intracranial pressure.
      e. Drugs (overdose).
         *1.* Heroin.
         2. Morphine.
         3. Aspirin.
         4. Intravenous iodinated contrast material (allergic reaction).
      f. Inhalational injury.
         *1.* Often delayed appearance of edema.
         2. Smoke.
         3. Carbon monoxide.
         4. Hydrocarbons.
      g. Near-drowning.
      h. Transfusion reaction.

i. ARDS.
   1. "Capillary leak."
   2. Posttraumatic.
   3. Postinfectious.
j. Liver disease (hypoproteinemia).
   1. Cirrhosis.
   2. Biliary atresia.
   3. Metabolic.

---

**Imaging** Three possible appearances.
1. Redistribution of pulmonary blood flow (earliest sign of pulmonary edema).
   - Greater than 10 mm Hg (normal is 5 to 10 mm Hg).
   - Vascular channels are recruited in upper lung zones, where pressures are relatively low, resulting in regional dilatation of upper zone vessels.
   - Perivascular edema and distended lymphatics result in dilatation and blurring of central and lower zone vessels.
2. Interstitial edema.
   - Pulmonary venous pressure is greater than 20 to 25 mm Hg.
   - Transudative fluid starts leaking into interstitial spaces, resulting in interstitial edema.
   - Interstitium of alveolar walls and interlobular septa become swollen with fluid; present as increased interstitial markings and septal lines (horizontal Kerley B lines along lateral lower margins of thorax).
3. Alveolar edema.
   - Overwhelming increase in pulmonary venous pressure can result in alveolar edema (greater than 25 mm Hg).
   - Edematous fluid first fills interstitial spaces, then spills over into alveolar air spaces, causing patchy air space. Central consolidation from alveolar pulmonary edema results in "bat-wing" pattern, so named for its bilateral perihilar distribution.

---

B. Pulmonary vessel abnormalities.
   1. Arterial.
      a. Absent.
         1. Pseudotruncus.

2. Bronchial collateral flow to lung.
 b. Hypoplastic.
   1. Associated with hypogenetic lung (scimitar syndrome).
   2. Associated with Swyer-James syndrome (bronchiolitis obliterans).
 c. Aneurysms.
   1. Rare.
   2. "Aneurysmal" dilatation of pulmonary artery can be seen with absent pulmonary valve.
 d. Pulmonary hypertension.
   1. Idiopathic.
     a. Rare.
     b. Found more commonly in females than in males.
   2. Precapillary (arterial).
     a. Eisenmenger complex (reversal of flow in patient with left-to-right shunt).
     b. Chronic lung changes.
       1) Cystic fibrosis.
       2) Langerhans cell histiocytosis.
     c. Chronic pulmonary emboli (sickle cell anemia).
     d. Chronic airway obstruction (enlarged tonsils and adenoids, which can lead to obstructive sleep apnea).
   3. Postcapillary (venous).
     a. Venous obstruction or venoocclusive disease.
     b. Left heart problems such as mitral or aortic stenosis.
   4. Persistent pulmonary hypertension of the newborn (see Chapter 2).

**Imaging** Classic chest radiographic finding is "pruned-tree" look, with rapid tapering of pulmonary arteries. Look for coexisting lung disease or heart disease.

2. Venous.
 a. Total anomalous pulmonary venous return.
   1. Supracardiac.
     a. Most common.
     b. Pulmonary venous return is to superior vena cava.
   2. Cardiac.
     a. Venous return is to right atrium or coronary sinus.
   3. Infradiaphragmatic.
     a. "Obstructive" type.
     b. Pulmonary venous return is to vessel below diaphragm, such as inferior vena cava.

b. Partial anomalous venous return.
   1. Associated with atrial septal defect (ASD), in particular, sinus venosus.
   2. Associated with hypogenetic lung, scimitar syndrome, or venolobar syndrome.
   3. Extralobar sequestration.
      a. Aberrant budding of foregut.
      b. Abnormal pulmonary tissue with separate pleural lining and no bronchial connection.
      c. Systemic venous drainage of aberrant segment with arterial flow being either pulmonary or systemic (aortic) collaterals.
c. Pulmonary varix.
d. "Meandering" pulmonary veins.
   1. Anomalous pulmonary veins still connect to left atrium, only via abnormal route.
   2. Can be isolated finding; is usually associated with hypogenetic right lung or scimitar syndrome.
3. Arteriovenous malformation (AVM).
   a. Between pulmonary artery and vein, abnormal connection that does not cross capillary bed.
   b. Pulmonary AVM can be solitary or multiple; lower lobes predominate, usually unilateral.
   c. Associated with Rendu-Osler-Weber syndrome.
      1. Autosomal dominant.
      2. Multiple AVMs.

**Imaging** Well-circumscribed, often peripheral nodule can be seen on chest radiograph. Look for large central vessels that "enter and leave" nodule. Multiple such nodules may be present.

C. Pulmonary thromboembolic disease.
   1. Pulmonary embolic events are rare in pediatrics.
   2. Predisposing factors.
      a. Indwelling venous catheters or intravascular clot.
      b. Hypercoagulable states.
         1. Sickle cell anemia.
         2. Nephrotic syndrome.
         3. Protein C deficiency.
      c. Trauma.
         1. Fat emboli (femur or tibia fracture).
         2. Vessel damage.
            a. Endothelial lining damage.

   *b.* Can lead to emboli formation.
  d. Bed-ridden state.
3. Septic emboli.
  a. Can arise from any infected site.
  b. Venous catheters.
  c. Heart valves.
  d. Site of osteomyelitis.

> **Imaging** Chest radiograph is commonly normal. Peripheral, scattered pulmonary nodules can be seen in septic emboli. Alveolar consolidation with pleural effusion can also be present. Nuclear medicine (ventilation-perfusion) scans may be helpful to diagnose presence of pulmonary embolus (look for mismatched defect, indicative of ventilation but no perfusion to affected lung lobe).

## SUGGESTED READINGS

Batra P: The fat embolism syndrome. *J Thorac Imaging* 1987; 2:12-17.

Budorick NE, McDonald V, Flisak ME, Moncada RM: The pulmonary veins. *Semin Roentgenol* 1989; 24:127-149.

Burke CM, Safai C, Nelson DP, Raffin TA: Pulmonary AVM: Critical update. *Am Rev Respir Dis* 1986; 134:334-339.

Effman EL, Merten DF, Kirks DR: Adult respiratory distress syndrome in children. *Radiology* 1985; 157:69-74.

Ellis K: Developmental abnormalities in the systemic blood supply to the lungs. *AJR* 1991; 156:669-679.

Fein IA, Rackow EC: Neurogenic pulmonary edema. *Chest* 1982; 81:318-320.

Higgins CB, Wexler L: Clinical and angiographic features of pulmonary arteriovenous fistulas in children. *Radiology* 1976; 119:171-175.

Kriss VM, Woodring JH, Cottrill CM: "Meandering" pulmonary veins: Report of a case in an asymptomatic 12 year old girl. *J Thorac Imaging* 1995; 10:142-145.

Milne ENC, Pistolesi M, Miniati M: The radiologic distinction of cardiogenic and non-cardiogenic edema. *AJR* 1985; 144:879-894.

Moes CAF, Freedom RM, Burrows PE: Anomalous pulmonary venous connections. *Semin Roentgenol* 1985; 20:134-150.

Putman CE, Tummilo AM, Myerson DA, Myerson PJ: Drowning: Another plunge. *AJR* 1975; 125:543-548.

Woodruff WW, Merten DF, Wagner ML: Chronic pulmonary embolism in children. *Radiology* 1986; 159:511-514.

# 5
# Congenital Lung Lesions

## Key Concepts

1. There are six general types of congenital lung abnormalities:
   a. Congenital lobar emphysema (CLE).
   b. Cystic adenomatoid malformation (CAM).
   c. Bronchogenic cysts.
   d. Sequestration.
   e. Pulmonary arteriovenous malformation (AVM).
   f. Venolobar (hypoplastic lung–scimitar syndrome).
2. Congenital pulmonary abnormalities are considered to be a spectrum, a "continuum of maldevelopment," involving abnormal differentiation of pulmonary parenchyma, pulmonary vessels, or both.
3. One end of the spectrum is CLE (abnormal lung supplied with normal pulmonary vessels); at the other end of the spectrum is AVM (normal lung tissue supplied by abnormal pulmonary vessels).
4. Clinical presentations vary and include neonatal respiratory distress (CLE and CAM), airway compression (bronchogenic cyst), recurrent infections (sequestrations), and cyanosis (AVM). Occasionally, congenital lung lesions can be an incidental finding on chest radiograph.

A. Congenital lung lesions.
   1. CLE.
      a. Progressive hyperaeration of lung lobe.
      b. Seen predominantly in upper lobes, in left more so than in right. Next most common area of involvement is right middle lung (RML). Rarely seen in lower lobes.
      c. Pulmonary vasculature is normal.
      d. Possible etiologies.
         *1.* Deficient bronchial cartilage or redundant mucosa causing air trapping.
         *2.* External obstruction, such as cysts or lymph nodes.
      e. Symptoms occur within the first 6 months of life (80% of cases).
      f. Cases in males predominate (2:1).
      g. From 10% to 30% are associated with congenital heart disease (CHD), especially ventricular septal defect and patent ductus arteriosus.

   **Imaging** Hyperlucent lung lobe can be seen on chest radiograph with progressive air trapping, often with mediastinal shift. Compressive atelectasis of adjacent lobes is often present. CLE can initially appear solid in newborn, owing to fluid retained in abnormal lobe.

   2. CAM.
      a. Multicystic, hamartomatous pulmonary tissue with abnormal overgrowth of bronchial structures. Normal pulmonary vessels are present.
      b. Equal frequency in all lobes except in RML and lingula, which are rare.
      c. Most (66%) are symptomatic (respiratory distress) within first month of life.
      d. Three histologic types: (see Fig. 2-1).
         *1.* Type 1.
            *a.* Single or multiple large cysts, greater than 2 cm.
            *b.* Most common (60%), best prognosis.
         *2.* Type II.
            *a.* Multiple small uniform cysts, less than 2 cm.
            *b.* About 35% of CAM.
            *c.* May be associated with other anomalies like CHD or pulmonary sequestration.
         *3.* Type III.
            *a.* Solid parenchymal mass made up of tiny cysts.
            *b.* Associated with hydrops and anasarca.
            *c.* Uncommon (5%), poor prognosis.

> **Imaging** "Bubbly" cystic mass can be seen on chest radiograph, often causing mediastinal shift. Can appear solid in first days of life (fluid-filled). In infants, multiple air-filled cysts of CAM have radiographic appearance similar to diaphragmatic hernia; however, bowel gas pattern is normal in children with CAM. CAM may be discovered on prenatal ultrasound as cystic intrathoracic mass.

3. Bronchogenic cysts.
   a. Embryology.
      1. Abnormal lung bud from developing foregut.
      2. Contains tissue normally found in trachea or bronchus, such as smooth muscle and cartilage.
   b. Two forms.
      1. Mediastinal.
         a. Usually asymptomatic.
         b. No bronchial communication.
         c. Presents later in life.
            1) As incidental radiographic finding.
            2) Mass effect on adjacent trachea (due to gradual expansion over time, since there is no outlet for mucus that continues to be secreted).
         d. Often subcarinal in location.
         e. Can be mistaken for esophageal duplication cyst.
      2. Intrapulmonary.
         a. Has bronchial communication; therefore, can present with recurrent pneumonias.
         b. Often found in lower lobes.
   c. Treatment is surgical resection, even of asymptomatic lesions, because of potential risk of airway obstruction or infection.

> **Imaging** Chest radiograph can show well-demarcated, smooth, oval, dense mass in pulmonary parenchyma or in middle mediastinum. Can mimic pulmonary sling when cyst is positioned between trachea and esophagus.

4. Bronchopulmonary sequestration.
   a. Mass of nonfunctioning lung tissue with aberrant vasculature.
   b. Intralobar.
      1. Does not have separate pleural lining.
      2. Vasculature is systemic (aortic) arterial supply with normal pulmonary venous drainage (into left atrium).
      3. Often asymptomatic, but can present with recurrent infection.
      4. Location.

a. Majority present on left (60%).
b. Usually posterior basal segment.
5. Usually does not have associated anomalies, and is uncommon in newborns. Usually discovered later in life, raising question of acquired etiology such as infectious.

**Imaging** Round, smooth opacity usually at lung base is seen on chest radiograph, often surrounded by aerated lung. Concomitant pneumonia may be present.

c. Extralobar.
   1. Separate pleural lining.
   2. Etiology probably related to supernumery lung bud arising caudal to normal lung bud; therefore, increased incidence in lower lobe.
   3. Majority found on left (80% to 90%); more common in males (80%) than in females.
   4. Arterial supply is usually systemic (but can be pulmonary) with systemic venous drainage (azygous or hemiazygous).
   5. Associated with other congenital abnormalities and diaphragmatic hernias.

**Imaging** Chest radiograph shows triangular density at lung base (posteromedial). Contrast computed tomography, magnetic resonance imaging, or angiography can demonstrate aberrant blood supply of both intralobar and extralobar sequestrations.

5. Pulmonary AVM.
   a. Congenital vascular connection between pulmonary artery and pulmonary veins without intervening capillary bed (right-to-left shunt).
   b. Presentation.
      1. About 50% are symptomatic with cyanosis.
      2. Paradoxical emboli (particularly septic emboli to brain).
   c. Usually found in lower lobes; no side predilection.
   d. Pulmonary AVM types.
      1. Solitary lesion (50%); bilateral (15% to 20%).
      2. Multiple, discrete lesions with one dominant lesion.
      3. Multiple discrete fistulas.
      4. Diffuse "telangiectatic" lesions.
   e. Strong association with Rendu-Osler-Weber syndrome (60%).
      1. Autosomal dominant.
      2. Characterized by telangiectatic lesions, hemangiomas, and pulmonary AVMs.

    f. Because of subpleural location of AVM nodule, AVMs are readily accessible to surgical resection.

> **Imaging** Chest radiograph may demonstrate focal pulmonary "nodules," often with dense, linear connection to hilum. Angiography is diagnostic and may be therapeutic, if transcatheter embolization is performed.

  6. Hypogenetic lung (venolobar or scimitar syndrome).
     a. Partial anomalous pulmonary venous return associated with ipsilateral lung hypoplasia.
     b. Hypoplastic lung associated with small pulmonary artery. Anomalous venous return usually to inferior vena cava (scimitar vessel, which is small left-to-right shunt).
     c. Right-sided lesion; therefore, often see cardiac dextroposition with increased incidence of CHD (often atrial septal defect).

> **Imaging** Chest radiograph shows small right hemithorax with mediastinal shift to right (often significant). Small right hilum with large vessel often paralleling right heart border (scimitar or anomalous vessel).

B. Secondary hypoplastic lung.
  1. Lungs initially form normally, but abnormal compressive forces cause limited lung development.
  2. Etiologies include.
     a. Oligohydramnios (due to renal problems such as failure, agenesis, or obstruction).
     b. Diaphragmatic hernia.
     c. Thoracic bony cage abnormalities.
        *1.* Can result in restrictive lung changes because of severely limited thoracic bony cage.
        *2.* Congenital thoracic cage abnormalities.
           *a.* Asphyxiating thoracic dystrophy.
           *b.* Jeune syndrome.
           *c.* Ellis-van Creveld syndrome.
           *d.* Thanatophoric dwarfism.

**SUGGESTED READINGS**

Boothroyd AE, Carty H, Arnold R: Shoe, scimitar and sequestration: A shifting spectrum. *Pediatr Radiol* 1995; 25:652-653.

Burke CM, Safai C, Nelson DP, Raffin TA: Pulmonary arteriovenous malformations: A critical update. *Am Rev Respir Dis* 1986; 134:334-339.

Felson B: Pulmonary sequestration revisited. *Med Radiogr Photogr* 1988; 64:1-27.

Heithoff KB, Sane SM, Williams HJ: Bronchopulmonary foregut malformations: A unifying etiological concept. *AJR* 1975; 126:46.

Kennedy CD, Haibibi P, Matthew DJ: Lobar emphysema: Long-term imaging work-up. *Radiology* 1991; 180:189-193.

Mata JM, Caceres J, Lucaya J: CT of congenital malformations of the lung. *Radiographics* 1990; 10:651-674.

Panicek DM, Heitzman ER, Randall PA, Groskin SA, Chew FS, Lane EJ, Markarian B: The continuum of pulmonary developmental anomalies. *Radiographics* 1987; 7:747-772.

Rosado-de-Christenson ML, Stocker JT: Congenital cystic adenomatoid malformation. *Radiographics* 1991; 11:865-886.

Sade RM, Clouse M, Ellis FH: The spectrum of pulmonary sequestration. *Ann Thorac Surg* 1974; 18:644-658.

Stigers KB, Woodring JH, Kanga JF: The clinical and imaging spectrum of findings in patients with congenital lobar emphysema. *Pediatr Pulmonol* 1992; 14:160-170.

Takahashi M, Ohno M, Mihara K: Pulmonary sequestration. *Radiology* 1975; 114:543.

Woodring JH, Howard TA, Kanga JF: Congenital pulmonary venolobar syndrome revisited. *Radiographics* 1994; 14:349-370.

# 6
# Chronic Lung Disorders

---

**Key Concepts**

1. With the exception of asthma and cystic fibrosis, chronic lung disorders are unusual in children (probably related to the lack of long-term exposure to smoking and other environmental hazards). Similarly, primary pulmonary neoplasms are also exceedingly rare in children.
2. Asthma is called reactive airway disease (RAD) in children less than 2 years of age, and often improves with time.
3. Cystic fibrosis should be suspected in any child with multiple, unexplained pneumonias.
4. Langerhans cell histiocytosis, (previously known as eosinophilic granuloma) although usually seen as bone lesions, can occur in the lung, often resulting in pulmonary fibrosis.

A. Asthma.
   1. Asthma is recurrent pulmonary disorder characterized by bronchospasm, resulting in labored breathing, wheezing, and coughing.
   2. Asthma can affect children of all ages, although it is often called RAD in children less than 2 years of age.
   3. Asthma is clinical diagnosis; not all wheezing is asthma. In infants and young children, chest radiography and contrast upper gastrointestinal examination may be necessary to exclude.
      a. Aspirated foreign body.
      b. Developmental abnormality of airway.
         *1.* Vascular ring.
         *2.* Tracheoesophageal fistula.
   4. Many children have atopic (allergic) backgrounds and recurrent pneumonias.
   5. Chest radiograph is obtained for atypical clinical picture.
      a. Unequal breath sounds.
         *1.* Atelectasis.
         *2.* Pneumonia.
      b. Fever, congestion, or rales (more than just wheezing).
      c. Dyspnea, chest pain.
      d. Unresponsive to normal therapy.
   6. Complications of asthma.
      a. Pneumonia.
      b. Atelectasis.
      c. Air leak.
         *1.* Pneumothorax.
         *2.* Pneumomediastinum.
      d. Allergic bronchopulmonary aspergillosis.

> **Imaging** Chest radiographs, following findings can be seen:
> - Normal.
> - Hyperaeration (most consistent finding).
> - Increased peribronchial secretions and edema ("cuffing").
> - Shifting atelectasis (mucus plugging), especially in right middle lung.
> - Mucoid impaction of bronchi ("finger-in-glove" appearance).

B. Cystic fibrosis (also known as mucoviscidosis).
   1. Inherited (autosomal recessive) error in chloride ion transport, resulting in thick, tenacious mucus (exocrine gland dysfunction that is hallmark of condition).

2. Affects approximately 1:2000 individuals, mostly in Caucasian population.
3. "Sweat test" (chemical analysis of chloride concentration) is screening test for cystic fibrosis (CF).
4. CF should be suspected in any child with unexplained episodes of pneumonia or failure to thrive.
5. Clinical manifestations.
    a. Pulmonary.
        1. Major cause of morbidity and mortality in child with CF.
        2. Bronchiectasis: bronchial wall dilatation.
            a. Viscous mucus is poorly cleared from airways and obstructs bronchioles. Postobstructive infection may occur; most commonly caused by *Staphylococcus aureus* and *Pseudomonas aeruginosa*.
            b. Persistent and recurrent infections impair mucociliary clearance.
            c. Recurrent pneumonias weaken and eventually dilate bronchial walls, leading to further inspissation and pneumonias.
        3. Lung abscesses can form in bronchiectatic cavities, leading to pulmonary destruction and fibrosis.
        4. Air trapping is also seen, consequence of multiple, segmentally obstructed bronchi.
        5. Cyclical airway obstruction and infection produce pulmonary fibrosis and pulmonary arterial hypertension.
        6. Cor pulmonale (right heart failure with right ventricular hypertrophy, secondary to lung disease) is common cause of death.
        7. Common complication.
            a. Hemoptysis from bronchial artery hemorrhage.
            b. When massive, may be treated with embolization.
        8. Treatment for CF.
            a. Preventive maintenance.
                1) Pulmonary percussion to prevent mucoid impactions.
                2) Proper antibiotic coverage for various pneumonias.
            b. New treatment options.
                1) Proteinase to break down mucus.
                2) Lung transplantation.
                3) Gene therapy.
                    a) Introduce missing gene via virus vector.
                    b) Therefore, incorporate missing gene into host genome.
    b. Gastrointestinal.
        1. Meconium ileus.

*a.* Presents in utero or at birth.
   *b.* Occurring in about 10% of children with CF.
   *c.* Thick meconium inspissates in terminal ileum and colon.
   *d.* Presents as bowel obstruction or meconium peritonitis.
 2. Meconium ileus equivalent.
   *a.* Older child or adolescent that presents with clinical signs of obstruction or appendicitis.
   *b.* Patient often needs cleansing enemas or oral Golytely to remove thick obstructing mucus and stool.
 3. Malabsorption.
   *a.* Dysfunctional pancreatic digestive enzymes.
   *b.* Pancreatic atrophy with fatty replacement.
   *c.* Rarely develops into diabetes, except in older adult survivors.
 4. Gallbladder sludge or cholelithiasis.
 5. Fatty liver.
   *a.* From malabsorption.
   *b.* Portal hypertension picture can develop in older children and adults.
     *1)* Splenomegaly.
     *2)* Ascites.
     *3)* Variceal bleeding.

> **Imaging** On chest radiograph, early CF can be seen as hyperaeration and bronchial wall thickening ("cuffing"). Mucoid impaction can be seen as fingerlike densities radiating from hilum. Bronchiectasis (dilated bronchi from repeated infection or injury) has been described as "tram tracks," also radiating from hilum. Eventually, these bronchiectatic cavities fill with fluid and can form abscesses. Pneumothorax is common end-stage complication. Hilar enlargement may be present, possibly owing to centrally dilated hypertensive pulmonary arteries.

C. Langerhans cell histiocytosis (LCH).
  1. Previously known as "histiocytosis X."
  2. Three types.
    a. Eosinophilic granuloma.
      *1.* Bony lesions.
      *2.* No pulmonary manifestations.
    b. Hand-Schüller-Christian syndrome.
      *1.* Chronic, disseminated form, often with pulmonary involvement.

         2. Bone lesions may also be present.
      c. Letterer-Siwe disease.
         1. Fulminant course with high mortality.
         2. Hepatosplenomegaly.
         3. Adenopathy.
         4. Bone marrow involvement.

> **Imaging** Chest radiographic appearance in LCH can demonstrate variety of abnormalities. Hyperaeration may be early finding. Reticulonodular pattern with upper lobe predominance may be present, caused by tiny parenchymal granulomas and lung cysts. Finally, honeycomb pattern (characteristic of end-stage lung disease) may develop. Pneumothorax can complicate end-stage LCH.

D. Collagen vascular.
   1. Types.
      a. Rheumatoid arthritis.
      b. Scleroderma.
      c. Systemic lupus erythematosis.
      d. Ankylosing spondylitis.
   2. Uncommon in pediatric population.
   3. Most common type in children is juvenile rheumatoid arthritis (JRA); still rarely has chest involvement.

> **Imaging** Often normal chest radiograph in early stages of disease. Reticular interstitial pattern can appear that can progress into pulmonary fibrosis (honeycomb lung). Pneumothorax can occur. Pleural and pericardial effusions can be seen with lupus and rheumatoid arthritis (also characterized by pulmonary nodules).

E. Sarcoid.
   1. Noncaseating granulomas of unknown etiology.
   2. Rare in children; can be seen in young African-American women.
   3. Multiorgan involvement.
      a. Bones.
         1. "Lacy," punctate lesions or granulomas.
         2. Especially in hands and feet.
      b. Eyes.
         1. Uveitis.
         2. Retinitis.
         3. Lacrimal gland involvement.

    c. Skin nodules.
    d. Lung.

> **Imaging** Chest radiograph can be normal. Hilar and mediastinal adenopathy are earliest radiographic manifestations of disease. Progressive disease involves pulmonary interstitium, which can present as reticulonodular pattern (often with upper lobe predominance). Finally, pulmonary involvement can progress to end-stage fibrosis (honeycomb lung). Hilar and mediastinal adenopathy often regress with progressive pulmonary involvement.

F. Pulmonary hemosiderosis (hemorrhage).
  1. Idiopathic pulmonary hemorrhage.
     a. Most common type in children.
     b. Usually occurs in children less than 10 years of age.
  2. Autoimmune disorders.
     a. Goodpasture's syndrome.
     b. Antiglomerular basement membranes.
  3. Pulmonary vasculitis.
     a. Rare in children.
     b. Types.
        *1.* Wegener granulomatosis.
        *2.* Allergic alveolar granulomatosis or Churg-Strauss syndrome.

> **Imaging** Initially appears as alveolar opacities on chest radiograph, usually near hilum. Can mimic pulmonary edema. After multiple episodes of hemorrhage, pulmonary fibrosis may result.

G. Alveolar proteinosis.
  1. Characterized by alveolar deposition of material high in lipids.
  2. Etiology is unknown; some physicians have suggested that it could be caused by deficiency of surfactant B (subunit of surfactant).
     a. Surfactant (reduces alveolar tension) has four important protein components.
     b. Genetic loss of subtype B leads to alveolar proteinosis.
     c. Can present at any time from newborn to adult (depends on amount of surfactant subunit B that can be produced by faulty Type II pneumatocytes).
     d. Consider diagnosis in full-term neonate who requires persistent surfactant therapy.
  3. Grim prognosis, especially in early presentation (less than 1 year).
  4. Treatment includes bronchoalveolar lavage.

> **Imaging** Chest radiograph reveals alveolar opacities with air bronchograms that resemble surfactant deficiency disorder in neonates.

H. Pulmonary tumors.
  1. Primary pulmonary neoplasms are rare in children.
  2. Hamartoma.
     a. Benign lesion.
     b. Probably arise from embryonic rests.
     c. Can contain pulmonary, bronchial, and cartilagenous components.

> **Imaging** Well-circumscribed pulmonary lesion is seen on chest radiograph; often lobulated with classic "popcorn calcifications."

  3. Askin tumor.
     a. Aggressive, destructive tumor that originates in soft tissues of chest wall or lung.
     b. "Small blue cells" of this primitive neuroectodermal tumor resemble those of Ewing sarcoma.

> **Imaging** Chest wall mass (often large), causing rib destruction with pleural and parenchymal invasion and effusions can be seen on chest radiograph.

  4. Pulmonary blastoma.
     a. Extremely rare.
     b. Thought to be derived from embryonal pulmonary tissue, hence designation of blastoma.

> **Imaging** Chest radiograph demonstrates well-circumscribed, often peripheral mass in pulmonary parenchyma. Usually not symptomatic; can be incidental finding on chest radiograph (can mimic round pneumonia). Can be quite large at presentation.

  5. Metastatic.
     a. Sarcomas.
        *1.* Osteogenic sarcoma.
        *2.* Ewing sarcoma.
        *3.* Rhabdomyosarcoma.
     b. Wilms tumor.
     c. Neuroblastoma.

> **Imaging** Chest radiograph may reveal round, smooth opacities scattered throughout lung fields. Computed tomography

scan of chest, however, is more sensitive study for pulmonary metastatic disease.

**SUGGESTED READINGS**

Amodia JB, Berdon WE, Abramson S, Baker D: Cystic fibrosis in childhood: Pulmonary, paranasal sinus and skeletal manifestations. *Semin Roentgenol* 1987; 22:125-135.

Askin FB, Rosai J, Sibley RK, Dehner LP, McAlister WH: Malignant small cell tumor of the thoracopulmonary region in childhood: A distinctive clinico pathologic entity of uncertain histogenesis. *Cancer* 1979; 43:2438-2451.

Bassett F, Corrin B, Spencer H, Lacronique J, Roth C, Soler P, Battesti JP, Georges R, Chretien J: Pulmonary histiocytosis X. *Am Rev Respir Dis* 1978; 118:811-820.

Eggli KD, Newman B: Nodules, masses and pseudomasses in the pediatric lung. *Radiol Clin North Am* 1993; 31:651-666.

Kirkpatrick JA, Harris GBC: Pulmonary manifestations of cystic fibrosis in the adolescent and young adult. *Contemp Diagn Radiol* 1981; 4:1-6.

Levy J, Wilmott RW: Pulmonary hemosiderosis. *Pediatr Pulmonol* 1986; 2:384-391.

McCook TA, Kirks DR, Merten DF, Osborne DR, Spock A, Pratt PC: Pulmonary alveolar proteinosis in children. *AJR* 1981; 137:1023-1027.

Merten DF, Kirks DR, Grossman H: Pulmonary sarcoidosis in childhood. *AJR* 1980; 135:673-679.

Orenstein DM, Bowen A: Cystic fibrosis: Clinical update for radiologists. *Radiol Clin North Am* 1993; 31:617-630.

Rebuck AS: Radiologic aspects of asthma. *Australas Radiol* 1970; 14:264-268.

Sumner TE, Phelps CR, Crowe JE, Poolos SP, Shaffner LD: Pulmonary blastoma in a child. *AJR* 1979; 133:147-148.

Yousefzadeh DK, Fishman PA: The triad of pneumonitis, pleuritis and pericarditis in juvenile rheumatoid arthritis. *Pediatr Radiol* 1979; 8:147-150.

# 7
# Mediastinal Masses

---

### Key Concepts

1. Mediastinal masses in children comprise a variety of developmental abnormalities and neoplasms (one third of which are neurogenic tumors).
2. Mediastinal masses can be incidental findings on a chest radiograph. This probably explains why many of these tumors are large at presentation. However, some mediastinal masses produce symptoms from mass effect on the airway (dyspnea, cough, stridor, or wheezing) or spinal cord (focal neurologic signs).
3. Differential diagnosis of a mediastinal mass is based on its location in the anterior, middle, or posterior compartments (Figs. 7-1 and 7-2).
4. Mneumonic for mediastinal masses:
   a. Anterior mediastinal mass: "Terrible Ts."
   b. Middle mediastinal mass: "A,B,C's."
   c. Posterior mediastinal mass: "Neurogenic."

A. Anterior mediastinal masses.
   1. Comprise 30% of mediastinal tumors.
   2. Contents of anterior mediastinum.
      a. Thymus.
      b. Lymph nodes.

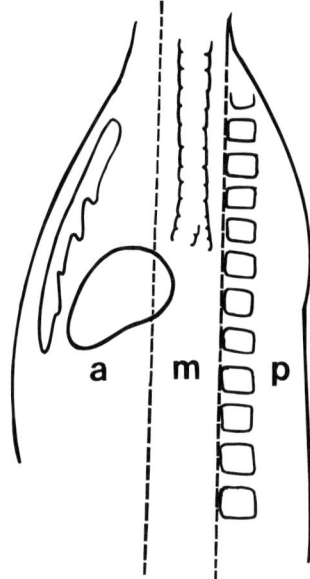

**Fig. 7-1** Lateral chest film separated into compartments (*a*, anterior; *m*, middle; *p*, posterior).

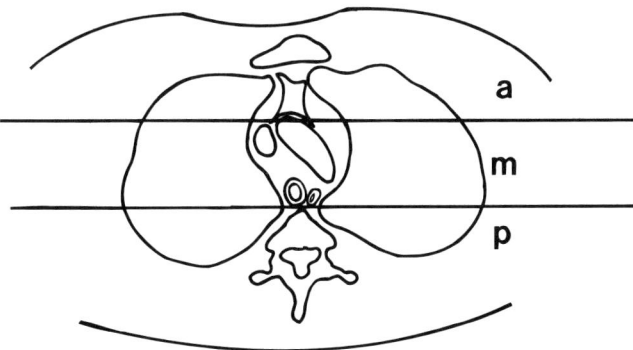

**Fig. 7-2** CT of chest separated into compartments (*a*, anterior; *m*, middle; *p*, posterior).

c. Anterior portion of heart and pericardium.
   d. Main pulmonary artery.
   e. Proximal ascending aorta.
   f. Phrenic nerve.
3. Anterior mediastinal mass differential diagnosis: ("Terrible Ts").
   a. Thymic hyperplasia.
   b. Thymic tumor (rare).
   c. Teratoma (germ cell tumors).
   d. Thyroid tumor (rare).
   e. "Terrible" lymphoma (T cell).
4. Thymus.
   a. Bilobed, pyramidal structure in anterior or superior mediastinum; can extend into posterior or middle mediastinum.
   b. Thymus is most conspicuous on chest radiographs of children in first 2 to 3 years of life, even though thymus reaches maximum size during adolescence.
   c. Hypoplastic thymus (consider immunodeficiency, since thymus normally produces T lymphocytes).
   d. Aplastic thymus.
      1. DiGeorge syndrome.
      2. Third or fourth pharyngeal pouch abnormality.
   e. Thymus can involute.
      1. Stress.
      2. Steroids.
      3. Illness.
   f. Thymic hyperplasia or pseudotumor.
      1. Physiologic enlargement ("rebound" hypertrophy).
      2. Occurs after stress involution.
   g. Thymic tumors.
      1. Rare.
      2. Types.
         a. Thymoma.
            1) Classic association of thymoma and myasthenia gravis in adults (approximately 50% of patients with thymoma have myasthenia gravis, while 15% of patients with myasthenia gravis have thymoma).
            2) This association is rarely found in children.
         b. Thymic cyst.
         c. Thymolipoma.
         d. Thymic enlargement with leukemic invasion.
   h. If diagnosing thymic hyperplasia versus other pathology, one can re-image to confirm stability and/or involution.

> **Imaging** On chest radiograph, widened mediastinum is present, often with "sail sign," "thymic wave," or "cardiothymic notch." Often difficult to ascertain true heart size on frontal radiograph because of normal infant or toddler thymus. On computed tomography (CT), thymus appears as concave, homogeneous, anterior mediastinal soft-tissue density that can be seen well into adulthood. Mediastinal shift or mass effect on other mediastinal structures is never seen with prominent thymus, even in its rebound or hypertrophied stage. Thymus might appear as lobulated mass in anterior mediastinum on both chest radiograph and CT.

 5. Germ cell tumor.
    a. Can arise from ectopic gonadal tissue that failed to migrate properly from urogenital ridge to gonads during embryogenesis.
    b. Found commonly in pelvis.
    c. Types.
        1. Teratoma (benign and malignant).
        2. Teratocarcinoma.
        3. Choriocarcinoma.
        4. Seminoma.
        5. Endodermal sinus (yolk sac).
        6. Mixed germ cell tumor.
    d. Teratoma.
        1. Next to hyperplastic (rebound) thymus, most common anterior mediastinal mass in children.
        2. Comprises 80% to 90% of germ cell tumors.
        3. Composed of all three germ layers: endoderm, ectoderm, and mesoderm.
        4. Benign.
            a. Often well-defined lobulated mass.
            b. Solid and/or cystic mass which may contain fat, teeth, calcifications, or skin.
            c. Can not be clearly differentiated from malignant variety based on radiographic appearance alone.
        5. Malignant.
            a. Teratoma or teratocarcinoma.
            b. Rare, solid mass; usually found in males.
            c. Increased alpha-fetoprotein (AFP) and human chorionic gonadotropin.
    e. Seminoma.

1. Normal AFP level.
2. Survival better than other malignant germ cell tumors.
3. Radiosensitive tumor.
4. Must exclude testicular primary (although metastatic disease usually goes to retroperitoneal lymph nodes).
   f. Endodermal sinus (yolk sac).
      1. Rare, very malignant tumor; often presents with metastatic disease.
      2. Not really germ cell tumor; derived from intraplacental perivascular tracts known as endodermal sinuses of Duval (hence name). Can also originate in yolk sac endoderm.
      3. Increased AFP levels.

> **Imaging** Chest radiograph and CT may demonstrate lobulated, anterior mediastinal mass (often large with tracheal displacement). Calcifications may be present (particularly in benign teratoma). Displacement of adjacent structures and tissue inhomogeneity distinguish this group of lesions from more common thymic hyperplasia.

6. Lymphoma.
   a. Lymphoma or leukemia is most common neoplasm in children, followed by central nervous system (CNS) tumors.
   b. About 60% are non-Hodgkin lymphoma (NHL); peak age range 7 to 11.
   c. About 40% are Hodgkin lymphoma (HL); peak age range 13 to 17.
   d. NHL.
      1. Usually disseminated disease (70%); close overlap with acute lymphocytic leukemia.
      2. Predominant primary site.
         a. Extranodal, especially in abdomen.
         b. In contrast to adult NHL and HL, mediastinal involvement occurs in only 25% of pediatric patients.
      3. Classification of NHL.
         a. Cell types.
         b. Cell markers.
         c. Degree of differentiation.
      4. Types of NHL.
         a. Lymphoblastic.
            1) From 30% to 35% of NHL types.
            2) Supradiaphragmatic (mediastinal mass).
            3) Can have head or neck adenopathy, usually T cell.
         b. Undifferentiated, non-Burkitt type.

1) From 25% to 30% of NHL types.
   2) Found in abdomen, particularly ileocecal region.
   c. Undifferentiated, Burkitt type.
      1) From 20% to 25% of NHL types.
      2) Monoclonal B cell lineage.
      3) African variety.
         a) Associated with Ebstein-Barr virus.
         b) Predominantly head and neck lesions.
      4) North American variety.
         a) Found more commonly in abdominal region.
         b) Poor prognosis.
   d. Histiocytic or large cell.
      1) From 15% to 20% of NHL types.
      2) Varying sites (including orbit and bone); infrequently presents as mediastinal mass.
e. HL.
   1. Ten percent of all HL occurs in children, mostly in adolescents.
   2. Clinical features, treatment, sites, and prognosis are identical to adult form.
      a. Stage I: disease limited to one lymph node (LN) region.
      b. Stage II: disease limited to one side of diaphragm, but two or more LN chains.
      c. Stage III: LN chains on both sides of diaphragm.
      d. Stage IV: diffuse involvement of LN, lungs, liver, bone marrow, CNS.
   3. Cervical adenopathy most common mediastinal nodes (85%).
   4. Types.
      a. Nodular sclerosis (60% to 70%).
      b. Mixed cellularity (15% to 25%).
      c. Lymphocytic predominance (10% to 15%).
      d. Lymphocytic depletion (1% to 5%).

**Imaging** Widened mediastinum is seen on chest radiograph, occasionally with hilar nodes as well. CT reveals heterogenous anterior mediastinal mass, often lobulated without calcifications. Lesion can be quite large, displacing mediastinal structures such as trachea and great vessels. Can infiltrate and enlarge thymus as well. After treatment, lesion can calcify.

B. Middle mediastinal masses (30%).
   1. Contents of middle mediastinum.
      a. Posterior heart and pericardium.
      b. Aortic arch and great vessels.

c. Pulmonary arteries.
   d. Trachea.
   e. LNs.
   f. Esophagus.
2. Middle mediastinal masses are almost always benign; lymphoma is one exception.
3. Differential list of middle mediastinal masses ("A,B,C's").
   a. *A*denopathy.
   b. *A*orta.
   c. *B*ronchogenic cyst.
   d. *C*ysts (developmental cysts, neurenteric).
   e. *C*ardiac masses.
4. Adenopathy.
   a. Almost always infectious or inflammatory.
      *1.* Tuberculosis (TB).
      *2.* Histoplasmosis.
      *3.* Mononucleosis.
      *4.* Sarcoid (rare in children).
   b. Neoplastic adenopathy.
      *1.* Lymphoma (also look for anterior mediastinal mass).
      *2.* Other lymphoproliferative disorders such as Castleman disease.
         *a.* Giant LN hyperplasia (massive LNs often seen in anterior mediastinum).
         *b.* Benign, uncommon entity; usually found in young women or adolescents.
      *3.* Rarely neoplastic or metastatic nodes.

> **Imaging** Middle, mediastinal (often hilar) soft-tissue lobulated masses can be seen on chest radiographs and on CT. Symmetric adenopathy may be present.

5. Aorta.
   a. Aneurysm (rare in children).
   b. Aortic dissection.
      *1.* Increased incidence with Marfan syndrome, Turner syndrome, and Noonan syndrome.
   c. Aortic transection.
      *1.* Motor vehicle accident.
         *a.* Acceleration or deceleration injury.

> **Imaging** Widened mediastinum on chest radiograph. When considering aortic leak, look for pleural effusion, apical

capping, and indistinct aortic knob. Contrast CT, magnetic resonance imaging (MRI), or angiography can better delineate extent of aortic injury.

6. Bronchogenic cyst.
   a. Bronchopulmonary foregut malformation caused by abnormal budding of developing foregut.
   b. Usually found in middle mediastinum (often near trachea or carina), but can be found anywhere in chest. Can also be peripheral lesion.
   c. Can be located between trachea and esophagus and mimic pulmonary sling.
   d. Lesion grows over time.
      *1.* Continues to secrete mucus with no outlet connection to either the trachea or esophagus.
      *2.* Can eventually cause mass effect and obstruct airway.

**Imaging** Chest radiograph demonstrates sharply marginated, smooth, round lesion. CT can confirm fluid nature of lesion. Can cause mass effect upon adjacent structures.

7. Cysts (developmental).
   a. Gastrointestinal duplication cyst (esophageal).
      *1.* Caused by faulty canalization of esophagus.
      *2.* Does not communicate with gut; consequently, intraluminal secretions accumulate, and size of lesion usually increases over time.
   b. Neurenteric cyst.
      *1.* Caused by faulty neural tube closure with continued neural (ectoderm) connection with endoderm.
      *2.* Resulting abnormal mesenchyme adjacent to neural tube leads to abnormal vertebral body formation (segmentation anomalies such as hemivertebrae or butterfly vertebrae).
      *3.* Found most commonly in thoracic spine with actual cyst located within mediastinum.
   c. Lymphangioma-hemangioma.
      *1.* Lymphangiomatous malformation, often with hemangiomatous component.
      *2.* Cystic hygroma (term used if large cystic spaces are present).
      *3.* These lesions are often infiltrative, making them difficult to completely resect; commonly recur.
      *4.* Associated with Turner syndrome, Noonan syndrome, and Down syndrome.

> **Imaging** Chest radiograph and CT show smooth, well-demarcated, fluid-filled lesion with thin wall. Internal septations may be present.

8. Cardiac masses.
   a. Uncommon.
   b. Fibroma.
      1. Myocardial mass, often of left ventricle or septum.
      2. Malignant counterpart (fibrosarcoma) is rare.
   c. Rhabdomyoma.
      1. Associated with tuberous sclerosis (50%).
      2. Often multiple lesions.
      3. Myocardial tumor that usually projects into ventricle.
      4. Malignant counterpart (rhabdomyosarcoma) is rare and not associated with tuberous sclerosis.
   d. Myxoma.
      1. Rare; 75% are left atrial.
      2. Subendocardial in origin; found more commonly in females than in males.
   e. Pericardial cyst.
   f. Be aware of possible intrinsic cardiac causes that can mimic mass, such as hypertrophy, pericardial effusion, or aneurysm.

> **Imaging** Chest radiograph can show abnormal cardiac silhouette, often with unusual bulge.

9. Esophageal.
   a. Esophageal masses or pathology are rare in children.
   b. One exception is hiatal hernia.
      1. Can be seen as isolated abnormality in children (as in adults).
      2. Sequelae of Nissen fundoplication.

> **Imaging** Soft-tissue mass seen posterior to heart (best seen on lateral chest radiograph). Air-fluid level is often present.

C. Posterior mediastinal masses.
  1. Forty percent of all mediastinal masses.
  2. Contents of posterior mediastinum.
     a. Thoracic duct.
     b. Descending aorta.
     c. Azygous and hemiazygous.
     d. Spine and nerve roots.
     e. Paravertebral sympathetic chain.
  3. Differential list of posterior mediastinal masses ("Neurogenic").

a. Nerve sheath (neurofibroma or schwannoma).
   b. Sympathetic nervous system (neuroblastoma, ganglioneuroblastoma, ganglioneuroma).
   c. Paraganglionic cell (pheochromocytoma or chemodectoma).
   d. Meningocele.
   e. Extramedullary hematopoiesis (rare).
4. Neurofibroma.
   a. Benign tumor of nerve sheath (schwannoma).
   b. Associated with neurofibromatosis; can arise in any nerve.
   c. Posterior mediastinum is common site for neurofibromas that arise from nerve roots exiting neural foramina.
   d. Can cause scoliosis, posterior rib erosion, or neuroforaminal widening.
   e. Can rarely be malignant (neurofibrosarcoma).

**Imaging** Chest radiograph may show paraspinal mass, neuroforaminal widening, scoliosis, rib erosion, or rib notching (if neurofibroma involves intercostal nerve). CT or MRI can demonstrate dumbbell-shaped, soft-tissue lesion in posterior mediastinum, extending through neural foramina.

5. Neuroblastoma.
   a. From 10% to 15% of neuroblastomas are located in thorax.
   b. Derived from primitive, sympathetic neuroblasts from neural crest.
   c. Tumor presents as smooth, often lobulated paraspinal mass.
   d. Osseous changes include rib erosions and destruction.
   e. Prognosis.
      *1.* More favorable prognosis for mediastinal neuroblastoma as compared with abdominal (adrenal) type.
      *2.* Prognosis is complex and dependent on many factors.
         *a.* Age (better prognosis if less than 1 year of age).
         *b.* Stage.
         *c.* n-*myc* gene copies.
         *d.* Shimada classification.
   f. Evidence of metastatic disease at presentation (60%).
      *1.* Skeletal.
         *a.* Focal lytic lesions.
         *b.* Lucent metaphyseal bands.
         *c.* Vertebral body collapse.
         *d.* Bone marrow involvement.
      *2.* Lymphadenopathy.
      *3.* Liver metastases.

            *4.* Skin lesions.
     g. Intraspinal invasion is more common with neuroblastoma in chest, as compared with neuroblastoma in abdomen.
     h. Staging.
          *1.* Stage I.
               *a.* Tumor confined to organ of origin.
               *b.* Survival greater than 90%.
          *2.* Stage II.
               *a.* Tumor extending beyond organ of origin, but not crossing midline.
               *b.* Ipsilateral lymph nodes may be involved.
          *3.* Stage III.
               *a.* Tumor extends across midline.
          *4.* Stage IV.
               *a.* Metastatic disease.
               *b.* Survival rate can drop to less than 20%.
          *5.* Stage IV S (s for "special").
               *a.* Patients who would be stage I or II but have remote disease to one or more of following: liver, skin, or bone marrow (but no bony metastasis).
               *b.* Excellent prognosis for those children who are less than 1 year of age.
     i. Interesting note: rare but well-documented incidence of malignant neuroblastoma "maturation" to well-differentiated benign neoplasm (ganglioneuroma). Spontaneous transformation occurs 1 to 2:1000.

> **Imaging** Chest radiograph demonstrates often inhomogeneous, posterior mediastinal soft-tissue mass, located adjacent to spine. CT is helpful for evaluation of extent of disease (distant metastases), while MRI can evaluate for vertebral or spinal canal invasion (via neural foramina). Calcifications are often present within inhomogeneous lesion. Nuclear medicine scan (metaiodobenzylguanidine or MIBG) can show tracer uptake in cells of neural crest origin; therefore, can assist in staging of disease.

6. Ganglioneuroma.
    a. Benign tumor of differentiated neural crest cells.
    b. Age 6 and older.
    c. Often seen extending along nerve roots into foramina (dumbbell-shaped lesion). Slow growing; compresses local structures.
    d. Malignant counterpart.
         *1.* Ganglioneuroblastoma.

2. Contains features of both ganglioneuroma and neuroblastoma (has undifferentiated neuroblasts and mature ganglion cells).

> **Imaging** Well-circumscribed, posterior paravertebral mass can be seen on chest radiograph. CT or MRI can often show mass arising from neural foramina, but can not differentiate between two types (ganglioneuroma and ganglioblastoma) radiographically. However, presence of calcifications is more ominous sign. Bony erosion may be present.

7. Meningocele.
   a. Neural tube defect can result in anterior or lateral meningocele.
   b. Rare; can be seen in neurofibromatosis.

> **Imaging** Posterior cystic mass continuous with thecal sac; can be seen on CT or MRI; look for adjacent abnormal vertebrae.

8. Neurenteric cyst (see Chapters 9 and 43).
9. Extramedullary hematopoiesis.
   a. Posterior mediastinal masses (usually multiple) appear as result of recruited sites of extramedullary hematopoiesis in cases of severe anemia, such as sickle cell or osteopetrosis.
   b. Uncommon in pediatrics because liver, spleen, and bone marrow are recruited first, when extra hematopoiesis is needed.

> **Imaging** Lobulated, often symmetric, paravertebral masses in posterior thorax on chest radiograph.

## SUGGESTED READINGS

Armstrong EA, Harwood-Nash DCF, Fitz CR: CT of neuroblastomas and ganglioneuromas in children. *AJR* 1989; 139:571-576.

Aterman K, Schneller TV, Wigger MJ: Maturation of neuroblastoma to ganglioneuroma. *Am J Dis Child* 1970; 120:217-222.

Cohen M, Hill CA, Cangir A, Sullivan MP: Thymic rebound after treatment of childhood tumors. *AJR* 1980; 135:151-156.

Drossman SR, Schiff RG, Kronfield GD, McNamara J, Leonidas JC: Lymphoma of the mediastinum and neck: Evaluation with Ga-67 imaging and CT correlation. *Radiology* 1990; 174:171-175.

Fox MA, Vix VA: Endodermal sinus tumor (yolk sac) of the anterior mediastinum. *AJR* 1980; 135:291-294.

Francis IR, Glazer GM, Bookstein FL: The thymus: Reexamination of age-related changes in size and shape. *AJR* 1985; 145:249-254.

Hamrick-Turner JE, Sarf MF, Power CI, Blumenthal BI, Royal SA, Iyer RV: Imaging of childhood non-Hodgkin lymphoma. *Radiographics* 1994; 14:11-28.

Kawashima A, Fishman EK, Kuhlman JE: CT of posterior mediastinal masses. *Radiographics* 1991; 11:1045-1067.

King MR, Telander RL, Smithson W: Primary mediastinal tumors in children. *J Pediatr Surg* 1982; 17:512-520.

Levitt RG, Husbond JE, Glazer HS: CT of primary germ cell tumors of the mediastinum. *AJR* 1984; 142:73-78.

Lund JT, Ehman RL, Julsrud PR: Cardiac masses: Assessment by MR imaging. *AJR* 1989; 152:469-473.

Merten DF: Diagnostic imaging of mediastinal masses in children. *AJR* 1992; 158:825-832.

Moon WK, Kim WS, Kim IO, Yeon KM, Han MC: Castleman disease in the child: CT and ultrasonographic findings. *Pediatr Radiol* 1994; 24:182-184.

Seigel MJ, Nadel SN, Glazer HS, Sagel SS: Mediastinal lesions in children: Comparison of CT and MR imaging. *Radiology* 1986; 160:241-244.

Taylor GE: Mediastinal masses. *Radiol Clin North Am* 1993; 31:677-691.

# SECTION II
## Gastrointestinal System

# 8
# Neonatal Abdomen: Bowel Obstruction and Masses

---

### Key Concepts

1. The normal neonatal radiograph should show air within the stomach by 15 minutes of age, with air reaching the colon by 24 hours. Bowel loops should be well distributed throughout the abdomen with nondistended, thin bowel walls; flanks should also be nondistended. Do not try to distinguish large bowel from small bowel in the neonate.
2. Distended neonatal bowel loops can be due to necrotizing enterocolitis (NEC), ileus (often from sepsis), or obstruction.
3. Four patterns of neonatal bowel obstruction.
    a. Gastric distension.
    b. "Double bubble."
    c. Proximal (a few dilated loops in the left upper quadrant).
    d. Distal (dilated loops throughout the abdomen).
4. Water-soluble enema for distal obstruction can be both diagnostic and therapeutic in the neonate. Look for the presence of a "microcolon."
5. Renal origin is the most common etiology for the abdominal mass in the neonate.

A. Bowel obstruction.
   1. Etiology of dilated bowel loops.
      a. NEC (see Chapter 12).
      b. Ileus.
         *1.* Often from sepsis.
         *2.* Seen in infants with intrauterine growth retardation.
      c. Obstruction (four bowel gas patterns).
         *1.* Distended stomach only (gastric outlet obstruction).
         *2.* "Double bubble" (dilated stomach and proximal duodenal).
         *3.* Proximal small bowel (few dilated loops in left upper quadrant).
         *4.* Distal small or large bowel (multiple dilated loops of bowel filling abdomen).
   2. Gastric distension only.
      a. Hypertrophic pyloric stenosis (HPS).
         *1.* Hypertrophy of circular musculature of pylorus causes obstruction.
         *2.* Occurs between third and sixth weeks of life.
         *3.* Incidence is 1:1000; found more commonly in males than in females (4:1).
         *4.* Presents with projectile, nonbilious vomiting.
         *5.* "Palpable olive" (hypertrophied pylorus).
         *6.* Be aware of pylorospasm that can mimic pyloric stenosis. However, pylorospasm usually lasts less than 5 minutes.
         *7.* Surgical pyloromyotomy is curative.

> **Imaging** Abdominal radiograph may demonstrate distended stomach; however, radiograph is often normal. Elongated pylorus ("string sign") with mass effect upon duodenal bulb ("shouldering") can be seen on upper gastrointestinal (UGI) examination. Also look for delayed gastric emptying time (can be due to either HPS or pylorospasm). Ultrasound (US) will show thickened hypoechoic muscular wall (measures greater than 3 mm in transverse dimension), with elongated pyloric channel (greater than 15 to 17 mm). When US is equivocal (measurement 2 to 3 mm), consider glucose and water meal to evaluate pyloric function (Fig. 8-1).

      b. Other gastric outlet abnormalities.
         *1.* Antral or pyloric atresia.
            *a.* Extremely rare.
            *b.* Gastrointestinal atresias are usually caused by ischemic events (except for duodenal atresia); therefore, they are rare in stomach, because of its redundant vascular supply.

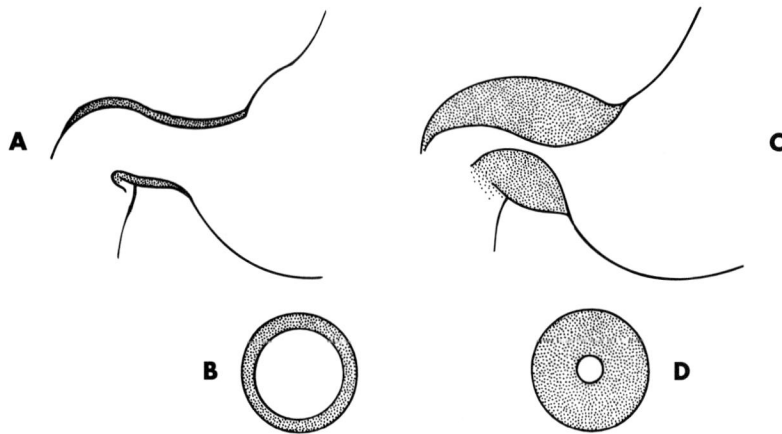

**Fig. 8-1** Ultrasound of pyloric muscle (stippled area represents muscular layer). **A,** Normal longitudinal view. **B,** Normal transverse view. **C,** Hypertrophic pyloric stenosis (longitudinal view). **D,** Hypertrophic pyloric stenosis (transverse view).

    2. Congenital antral webs or diaphrams.
       *a.* Rare.
       *b.* Variable in size and obstructive potential.

> **Imaging** Can appear as linear filling defects near antrum or pylorus on UGI examination.

    3. Volvulus.
       *a.* Causes outlet obstruction, sometimes with vascular compromise.
       *b.* Rare.
       *c.* Types.
          *1)* Mesenteroaxial.
          *2)* Organoaxial.

> **Imaging** UGI examination can show rotated stomach with total or partial gastric outlet obstruction. Look for presence of hiatal hernia (often seen with organoaxial volvulus) or bowel malrotation (can be seen with mesenteroaxial volvulus).

    c. Lactobezoar.
       *1.* Improperly mixed formula can precipitate out in stomach, causing formation of lactobezoar.
       *2.* This foreign body can obstruct gastric outlet.

> **Imaging** Look for irregular, persistent, often floating, filling defect on UGI examination.

   d. Prostaglandin administration.
      *1.* Antral thickening and/or gastric outlet obstruction can occur, following prostaglandin administration (keeps patent ductus arteriosus open in treatment of congenital heart disease [CHD] such as pulmonary atresia or aortic coarctation).
      *2.* Gastric distension and obstruction resolve upon cessation of prostaglandin therapy.
3. "Double bubble."
   a. Duodenal atresia or stenosis.
      *1.* Atresia is much more common than stenosis.
      *2.* Incidence is 1:6000; 30% of patients have Down syndrome.
      *3.* Etiology (Fig. 8-2).
         *a.* Faulty recanalization of bowel.
         *b.* Look for polyhydramnios.
      *4.* Be aware that presence of distal bowel gas does not rule out duodenal atresia. Bowel gas can be seen distal to duodenal atresia, owing to anomalous pancreatic ducts.

> **Imaging** Abdominal radiograph demonstrates distension of stomach and proximal duodenum (causing double bubble). Prenatal US can also make this diagnosis. Polyhydramnios may be present.

   b. Midgut volvulus.
      *1.* Surgical (and therefore radiologic) emergency.
      *2.* Abnormally positioned small bowel (malrotation) predisposes to twisting (volvulus) because of short mesentery. Resulting vascular compromise (obstruction of superior mesenteric artery [SMA]) can infarct bowel.
      *3.* Presents with bilious vomiting and/or pain in older children.
      *4.* Malrotation is not synonomous with midgut volvulus.
         *a.* There are many patterns of malrotation, of which only few are at high risk for midgut volvulus (see Chapter 10).
         *b.* Malrotation type IIIa.
            *1)* Midline duodenum and cecum results in short mesentery.
            *2)* Most common malrotation pattern to cause midgut volvulus.
      *5.* Ladd bands (see Chapter 10).

*a.* Right upper quadrant peritoneal bands that originate from malfixation of colon.
  *b.* Cecum malposition and lack of hepatic flexure fixation.
  *c.* Ladd bands can cross over duodenum and obstruct lumen.

**Imaging** Abdominal radiograph can show gastric distension with paucity of distal gas. UGI contrast examination can show corkscrew appearance of duodenum, as gut twists around SMA. However, with actual midgut volvulus, bowel obstruction will occur, and very little contrast will be seen beyond second portion of duodenum. Although UGI is examination of choice for this entity, US findings of malrotation or midgut volvulus have been described: reversal of normal superior mesenteric artery and superior mesenteric vein orientation can be seen on midline transverse images.

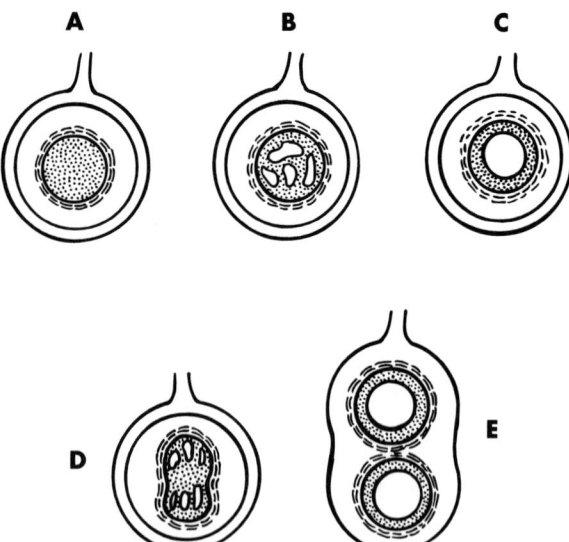

**Fig. 8-2** Canalization of bowel (etiology of duodenal atresia and duplication cysts). **A,** Solid lumen of bowel prior to canalization (failure of development at this level results in atresia). **B,** Vacuoles forming. **C,** Coalescing vacuoles eventually form bowel lumen. **D,** Abnormal vacuole formation without coalescing. **E,** Results in more than one bowel lumen (one of which is true lumen and other is duplication cyst).

c. Annular pancreas.
  1. Pancreatic tissue encircles second portion of duodenum, near ampulla of Vater.
  2. Rare.
  3. Etiology.
    a. Failure of ventral pancreatic anlage to migrate dorsally and fuse with dorsal pancreas during development.
    b. Age of presentation depends on degree of obstruction by constricting pancreas.

**Imaging** UGI examination will reveal constricting lesion of duodenum that causes either partial or complete obstruction.

d. Preduodenal portal vein.
  1. Rare.
  2. Embryology.
    a. Vitelline veins are early embryologic drainage of gut with three anastomotic channels. Normally, middle channel persists as portal vein (posterior to duodenum).
    b. Persistence of inferior channel results in anteriorly positioned portal vein (preduodenal).
  3. Anomalous position of preduodenal portal vein can produce duodenal obstruction.
  4. Association with other anomalies (85%).
    a. Midgut malrotation.
    b. Duodenal atresia.
    c. Annular pancreas.
    d. Biliary atresia.
4. Proximal small bowel obstruction.
  a. Jejunal atresia or stenosis.
    1. Most atresia or stenosis is due to ischemia.
    2. Atresia is much more common than stenosis.
    3. Proximal obstruction results in colon of normal caliber (rather than microcolon), since bowel distal to obstruction continues to produce enough secretions to normally distend colon.

**Imaging** Abdominal radiograph reveals few bowel dilated loops in left upper quadrant.

5. Distal small or large bowel obstruction.
  a. Clinical presentation is distended abdomen, often with failure to pass meconium. Initial radiographic findings of multiple dilated bowel loops throughout abdomen suggest distal bowel obstruction.

b. Start evaluation with simple question: "Is there an anus?"
c. If no anus is present, diagnosis is: Imperforate anus.
   1. Incidence is 1:5000; found more commonly in males than in females.
   2. Types.
      a. High.
         1) Rectal pouch terminates above levator sling.
         2) Maintaining rectal continence is of concern in this group because of poorly developed levator sling.
         3) Result: infants with high imperforate anus have diverting colostomy until levator sling matures and definitive repair of anus can be performed (usually during the first year of life).
         4) Increased incidence of genitourinary (GU) fistulas.
      b. Low.
         1) Rectal pouch passes through levator sling.
         2) Often perineal dimple or perineal fistula is present.
         3) Because levator sling is well developed, pull-through procedure or anoplasty at birth can be performed.
   3. Associated with VACTERL:
      a. Vertebral anomalies (segmentation abnormalities).
      b. Anal atresia.
      c. Cardiac abnormalities.
      d. TracheoEsophgeal fistula.
      e. Renal.
      f. Limb anomalies.
   4. Urinary tract abnormalities are commonly seen.
      a. Incidence of low anal atresia (25%).
      b. Incidence of high anal atresia (40%).

**Imaging** Abdominal radiographs show multiple dilated bowel loops. US can elucidate level of pouch: low atresia is pouch located less than 5 mm from perineal surface; treat anything greater than 5 mm as high atresia. Voiding cystourethrogram (VCUG) can be done to look for commonly associated GU fistula (from rectal pouch to bladder, urethra, or vagina), especially in infants with high anal atresia.

d. If anus is present, proceed to water-soluble enema.
   1. Can be therapeutic (for removal of meconium plugs) as well as diagnostic.
   2. Contrast should be allowed to flow into colon by gravity; using syringe is not recommended, since it is difficult to

estimate intraluminal pressure generated by injection; could cause perforation of already compromised bowel.
        3. Entire colon should be visualized with contrast refluxed into distal ileum.
        4. Contents and caliber of colon should be evaluated.
    e. If normal caliber colon is present.
        1. Meconium plug syndrome.
            a. Multiple filling defects are noted in colon (meconium plugs).
            b. Most common cause of distal bowel obstruction in neonate.
            c. Also known as "small left colon syndrome" and "colonic inertia syndrome."
            d. Often seen in infants of diabetic mothers with poor, slow initial emptying of colon.
            e. Once meconium is removed.
                1) Normal function is restored.
                2) No further treatment or follow-up is needed (although some physicians advocate rectal biopsy to rule out Hirschsprung disease).
            f. Occasionally, repeat therapeutic enema is needed.

> **Imaging** Normal caliber colon is present on water-soluble enema. However, multiple filling defects are noted along course of colon consistent with meconium plugs. Look for characteristic mild narrowing of left colon.

        2. Hirschsprung disease.
            a. Also known as aganglionosis of colon.
                1) Disruption of orderly migration of ganglion cells from neural crest to bowel results in bowel segments with missing ganglion cells.
                2) Migration of ganglion cells proceeds caudally in hindgut.
                3) Further ganglionic migration terminates at point of disruption; no "skip" segments of normally innervated bowel occur beyond this level.
            b. Present as neonates (80%).
                1) Constipation.
                2) Abdominal distension.
                3) May have vomiting.
            c. Incidence is greater in males than in females (except for total colonic Hirschsprung disease, which is more common in females).
            d. Total colonic Hirschsprung disease.

1) Rare (3% to 5%).
2) More common in girls.
3) Difficult radiographic diagnosis when whole colon is involved, since no "transition zone" can be elicited; often entire colon appears normal.
     e. No bowel preparation or rectal manipulation prior to enema because they can eradicate transition zone (see Imaging).
     f. Location of transition zone.
        1) In rectosigmoid area (65%).
        2) In descending colon (14%).
        3) In rectum (8%).
        4) In colon proximal to splenic flexure (10%).
     g. Easy diagnosis to miss.
        1) Particularly "ultrashort" segment Hirschsprung disease.
        2) Rectal biopsy often warranted.
     h. Complications.
        1) Enterocolitis.
        2) Chronic constipation (when diagnosis is missed in infancy).

**Imaging** Abdominal radiograph demonstrates multiple dilated distal loops. On enema study, look for transition zone (difference in caliber between small distal bowel and dilated proximal bowel (most common in rectosigmoid area). Evaluate rectosigmoid ratio. In normal children, look for at least 1:1 ratio between width of rectum and sigmoid on anteroposterior film. (If rectum is smaller than sigmoid, Hirschsprung disease is suspected.) Additional imaging findings in diagnosis of Hirschsprung disease include "saw-tooth" contractions of bowel (due to denervation spasticity) and pneumatosis in full-term infant.

  3. Bowel dysgenesis (segmental ileal dilatation).
     a. Poorly functioning bowel loop (usually ileal).
        1) Presumably due to poorly functioning myenteric plexus.
        2) Lack of peristalsis results in nonmechanical obstruction ("pseudoobstruction").
     b. Must be differentiated from bowel loop with limited function from prior episode of NEC.

**Imaging** Delayed transit time can be seen on contrast study with evidence of poorly functioning, yet nonobstructive loop (often seen as persistent "bulbous bowel loop").

f. If microcolon is present (colon of narrow caliber resulting from chronic distal small bowel obstruction), insufficient intraluminal secretions are produced in distal small bowel obstruction, distending colon and resulting in narrow, stringlike colon caliber.
1. Meconium ileus.
   a. Viscous, inspissated meconium in distal ileum causes obstruction in right lower quadrant.
   b. Strong association with cystic fibrosis.
      *1)* Need to obtain sweat test.
      *2)* Children with cystic fibrosis sometimes present with meconium ileus (10%).
   c. Water-soluble enema can be therapeutic.
      *1)* Disimpact thick, tenacious meconium.
      *2)* Multiple enemas often required.
      *3)* If enema is not successful in clearing obstructive meconium, surgery is needed.

**Imaging** Abdominal radiograph can show distal bowel obstruction pattern; in about half of cases, "soap-bubble" appearance is seen in right lower quadrant (resulting from swallowed air that reaches inspissated meconium). Water-soluble enema reveals microcolon with dilated terminal ileum, containing filling defects in distal ileum (meconium).

2. Ileal or distal jejunal atresia.
   a. Atresia is much more common than stenosis.
   b. Probably ischemic etiology. Most cases are idiopathic, although there may be association with maternal cocaine use (powerful vasoconstricting agent).
   c. Types of small bowel atresia (Fig. 8-3).
      *1)* Type I (web or thin diaphragm occludes lumen).
      *2)* Type II (two blind-ended loops connected by fibrous cord).
      *3)* Type III.
         *a)* Same as Type II but without fibrous cord.
         *b)* Instead, have V-shaped mesenteric defect.
         *c)* Includes "apple-peel" atresia (large V-shaped mesenteric defect with resulting blind-ended distal bowel wrapping around rudimentary mesentery).
      *4)* Type IV (multiple atresias).

**Imaging** Few dilated loops in left upper quadrant can be seen on abdominal radiograph (resulting from jejunal atresia),

*Continued*

> *Continued from previous page*
> versus many distal dilated loops (resulting from ileal or colonic atresia). Look for calcifications or free air that could indicate complicated meconium peritonitis (perforation). Microcolon may be present on enema study (water-soluble enema should be used because of possible free peritoneal communication at level of atresia, either resulting from anomalous development or bowel necrosis). Hint: the more normal the colon, the more proximal the obstruction. Contrast may also reflux into small, unused terminal ileal loops ("microileum") that are distal to area atresia.

   3. Colonic atresia.
      a. Probable ischemic etiology.
      b. Types.
         1) Type I.
            a) Occluded by diaphragm.
            b) Microcolon that ends in club shape.
         2) Type II (fibrotic cord bridges atretic bowel).
         3) Type III (atresia with V-shaped mesenteric defect).

> **Imaging** Contrast enema demonstrates microcolon with abrupt, persistent termination of contrast column, without reaching small bowel. Distal end may also be open to peritoneal cavity.

B. Meconium peritonitis.
   1. Results from in utero bowel perforation.
      a. Leakage of meconium causes aseptic, chemical peritonitis.
      b. Results in linear or punctate calcifications extending over serosal surfaces of abdominal viscera.
      c. Because of patent processus vaginalis, calcifications can extend into scrotum.
   2. Two forms.
      a. Uncomplicated.
         *1.* Abdominal calcifications are incidental findings, as intrauterine bowel perforation has sealed itself prior to birth.
         *2.* Does not require further imaging evaluation if bowel obstruction is not present.
      b. Complicated.
         *1.* Free air may be present in addition to abdominal calcifications, indicative of ongoing obstruction (and/or current perforation), as can be seen with volvulus or small bowel stenosis or atresia.

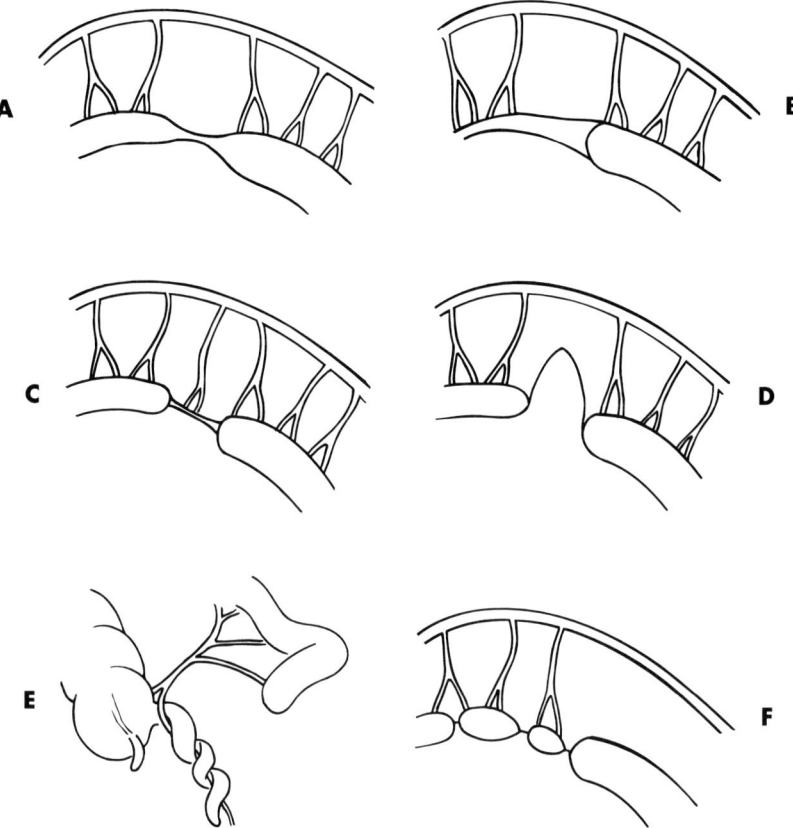

**Fig. 8-3** Bowel stenosis and atresia types. **A,** Stenosis. **B,** Atresia with thin web. **C,** Atresia with blind-ending loops, connected by fibrous cord. **D,** Atresia with blind-ending loops and mesenteric defect (no fibrous connection). **E,** Large mesenteric defect with atretic bowel wrapping around mesenteric remnant (apple peel). **F,** Multiple segments of atresia.

2. Significant number of complicated meconium peritonitis is due to cystic fibrosis, with viscous meconium, causing obstruction or perforation (meconium ileus).

**Imaging** Scattered calcifications can be seen anywhere in abdomen or pelvis on abdominal radiograph including scrotum (via patent processus vaginalis). Look for pneumoperitoneum, indicative of ongoing obstruction and perforation.

C. Abdominal masses.
  1. Need to determine organ in which mass originates.
     a. First imaging study to evaluate neonatal abdominal mass should be US.
     b. Renal origin for abdominal mass in infant is by far most common.
        *1.* If US determines mass to be of renal origin (hydronephrosis), VCUG may be helpful. (Intravenous pyelogram has limited

---

### Differential Diagnosis of Abdominal Mass in Neonate*

- Renal masses (55%).
  - Hydronephrosis or dilated renal collecting system (25%).
  - Multicystsic dysplastic kidney (15%).
  - Polycystic kidney disease (autosomal recessive).
  - Mesoblastic nephroma.
  - Renal ectopia.
  - Renal vein thrombosis.
  - Nephroblastomatosis (high risk for Wilms tumor).
- Genital masses (15%).
  - Hydrometrocolpos.
  - Ovarian cyst.
- Gastrointestinal masses (15%).
  - Duplication cyst.
  - Meconium ileus (dilated bowel loops).
  - Mesenteric or omental cyst.
- Nonrenal retroperitoneal masses (10%).
  - Adrenal hemorrage.
  - Neuroblastoma.
  - Teratoma.
- Hepatosplenobiliary (5%).
  - Hemangioendothelioma or hemangioma.
  - Hepatoblastoma.
  - Hepatic cyst.
  - Splenic hematoma.
  - Splenic cyst.
  - Choledochal cyst.
  - Gallbladder hydrops.
- Differential diagnosis of cystic mass in neonate (nonrenal).
  - Ovarian cyst.
  - Duplication cyst.
  - Choledochal cyst.
  - Omental or mesenteric cyst.

*Data from Kirks DR, Merten DF, Grossman H, Bowie JD: Diagnostic imaging of pediatric abdominal masses: An overview. *Radiol Clin North Am* 1981; 19:527-545.

value, because of decreased concentrating ability of neonatal kidney.)
        2. Computed tomography can be helpful in evaluation of solid masses or mixed solid and cystic masses.
  D. Anterior abdominal wall defects.
     1. Formation of anterior abdominal wall.
        a. Formed by circumferential folding of cephalic, caudal, and two lateral folds. Apices of these folds meet at umbilicus.
        b. Midgut physiologically develops extraabdominally and then returns to abdomen (sixth to tenth week of gestation), while these folds are forming.
     2. Incidence is 1:2000 to 4000.
     3. Types.
        a. Gastroschisis.
           *1.* Paraumbilical defect caused by defective formation of lateral abdominal fold.
              *a.* Usually right-sided.
              *b.* Normal umbilicus.
           *2.* Bowel loops remain outside abdomen without peritoneal covering (gut never returns to abdomen after physiologic herniation at sixth to tenth week of gestation).
           *3.* At birth, bowel is edematous and has abnormal motility (possibly owing to myenteric damage from prolonged amniotic fluid exposure).
           *4.* Associations.
              *a.* Prematurity.
              *b.* Malrotation.
              *c.* Bowel atresia.
        b. Omphalocele.
           *1.* Involves central abdomen and umbilicus.
           *2.* Caused by malformation of both lateral folds.
           *3.* Anteriorly protruded bowel and sometimes viscera (usually liver) are covered by sac (peritoneum-amnion).
           *4.* Umbilicus inserts directly on sac.
           *5.* Poor prognosis due to associated anomalies, such as CHD.
           *6.* Pentalogy of Cantrell.
              *a.* Further failure of cephalic fold to form.
              *b.* Pericardial and sternal defect with "uncovered" heart (ectopia cordis); usually with CHD.

**Imaging** Postpartum clinical diagnosis, although anterior wall defects can be diagnosed prenatally with US. Diagnostic imaging is predominantly done to look for associated anomalies, such as CHD.

## SUGGESTED READINGS

Abramson SJ, Baker DH, Amodio JB, Berdon WE: Gastrointestinal manifestations of cystic fibrosis. *Semin Roentgenol* 1987; 22:97-113.

Bair JH, Russ PD, Pretorius DM, Manchester D, Manco-Johnson ML: Fetal omphalocele and gastroschisis: A review of 24 cases. *Am J Roentgenol* 1986; 147:1047-1051.

Bell MJ, Ternberg JL, Bower RJ: Ileal dysgenesis in infants and children. *J Pediatr Surg* 1982; 17:395-399.

Berdon WE, Slovis TL, Campbell JB, Baker DH, Haller JO: Neonatal small left colon syndrome: Its relationship to aganglionosis and meconium plug syndrome. *Radiology* 1977; 125:457-462.

Hayden CK, Boulden TF, Swischuk LE, Lobe TE: Sonographic demonstration of duodenal obstruction with midgut volvulus. *AJR* 1984; 143:9-10.

Gaisle G, Odagiri K, Oh KS, Young LW: The bulbous bowel segment: A sign of bowel obstruction. *Radiology* 1980; 135:331-334.

Jaramillo D, Lebowitz RL, Hendren WH: The cloacal malformation: Radiologic findings and imaging recommendations. *Radiology* 1990; 177:441-448.

Johnson JF, Robinson LH: Localized bowel distension in the newborn: A review of the plain film analysis and differential diagnosis. *Pediatrics* 1984; 73:206-215.

Kirks DR, Merten DF, Grossman H, Bowie JD: Diagnostic imaging of pediatric abdominal masses: An overview. *Radiol Clin North Am* 1981; 19:527-545.

Kriss VM, Desai NS: Relation of gastric distension to prostoglandin therapy in neonates. *Radiology* 1997; 203:219-221.

Leonidas JC, Magid N, Soberman N, Glass TS: Midgut volvulus in infants: Diagnosis with US. *Radiology* 1991; 179:49-493.

O'Donovan AN, Habra G, Somers S, Malone DM, Rees A, Winthrop AL: Diagnosis of Hirschsprungs disease. *AJR* 1996; 167; 517-520.

Pantoja E, Nagy F, Thomas HA, Zambernard J, Bartley MC: Annular pancreas. *Med Radiogr Photogr* 1985; 61:2-9.

Ramsden WH, Arthur RJ, Martinez D: Gastroschisis: A radiological and clinical review. *Pediatr Radiol* 1997; 27:166-169.

Schmahmann S, Haller JO: Neonatal ovarian cysts: Pathogenesis, diagnosis and management. *Pediatr Radiol* 1997; 27:101-105.

Simpson AJ, Leonidas JC, Krasna IH, Becker JM, Schneider KM: Roentgen diagnosis of midgut malrotation: Value of upper gastrointestinal radiographic study. *J Pediatr Surg* 1972; 7:243-252.

White KS: Imaging of abdominal masses in children. *Semin Pediatr Surg* 1992; 1:269-76.

Winters WD, Weinberger E, Hatch EI: Atresia of the colon in neonates: Radiographic findings. *AJR* 1992; 159:1273-1276.

# 9
# Abnormalities of the Foregut (Esophagus and Stomach)

### Key Concepts

1. Esophageal atresia with distal fistula is the most common type of tracheoesophageal (TE) malformation followed by esophageal atresia (no tracheal fistula), and the H-type TE fistula.
2. Gastroesophageal reflux is common in the infant but should resolve by 18 months of age; reflux esophagitis can occur.
3. Common developmental cysts involving the foregut are bronchogenic, esophageal, or gastric duplication cysts and neurenteric cysts.
4. Congenital gastric malformations are rare because of the redundant nature of gastric vasculature.
5. Peptic ulcer disease (PUD) is uncommon in children. Predisposing conditions are often present such as medication-induced PUD.

## FOREGUT DEVELOPMENT

The embryologic foregut develops into a dorsal digestive portion (which later forms the esophagus and stomach) and a ventral respiratory portion (which becomes the trachea and the lungs). The dorsal and ventral portions of the foregut are separated by an esophageal and tracheal septum that forms by the fifth week of gestation (see Fig. 1-5). The stomach forms via fusiform dilatation of the foregut (distal to the esophageal and tracheal development) at approximately the fifth week of gestation (Fig. 9-1).

A. Congenital foregut malformations.
   1. Esophageal atresia and TE fistula.
      a. Caused by incomplete separation of dorsal and ventral portions of foregut.
      b. 1:3000 to 5000 live births.
      c. Associated with vertebral anomaly, anal atresia, cardiac abnormality, tracheoesophageal fistula, renal and limb malformations (VACTERL).
      d. Types (Fig. 9-2).
         *1.* Esophageal atresia without tracheal fistula (8%).
            *a.* Aberrant dorsal deviation of TE septum that results in separation of dorsal portion of foregut (esophagus) from rest of foregut.

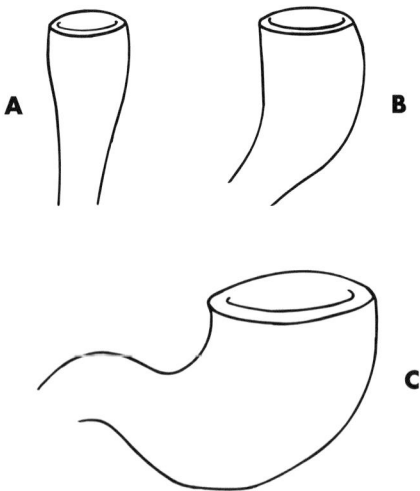

**Fig. 9-1** Gastric development. **A,** Developing distal aspect of foregut enlarges. **B,** Enlarged portion forms small turn. **C,** This enlarged portion of foregut eventually forms stomach.

b. Inability to pass nasogastric (NG) tube is often early clinical clue to diagnosis.
2. Esophageal atresia with distal tracheal fistula (most common form, 80%).
3. Esophageal atresia with proximal fistula (1%).
4. Esophageal atresia with proximal and distal tracheal fistulas (2%).
5. Tracheoesophageal fistula or H-type fistula.
   a. Six percent.
   b. Often presents late with recurrent pneumonias.
e. Treatment for esophageal atresia or fistula.
   1. Surgical repair (primary anastomosis if possible).
   2. Thoracotomy done on side opposite aorta (that is, right-sided thoracotomy is performed when left aortic arch is present).
f. Complications following repair.
   1. Leak at anastomosis.

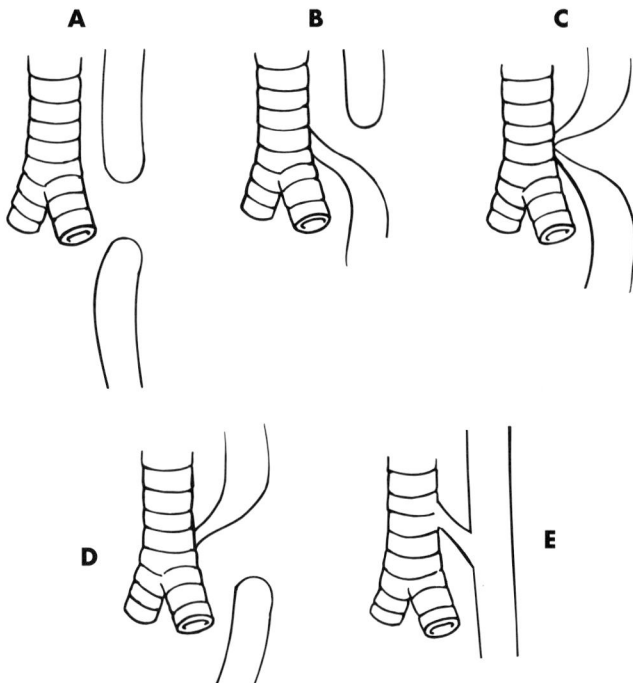

**Fig. 9-2** TE fistula types. **A,** Esophageal atresia without fistula. **B,** Esophageal atresia with distal fistula. **C,** Esophageal atresia with proximal and distal fistulas. **D,** Esophageal atresia with proximal fistula. **E,** H-type fistula.

2. Recurrent or missed fistula.
3. Strictures.

**Imaging** Diagnosis can often be made on clinical history and radiograph. Gasless abdomen will be present on abdominal radiograph in infants with pure esophageal atresia. Coiled NG tube often outlines atretic pouch and can characterize its borders; similarly, injected air can outline extent of esophageal atresia. These radiographic findings are also seen in children with esophageal atresia and tracheal fistula, except that in these children, air is present in distal gastrointestinal tract. Remember to look for elements of VACTERL listed above.

Evaluation of H-type fistula requires fluoroscopic contrast examination: gradual opacification of entire esophagus in oblique prone position, in order to locate fistula. In order to achieve sufficient opacification of esophagus, use nasoesophageal tube for contrast injection. Fistulous track can be quite small and subtle (look for track that often heads in cranial direction; N-type fistula would be more correct term than H-type).

Following surgical repair, contrast study usually reveals poor esophageal motility with intraesophageal reflux. Look for strictures (common, often not symptomatic) and recurrent fistulas or leaks at anastomatic site.

2. Laryngotracheoesophageal cleft (rare).
    a. Failure to complete proximal tracheal and esophageal separation with resulting proximal fistulous connection.
    b. Spectrum.
        1. Small defect (laryngeal cleft).
        2. Large defect (esophagotrachea with common tracheal and esophogeal lumen extending to carina).
    c. Presents with respiratory distress during feeds, often with recurrent aspiration pneumonia.

**Imaging** Contrast study demonstrates long segmental communication between proximal esophagus and trachea.

3. Esophageal bronchus.
    a. Aberrant lung bud arising directly from esophagus; develops into bronchus with anomalous esophageal connection.
    b. Usually lower lobe location with systemic arterial supply.
    c. Rare.
    d. Respiratory distress with feeds; chronic, persistent pulmonary infections are often present.

e. Endoscopy can reveal aberrant branch.

**Imaging** Contrast study of esophagus can demonstrate opacification of aberrant bronchus (usually lower lobe) and aberrant bronchial tree.

4. Developmental cysts.
   a. Bronchogenic cyst.
      1. Abnormal budding of ventral diverticulum results in thin-walled, smooth cyst with respiratory epithelium but no residual connection with tracheal or bronchial tree.
      2. Location.
         a. Middle mediastinum or hilum is most common.
            1) Can be seen between trachea and esophagus.
            2) Mimics pulmonary sling.
         b. Pulmonary (distal bronchi).
      3. Complications.
         a. Over time, bronchogenic cyst can compress and displace airway because of inspissated mucus; surgical removal is therefore indicated even in asymptomatic cases.
         b. Infection.

**Imaging** Chest radiograph may demonstrate round opacity in lungs (parenchymal bronchogenic cyst) or splaying of carina, due to middle mediastinal mass. Computed tomography (CT) better displays smooth, round, cystic structure.

   b. Neurenteric cyst.
      1. Caused by incomplete closure of primitive neurenteric canal (connection between yolk sac and amniotic cavities).
      2. Secretions produced by cyst mucosa can lead to increasing cyst size.
      3. Associated with vertebral anomalies (segmentation abnormality) resulting from disruption of normal somite or mesenchyme development.

**Imaging** Posterior mediastinal mass can be seen on chest radiograph. Look for adjacent vertebral abnormalities. Again, CT clearly demonstrates cystic nature of the lesion.

   c. Duplication (enteric) cysts.
      1. Location.
         a. Anywhere along gastrointestinal tract.
         b. Most common sites.
            1) Terminal ileum.
            2) Distal esophagus.

3) Stomach.
4) Duodenum.
 2. Spherical or tubular cystic structure.
    a. Causes smooth mass effect.
    b. Displaces bowel loops; can cause obstruction.
    c. Usually no communication with gastrointestinal tract.
 3. Etiology (see Fig. 8-2).
    a. Faulty recanalization of lumen.
    b. Occurs at approximately eighth week of gestation.
 4. Inspissated secretions lead to increasing cyst size. Resulting mass effect can cause partial or complete bowel obstruction.
 5. Surgical resection.

> **Imaging** Chest radiograph often shows smooth, round, middle or posterior mediastinal mass. CT demonstrates cystic mass with variable mass effect. CT appearance can also vary, depending on presence of hemorrhage, infection, or dense secretions.

B. Esophageal pathology.
 1. Gastroesophageal reflux disease (GERD).
    a. Common in first few weeks of life; should resolve by 18 months of age.
    b. Decreases with age; associated with hiatal hernia, cystic fibrosis.
    c. Presentation.
       1. Dysphagia.
       2. Stridor, apnea.
       3. Pneumonia.
    d. Commonly occurs in conjuction with defective esophageal motility, such as in postsurgical esophageal atresia.
    e. Treatment involves antireflux precautions.
       1. Smaller, more frequent feedings.
       2. Thickened feeds.
       3. Maintain upright position.
    f. Refractory cases.
       1. Failure to thrive.
       2. Recurrent pneumonias.
       3. Surgical option (Nissen fundoplication).

> **Imaging** Intermittant fluoroscopy during barium study can show reflux of contrast. Remember to rule out gastric outlet abnormalities as cause of repeated gastroesophageal reflux. Other means of diagnosing GERD is

nuclear medicine (Tc-99m sulfur colloid) and pH probe evaluation.

2. Esophagitis.
   a. Most commonly caused by gastroesophageal reflux.
   b. Can be infectious.
      1. Candidiasis.
      2. Cytomegalovirus.
      3. Herpes simplex virus.
      4. Acquired immunodeficiency syndrome.
   c. Epidermolysis bullosa.
      1. Disease of squamous epithelium.
      2. Mucosa irregularity and sloughing.
   d. Crohn disease.
      1. Aphthous ulcers.
      2. Disease predominantly located in distal bowel.
   e. Lye ingestion.
      1. Burns mouth, pharynx, and esophagus.
      2. Usually no gastric injury, since gastric acid neutralizes alkali.
      3. Long segment strictures of burned areas are common.
      4. Surgical treatment.
         *a.* Dilatation.
         *b.* Colonic interposition may be needed (depending on amount of esophageal damage).

**Imaging** Barium swallow reveals mucosal irregularity ("shaggy mucosa") and ulceration of esophagus. Esophageal motility is often delayed.

3. Foreign body.
   a. Most commonly occurs in normal toddler, or older children who are developmentally delayed or mentally compromised.
   b. Common foreign bodies include hot dogs, candy, or coins.
   c. Foreign body lodged in esophagus.
      1. Perforation or retropharyngeal abscess is serious complication; therefore, foreign body needs to be extracted.
      2. Look for adjacent edema that can compress or displace airway.

**Imaging** Radioopaque foreign bodies are readily visible. Barium swallow can be done for suspicion of nonradioopaque foreign body (look for esophageal filling defect).

4. Achalasia.
   a. Failure of relaxation of lower esophageal sphincter.

b. Rare in children; less than 5% of all achalasia cases.
c. Presentation.
   1. Dysphagia (associated with abnormal motility).
   2. Recurrent pneumonias from aspiration.
d. Endoscopic dilatation of distal esophagus can be helpful. Otherwise, surgical intervention may be required.

> **Imaging** Chest radiograph often reveals air-filled, dilated esophagus. Tight gastroesophageal junction results in persistent barium column with distal "beak."

5. Esophageal mass.
   a. Neoplasms are extremely rare in children.
   b. Leiomyomas, hemangiomas.
   c. Varices (portal hypertension).
   d. Foreign body.

> **Imaging** Filling defect can be seen on barium swallow.

C. Gastric pathology.
   1. Gastric atresia.
      a. Rare.
      b. Complete, fibrous, or membranous web (can be partially obstructing).
      c. Probably due to ischemic event; are rare therefore, due to redundant vascular supply of stomach.
      d. Associated with polyhydramnios.
   2. Gastric duplications.
      a. Seen along greater curvature, especially near antrum.
      b. Present with mass effect, vomiting.

> **Imaging** On contrast study, smooth mass effect can be seen along greater curvature of stomach. Ultrasound reveals cystic mass adjacent to stomach (look for hypoechoic rim of muscular layer).

   3. Peptic ulcer disease.
      a. Unusual in children, can present with chronic pain.
      b. Younger children often have predisposing conditions.
         1. Cystic fibrosis.
         2. Zollinger-Ellison syndrome (hyperacidity).
         3. Medication related.
            a. Children rarely receive aspirin today because of risk of Reye syndrome.
            b. Instead, can be seen with chronic ingestion of nonsteroidal antiinflammtory medications.

c. Gastritis can coexist.
   1. Nonspecific finding.
   2. Often infectious etiology, such as *Campylobacter pyloris*.

**Imaging** Contrast study can demonstrate ulcer "crater" and radiating folds. However, this finding may be subtle, and endoscopy may be needed for definitive diagnosis. Sometimes only gastritis can be seen (thickenened gastric rugal folds).

4. Hypertrophic pyloric stenosis (see Chapter 8).
5. Bezoar.
   a. Mass of undigested foreign material.
   b. Types.
      1. Trichobezoar (hair).
      2. Phytobezoar (undigested food, often vegetable matter).
      3. Lactobezoar.
         a. Improperly mixed infant formula.
         b. Can lead to precipitation of irregular mass that can cause gastric outlet obstruction.

**Imaging** Mottled intraluminal gastric mass can sometimes be seen on abdominal radiograph. Contrast study shows filling defect within stomach that can lead to gastric outlet obstruction or delay in gastric emptying.

6. Chronic granulomatous disease of childhood.
   a. Immunodeficiency resulting from dysfunctional granulocytes that phagocytize bacteria but can not destroy them.
   b. Presents with chronic pneumonias, esophageal dysmotility, antral gastritis.
   c. Complications include strictures of stomach and bowel.

**Imaging** Contrast study reveals narrowing and thickening of stomach antrum. Lymphoma of stomach can have similar appearance.

7. Gastric masses.
   a. Neoplasms are rare.
      1. Teratoma.
      2. Leiomyoma.
   b. Polyps (see Chapter 11).
      1. Gardner syndrome.
      2. Peutz-Jeghers syndrome.
   c. Ectopic pancreas.
      1. "Umbilicated" mass in gastric antrum.

2. Can prolapse through pylorus and cause obstruction.
   3. Seen as persistent filling defect in distal stomach on contrast study.
   d. Varices (from portal hypertension or splenic vein thrombosis).
8. Gastric volvulus.
   a. Rare in children.
   b. Abnormal twisting of stomach that causes gastric outlet and vascular obstruction.
   c. Two types.
      *1.* Organoaxial (less common).
      *2.* Mesoaxial (more serious because of potential vascular compromise).

**Imaging** Abnormal gastric outline can be seen on radiographs or contrast study; stomach can even be found in chest.

## SUGGESTED READINGS

Agha FP, Gabriele OF, Abdulla FH: Complete gastric duplication. *AJR* 1981; 137:406-407.

Bowen A, Gibson MD: Chronic granulomatous disease of childhood with gastric antral narrowing. *Pediatr Radiol* 1980; 10:119-120.

Cleveland RH, Kushner DC, Schwartz AN: Gastroesophageal reflux in children. *AJR* 1983; 141:53-56.

Drumm B, Rhoads JM, Stringer DA, Sherman PM, Ellis LE, Durie PR: Peptic ulcer disease in children: Etiology, clinical findings and clinical course. *Pediatrics* 1988; 82:410-414.

Fitch SJ, Tonkin ILD, Tonkin AK: Imaging of foregut duplication cysts. *Radiographics* 1986; 6:189-201.

Griscom NT, Martin TR: Trachea and esophagus after repair of esophageal atresia and distal fistula. *Pediatr Radiol* 1990; 20:447-450.

Heyman S: Esophageal scintigraphy (milk scans) in infants and children with esophageal reflux. *Radiology* 1982; 144:891-893.

Kilman WJ, Berk RN: The spectrum of radiographic features of aberrant pancreatic rests involving the stomach. *Radiology* 1977; 123:291-296.

Lalleman D, Quignodon JF, Courtel JV: Anomalous origin of bronchus from the esophagus: Report of three cases. *Pediatr Radiol* 1996; 26:179-182.

Starinsky R, Berlovitz J, Mores AJ, Versano D, Pajewsky M, Modai D: Infantile achalasia. *Pediatr Radiol* 1984; 14:113-115.

Stringer DA, Ein SH: Recurrent tracheoesophageal fistula: A protocol for investigation. *Radiology* 1984; 151:637-641.

Wilkinson AG, Mackenzie S, Hendry GMA: Complete laryngo-tracheo-esophageal cleft: CT diagnosis and associated abnormalities. *Clin Radiol* 1990; 41:437-438.

Ziprlowski MN, Teele RL: Gastric volvulus in childhood. *AJR* 1979; 132:921-925.

# 10
# Abnormalities of the Midgut (Small Bowel)

### Key Concepts

1. Midgut voluvulus is an emergency that can lead to bowel necrosis; it is associated with several types of malrotation patterns (especially type IIIa).
2. Duodenal hematoma is usually related to trauma; can be worrisome sign of nonaccidental trauma or child abuse.
3. Infectious gastroenteritis is common in children with nonspecific radiographic findings of multiple dilated bowel loops, often with air-fluid levels.
4. Inflammatory bowel disease (Crohn disease) is seen in the adolescent. It is characterized by transmural, noncaseating granulomas found most commonly in the terminal ileum.
5. Lymphoma in children can infiltrate, thicken, and encase bowel walls. Abdominal ascites is also often present.

## MIDGUT DEVELOPMENT

The midgut forms bowel from the duodenum (at the level of the bile duct orifice) to the distal third of the transverse colon. Initially, the midgut is a hollow tube that undergoes rapid growth and rotation (normal duodenal and colon rotation undergoes 270 degrees of counterclockwise rotation). By the sixth to tenth week of gestation, the midgut develops extraabdominally, and then returns to the abdomen to undergo a final rotation. Bowel development has been divided into the following stages (Fig. 10-1).

Stage I (less than sixth week of gestation).
- Duodeum rotates 90 degrees to lie to right of superior mesenteric artery (SMA).
- Cecum rotates 90 degrees to lie to left of SMA.

Stage II (sixth to tenth week of gestation).
- Bowel leaves abdomen.
- Duodenum rotates another 90 degrees to lie posterior to SMA.

Stage III (tenth week of gestation).
- Bowel returns to abdomen.
- Final 90 degrees of duodenal and 180 degrees of cecal rotation.

This pattern of rotation results in a ligament of Treitz or duodenal and

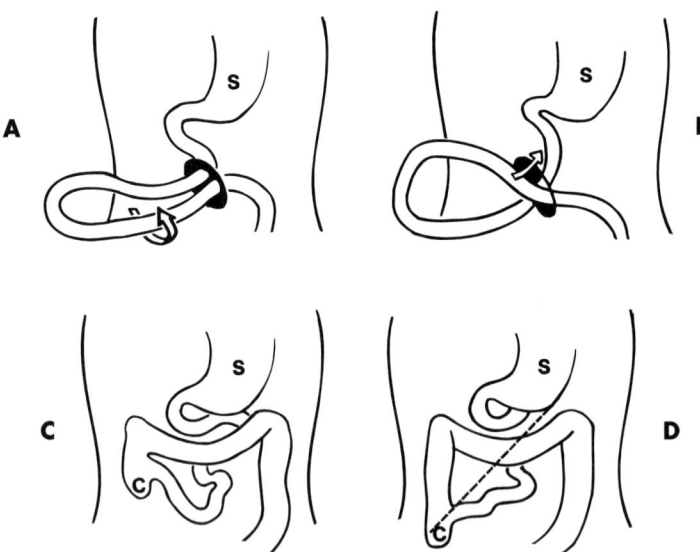

**Fig. 10-1** Midgut development: stomach *(s)*; cecum *(c)*. **A,** Extraabdominal bowel that undergoes rotation. **B,** Rotated bowel returns to abdomen. **C,** Duodenal and cecal rotation. **D,** Normally aligned bowel with DJJ in right upper quadrant and cecum in right lower quadrant, with broad mesenteric band *(dotted line)*.

jejunal junction (DJJ) lying to the left of midline at the level of the duodenal bulb, with the cecum positioned in the right lower quadrant (RLQ). A broad mesenteric root forms that extends from the DJJ to the ileocecal valve, fixing the position of the bowel, and thereby preventing volvulus (twisting of the bowel).
A. Midgut (small bowel) pathology: congenital.
   1. Malrotation (Fig. 10-2).

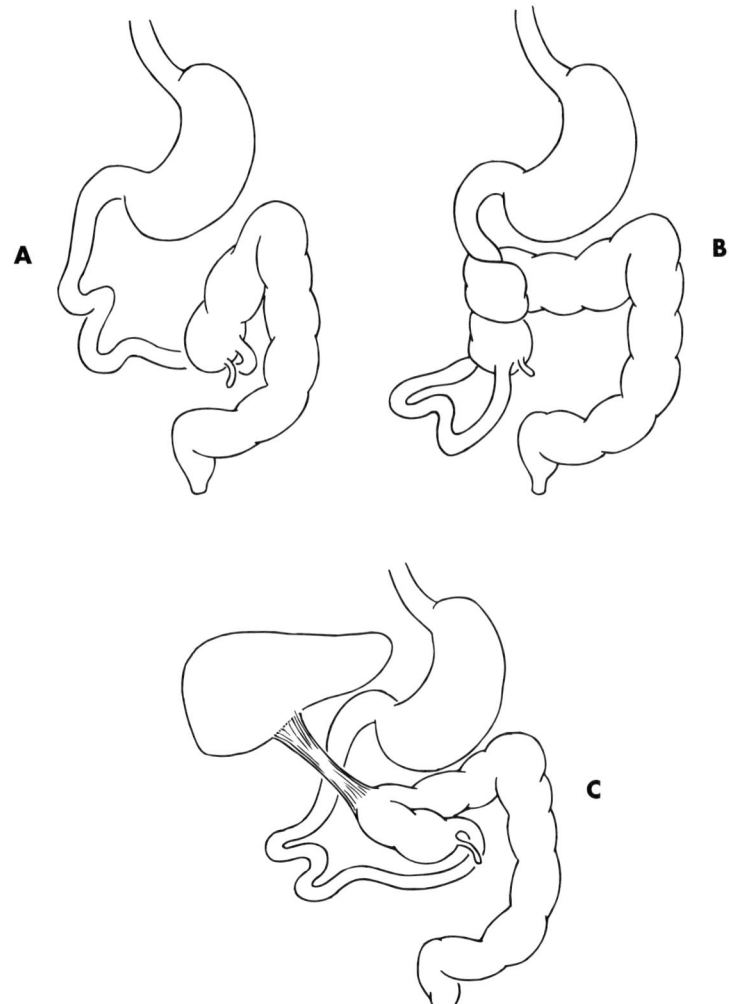

**Fig. 10-2** Common malrotation patterns. **A,** Nonrotation. **B,** Type IIIa (high risk of volvulus). **C,** Ladd bands.

a. Classified according to arrested stage of development.
b. Types of malrotation.
    1. Type I.
        a. Also known as nonrotation.
        b. Occurs prior to extraabdominal midgut development.
        c. Duodenum is positioned on right, and distal colon is positioned to left of midline.
        d. Small bowel usually has long mesentery; therefore, there is low risk of volvulus.
    2. Type II.
        a. Type IIa.
            1) Position of duodenum is abnormal with normally positioned colon.
            2) Ladd bands.
                a) Peritoneal attachments of small bowel in abnormal location because of malrotation.
                b) Can cause bowel obstruction.
        b. Type IIb.
            1) Reversed rotation.
            2) Duodenum is anterior to SMA, with colon posterior to SMA.
        c. Type IIc.
            1) Internal hernia.
            2) Duodenum position is anterior to SMA, and colon is anterior to duodenum.
            3) Small bowel can become encased in mesenteric sac known as paraduodenal hernia (appears as rounded mass of gas-filled loops).
    3. Type III.
        a. Type IIIa.
            1) Duodenum in midline with cecum overlying DJJ.
            2) Results in short mesentery with high risk of volvulus (gut twisting around SMA).
            3) Midgut volvulus.
                a) Surgical (and therefore, radiologic) emergency. Need to relieve acute obstruction and potential bowel ischemia.
                b) Can present with bilious vomiting and abdominal pain.
                c) Delay in surgery could result in infarction of large portions of bowel.
        b. Type IIIb.

*1)* Hepatic flexure is not fixed.
*2)* Ladd bands over malrotated bowel can cause obstruction.
   c. Type IIIc.
      *1)* Mobile cecum with incomplete attachment of cecum or mesocolon (14% of children).
      *2)* In absence of other findings, mobile cecum is not significant.
 c. Treatment.
   *1.* Most malrotation pattern types do not require treatment, unless associated with midgut volvulus or obstructing Ladd bands.
   *2.* In cases of high-risk malrotation (type IIIa), prophylactic fixation of bowel to prevent volvulus may be warranted.

---

**Imaging** (Fig. 10-3).
Upper gastrointestinal (UGI) examination.
- UGI examination is preferred first modality in evaluation of malrotation and midgut volvulus.
- Normally, DJJ should be lateral to left pedicle of spine, and should extend superiorly to about level of duodenal bulb (C loop).
- In cases of malrotation, DJJ remains on right, with corkscrew appearance of duodenum.

Enema: look for transverse colon to cross midline but then double back, so that cecum lies in midline.

Ultrasound (US).
- Can also demonstrate malrotation, but does not replace UGI examination.
- Look for reversal of normal SMA and superior mesenteric vein positons (see Chapter 8).

---

2. Duodenal atresia or stenosis.
   a. 1:6000 incidence.
   b. Ninety percent are atresia (50% atresia, 40% obstructing web); 10% are stenosis.
   c. Occurs near ampulla of Vater probably because of complex organogenesis in this region (pancreas, biliary system, and bowel development and rotation).
   d. Etiology is due to recanalization abnormality (see Fig. 8-2).
   e. Associations.
      *1.* Down syndrome (33%).
      *2.* Polyhydramnios.

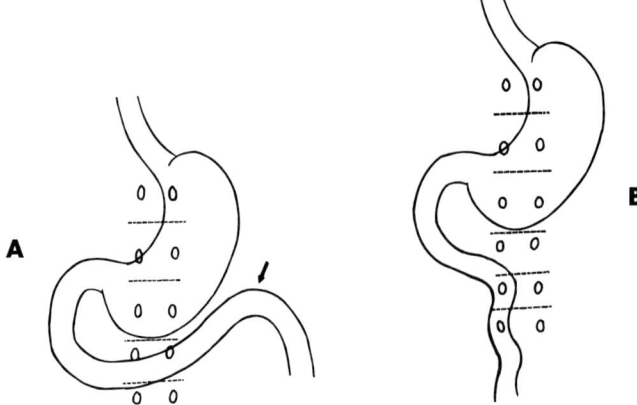

**Fig. 10-3** UGI examination. **A,** Normal C loop of duodenum; DJJ crosses left pedicle *(arrow).* **B,** IIIa malrotation. DJJ does not cross left pedicle; instead, reveals corkscrew pattern.

> **Imaging** Double bubble appearance is seen on abdominal radiograph because of dilated stomach and proximal duodenum. However, distal jejunal gas can be seen in duodenal atresia, if anomalous pancreatic ducts bypass atresia. In duodenal stenosis (which can present later in life), dilated duodenum ("windsock") can be seen on UGI examination with curvilinear lucency (stenotic web).

3. Jejunal or ileal atresia (see Chapter 8).
4. Patent omphalomesenteric (vitelline) duct (Fig. 10-4).
   a. Normal connection between primitive midgut and embryonic yolk sac that is usually obliterated by sixth week of gestation.
   b. Types.
      *1.* Fully patent omphalomesenteric duct.
         *a.* Rare.
         *b.* Presents as umbilical stool drainage in neonate.
      *2.* Vitelline cyst.
      *3.* Vitelline sinus tract.
      *4.* Meckel diverticulum.
         *a.* Persistent remnant of omphalomesenteric duct.
         *b.* Located near ileocecal valve, along antimesenteric border.
         *c.* Can present with gastrointestinal (GI) bleeding because of presence of gastric tissue.
         *d.* "Rule of 2s."

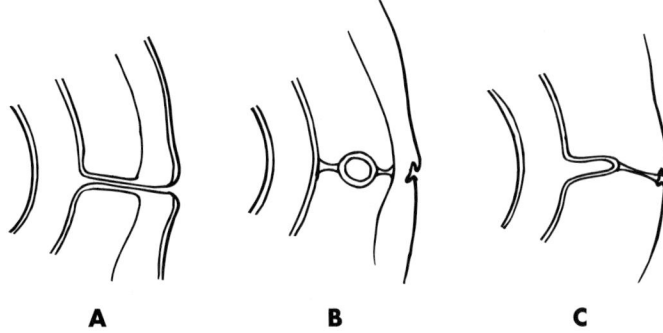

**Fig. 10-4** Omphalomesenteric (vitelline) duct types. **A,** Patent omphalomesenteric duct. **B,** Vitelline cyst. **C,** Meckel diverticulum.

    *1)* Two percent of population.
    *2)* Two percent develop complications.
    *3)* Complications occur before 2 years of age.
    *4)* Located within 2 feet of ileocecal valve.

> **Imaging** If patent duct is suspected, water-soluble contrast can be injected, via draining umbilical sinus, to demonstrate connection to bowel. Nuclear medicine (Tc-99m pertechnetate) can be useful because of tendency for Meckel diverticulum to have gastric mucosa and cause bleeding. Positive study is persistent uptake in RLQ (since Meckel diverticulum is usually found near distal ileum).

5. Cysts.
 a. Bowel duplication cyst.
  1. Due to bowel recanalization error that occurred early in gestation.
  2. Usually located near ileocecal valve or terminal ileum.
  3. Usually spherical but can be tubular.
  4. Can get quite large and cause obstruction.
  5. Does not communicate with bowel lumen.
 b. Mesenteric or omental cyst.
  1. Lymphangiomatous origin.
  2. Mesenteric cysts occur more commonly than omental cysts; both often present with abdominal distension or palpable mass.
  3. Often closely adherent to bowel (surgical resection of cyst may require bowel resection as well).

> **Imaging** Abdominal radiograph may show mass effect (depending on size of lesion). Computed tomography (CT) or US will demonstrate cystic lesion; lack of hypoechoic border (muscularis layer) differentiates mesenteric or omental cyst from bowel duplication cyst, which has muscularis layer.

B. Midgut (small bowel) pathology: acquired.
  1. Infectious gastroenteritis.
     a. Common infectious abnormalities.
        *1.* Viral (most common).
        *2.* Can be bacterial.
           *a.* Salmonella.
           *b.* Shigella.
           *c.* Escherichia coli.
        *3.* Parasites.
           *a.* Giardia.
           *b.* Ascaris.
           *c.* Entamoeba histolytica.
     b. Because of diarrhea and vomiting, severe dehydration (especially in infants) can be serious complication.

> **Imaging** Abdominal radiographs demonstrate nonspecific findings of multiple dilated loops of bowel, often with air-fluid levels. US may show small amount of free fluid in abdomen.

  2. Hematoma.
     a. Duodenal hematoma.
        *1.* Intramucosal hematoma caused by blunt trauma.
           *a.* Bicycle handlebars.
           *b.* Motor vehicle accident.
           *c.* Kicked or punched in abdomen (child abuse).
        *2.* Duodenum is more prone to traumatic injury because it is fixed in position within retroperitoneum, where it crosses spine.
     b. Jejunal or ileal hematomas.
        *1.* Usually due to bleeding dyscrasias.
        *2.* Henoch-Schönlein purpura.
           *a.* Vasculitis of small vessels (immune etiology).
           *b.* Occurs in children 3 to 10 years of age.
           *c.* Presentation.
              *1)* Purpuric rash.

2) About 50% to 60% have GI manifestations such as bleeding.
3) Can cause intussusception.

**Imaging** Bowel fold thickening ("stack of coins") with coiled spring appearance can be seen on UGI examination. Usually present in third portion of duodenum as it crosses spine. Thumbprinting from hemorrhage or edema of bowel wall can be present; obstruction can also be present. Thickened bowel walls can also be seen on US and CT.

3. Inflammatory bowel disease (IBD).
    a. Regional enteritis or Crohn disease.
    b. Usually presents in older children or adults (uncommon in children less than 10 years of age).
    c. Etiology.
        1. Transmural, noncaseating granulomas found most commonly in terminal ileum, but can be found anywhere in GI tract.
        2. No known cause (perhaps autoimmune?).
    d. Clinical presentation.
        1. Fever.
        2. Crampy, abdominal pain.
        3. Diarrhea.
        4. Elevated white blood count.
        5. Weight loss.
    e. Need to rule out infectious source of symptoms.
        1. *Yersinia.*
        2. *Campylobacter.*
        3. *Shigella.*
        4. *E. histolytica.*
    f. Treatment.
        1. Usually conservative management (steroids, asulfidine).
        2. Surgery is reserved for complications such as stricture or obstruction (yet, recurrence rate is over 90%).

**Imaging** On contrast study of bowel: aphthous ulcers, "cobblestone ulcerations," bowel wall thickening, bowel stenosis or obstruction (string sign), or fistulous connections (particularly perianal) are present; skip lesions with intervening normal bowel are also common.

4. Malabsorption.
    a. Often presents with weight loss and diarrhea.

b. Types.
   *1.* Celiac disease.
      *a.* Gluten enteropathy.
      *b.* Microvillus deficiency (similar entity to celiac disease without gluten abnormality).
   *2.* Milk allergy, lactose intolerance, disaccharidase deficiency.
   *3.* IBD (Crohn disease).
   *4.* Eosinophilic gastroenteritis.
   *5.* Intestinal lymphangiectasia.
      *a.* Congenital dilatation of bowel lymphatics that results in protein-losing enteropathy.
      *b.* Associated with Noonan syndrome.

> **Imaging** Contrast study of bowel often shows nonspecific pattern of mild small bowel dilatation and segmentation with variable bowel fold thickness. Flocculation of contrast agent (barium) has been described in past.

5. SMA syndrome.
   a. Etiology.
      *1.* Compression of third portion of duodenum as it crosses spine.
      *2.* Loss of intraabdominal fat in this region causes compression of duodenum between SMA and spine in supine patient.
   b. Often seen in thin, debilitated children, often after sudden weight loss (chemotherapy, orthopedic body cast).
   c. Presents with vomiting, especially after lying in supine position.
   d. Treatment.
      *1.* Condition can be acutely treated with direct placement of nasojejunal feeding tube.
      *2.* Sometimes positional therapy (such as prone position) can reduce symptoms.
      *3.* Long-term objectives include weight gain, in order to reform "buffer" zone between spine and duodenum.

> **Imaging** Contrast study demonstrates dilated duodenum and delayed emptying prior to bowel crossing spine. These findings often resolve in prone position.

6. Tumors.
   a. Lymphoma.
      *1.* Non-Hodgkin, often Burkitt type (B cell lymphoma).
      *2.* Bowel wall infiltration or encasement that can cause intussusception or bowel obstruction. Abdominal mass may also be present.
      *3.* Common location is RLQ, near ileocecal valve.

> **Imaging** Contrast study may demonstrate narrowed bowel lumen. US or CT can also show thickened bowel folds or wall with luminal narrowing. Abdominal ascites are commonly present as well.

    b. Other small bowel tumors are uncommon, and usually benign.
       *1.* Can act as lead point for intussusception.
       *2.* Types.
          *a.* Lipomas.
          *b.* Leiomyoma, leiomyosarcoma.
          *c.* Hemangiomas.
          *d.* Polyps (may be part of polyposis syndromes).
          *e.* Fibromas.
    c. Malignant (rare).
       *1.* Carcinoid.
       *2.* Metastasis (such as melanoma).

> **Imaging** On contrast study, appear as smooth filling defect. Target lesion has been described for metastases (melanoma).

## SUGGESTED READINGS

Berdon WE: Diagnosis of malrotation and volvulus in the older child and adult: A trap for radiologists. *Pediatr Radiol* 1995; 25:101-103.

Fink AM, Alexopoulou E, Carty H: Bleeding Meckel's diverticulum in infancy: Scintigraphic and ultrasound appearances. *Pediatr Radiol* 1995; 25:155-156.

Gaines PA, Saunders JS, Drake D: Midgut malrotation diagnosed by ultrasound. *Clin Radiol* 1987; 38:51-53.

Gaisle G, Curnes JT, Scatliff HJ, Croom RD, Vanderzalm T: Neonatal obstruction from omphalomesenteric duct remnants. *AJR* 1985; 144:109-112.

Glasier CM, Siegel MJ, McAlister WH, Shackelford GD: Henoch-Schönlein syndrome in children: Gastrointestinal manifestations. *AJR* 1981; 136:1081-1085.

Jabra AA, Fishman EK, Taylor GA: CT findings of inflammatory bowel disease in children. *AJR* 1994; 162:975-979.

Lizerbram EK, Mahour GH, Gilsanz V: Dual patency of the omphalomesenteric duct and urachus. *Pediatr Radiol* 1997; 27:244-246.

Long FR, Kramer SS, Markowitz RI, Taylor GE: Radiographic patterns of intestinal malrotation in children. *Radiograpics* 1996; 16:547-560.

Long FR, Kramer SS, Markowitz RI, Taylor GE, Liacouras CA: Intestinal malrotation in children: Tutorial on radiographic daignosis in difficult cases. *Radiology* 1996; 198:775-780.

Munns SW: Hyperalimentation for SMA (cast) syndrome following correction of spinal deformity. *J Bone Joint Surg Am* 1984; 66:1175-1177.

Riddlesberger MM: CT of complicated inflammatory bowel disease in children. *Pediatr Radiol* 1985; 15:384-387.

Ros PR, Olmsted WW, Moser RP, Dachman AH, Hjemstad BH, Sobin LH: Mesenteric and omental cysts: Histologic classification with imaging correlation. *Radiology* 1987; 164:327-337.

Siegel MJ, Shackelford GD, McAlister WH: Small bowel volvulus in children: Its appearance on the barium enema examination. *Pediatr Radiol* 1980; 10:91-93.

Stringer DA: Imaging inflammatory bowel disease in the pediatric patient. *Radiol Clin North Am* 1987; 25:93-113.

Teele RL, Henschke CT, Tapper D: The radiographic and ultrasonographic evaluation of enteric duplication cysts. *Pediatr Radiol* 1980; 10:9-14.

Vade A, Blane CE: Imaging of Burkitt lymphoma in pediatric patients. *Pediatr Radiol* 1985; 15:123-126.

Weizman Z, Stringer DA, Durie PR: Radiologic manifestations of malabsorption: A nonspecific finding. *Pediatrics* 1984; 74:530-533.

# 11
# Abnormalities of the Hindgut (Large Bowel)

---

### Key Concepts

1. Imperforate anus (anal atresia) is strongly associated with vertebral anomalies, anal atresia, cardiac malformations, tracheoesophageal fistula, and renal and limb anomalies (VACTERL). Look for the common genitourinary (GU) fistula (connecting the anus to the GU tract).
2. Hirschsprung disease is caused by an interruption in bowel innervation, and the denervated bowel can manifest as a "transition zone" on enema examination.
3. Searching for juvenile polyps in the child with rectal bleeding is one of the few indications in children for an air-contrast enema. Common location for these smooth, often pedunculated lesions is in the rectosigmoid area.
4. Ulcerative colitis is usually seen in children greater than 10 years of age. Contrast enema examination reveals mucosal irregularity, often with punctate ulcerations ("collar button"). A tubular and featureless appearance ("lead pipe") can also be present.
5. Lymphoid follicullar pattern is commonly present in the pediatric colon and can mimic colonic polyposis. The term "lymphoid hyperplasia" is reserved for larger lymphoid follicles, a condition seen with inflammatory changes, such as inflammatory bowel disease (IBD).

## HINDGUT DEVELOPMENT

The hindgut extends from the transverse colon to the anus, defined by its blood supply from the inferior mesenteric artery. Development and rotation of the hindgut occurs simultaneously with the midgut (see Chapter 10). The rectum and anus form from cloacal differentiation; development of the lower gastrointestinal, reproductive tract, and the lower urinary tract are closely related (see Chapter 22). By the third week of gestation, the distal portion of the hindgut establishes a connection with the cloaca (cavity lined with endoderm). The distal cloaca is in contact with the ectoderm, forming a cloacal membrane. By the fifth week of gestation, a wedge of mesoderm (the urorectal septum) grows caudally, separating the cloaca into ventral (urogenital) and dorsal (rectal) portions. At the seventh week of gestation, the urorectal septum passes through the cloacal membrane, dividing it into urogenital and anal membranes; this results in the formation of the perineum (Fig. 11-1).

The ventral portion of the cloaca will eventually form the GU structures, while the rectum and anus form from the dorsal portion.

Colonic innervation originates from ganglion cells of the neural crest, which migrate in a characteristic ordered progression from proximal to distal colon (during the seventh to twelfth week of gestation).

A. Hindgut (large bowel) pathology: congenital.
   1. Colonic atresia (see Chapter 8).
   2. Colonic duplications.
      a. Early in gestation, solid bowel canalizes to form lumen. Errors in canalization can result in duplication cysts.
      b. Can be tubular or round duplication cysts.
      c. Between 4% and 18% of all duplications involve colon; usually no connection with true colonic lumen.
      d. These cysts may enlarge, because of inspissated mucus secretion.
      e. Clinical presentation.
         *1.* Obstruction.

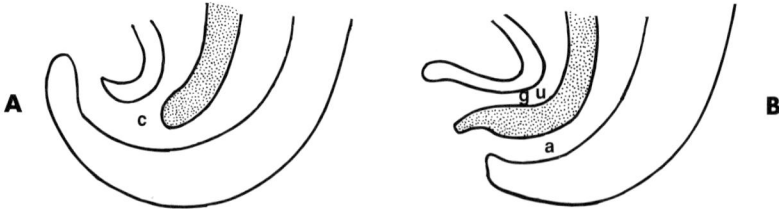

**Fig. 11-1** Development of hindgut. **A,** Early in development, cloaca *(c)* is present, common opening for both hindgut and genitourinary systems; urorectal septum *(stippled)*. **B,** Urorectal septum *(stippled)* divides cloaca into urogenital *(gu)* and anal *(a)* portions.

2. Constipation.
f. Types.
   1. Type I.
      a. Duplicates portion of colon.
      b. Spherical.
   2. Type II.
      a. Duplicates entire colon (tubular); ends in blind pouch.
      b. Duplication usually lies posterior to colon (presacral).
      c. Can have double anus with urogenital duplication (two bladders).

**Imaging** Abdominal radiograph may show mass effect or displacement of bowel; look especially for widening of rectosacral space. Duplications rarely communicate with true colonic lumen; therefore, enema may only demonstrate adjacent mass effect. Ultrasound (US) or computed tomography (CT) can demonstrate cystic abnormality.

3. Anorectal malformations (see Chapter 8).
   a. Anal atresia, also known as imperforate anus.
   b. 1:5000; found more commonly in males than in females.
   c. Types include: high, low, and intermediate.
   d. Associations.
      1. VACTERL.
      2. Sacral agenesis.
      3. Urinary tract abnormalities.
         a. Incidence of low malformation (25%); high malformation (40%).
         b. Most commonly have GU fistulous connection to rectal pouch.
         c. Crossed-fused ectopia.
         d. Renal agenesis.
         e. Pelvic or "horseshoe" kidney.
4. Hirschsprung disease (see Chapter 8).
   a. Interruption of caudal migration and/or development of ganglion cells in characteristic pattern of proximal to distal colon, produces distal bowel segment with limited peristalsis.
   b. Length of abnormally innervated bowel varies, but never contains areas of normal ganglion cells (that is, there are no skip lesions in Hirschsprung disease).
   c. 1:5000 incidence; usually presents in infants (80%).
   d. Transition zone usually occurs in anal, rectal, or sigmoid area (73%); descending left colon (14%); in more proximal bowel (10%).

e. Total colonic Hirschsprung disease is uncommon (3%), found usually in females.
5. Malfixed or malpositioned colon (see Chapter 10).
   a. Closely tied to midgut (small bowel) rotation.
   b. Abnormal rotation of small bowel can result in abnormally positioned colon.
   c. Ladd bands can form because of malpositioned colon; can cause obstruction.

B. Hindgut (colon) pathology: acquired.
  1. Pneumatosis intestinalis.
     a. Air in bowel wall.
     b. Usually, clinically significant finding.
     c. Causes.
        *1.* Neonatal necrotizing enterocolitis.
        *2.* Bowel obstruction.
        *3.* Infection.
           a. Enterocolitis.
           b. Can be seen with Hirschsprung disease.
        *4.* Vascular insult (ischemic colitis).
     d. Can be benign entity.
        *1.* Hirschsprung disease (in term infant).
        *2.* Steroids.
        *3.* Cow's milk intolerance.
        *4.* Dissection of air from barotrauma in chest.
           a. Pulmonary interstitial emphysema.
           b. Air leak (pneumothorax or pneumomediastinum).
           c. Cystic fibrosis.
        *5.* Collagen-vascular disorders.

> **Imaging** Abdominal radiograph shows multiple, linear lucencies within bowel wall (can be subtle). Commonly seen in right lower quadrant (involving distal small bowel and right colon).

  2. Juvenile polyps.
     a. Two possible causes.
        *1.* Most are probably inflammatory; caused by mucous gland hypertrophy and ductular obstruction.
        *2.* Some may be hamartomatous lesions; regardless, they are not precancerous.
     b. Commonly seen in 3 to 8 year olds; found more commonly in males than in females.
     c. Present with painless, rectal bleeding.

> **Imaging** Evaluation for polyps is one of few indications for air-contrast enema in children (with prior bowel cleansing). However, single-contrast enema can be used with careful attention to technique. Look for smooth, often pedunculated lesion located in rectosigmoid area (75% to 85%). Multiple lesions can be present.

3. Polyposis syndromes.
   a. Numerous (often innumerable) polyps are present within colon.
   b. Types.
      *1.* Familial polyposis coli.
         *a.* Autosomal dominant.
         *b.* "Carpet of polyps," can be confused with lymphoid follicular pattern (normal enema finding in colon).
         *c.* Risk of carcinomatous transformation.
      *2.* Gardner syndrome.
         *a.* Autosomal dominant.
         *b.* Adenomatous polyps (malignant risk).
         *c.* Desmoid tumors, fibromatosis.
         *d.* Osteomas.
      *3.* Peutz-Jeghers syndrome.
         *a.* Autosomal dominant.
         *b.* Hamartomatous polyps; low cancer risk.
         *c.* Mucocutaneous pigmentation (lips and buccal mucosa).

> **Imaging** Air-contrast or single-contrast enema can reveal multiple (often innumerable) polyps of varying sizes and shapes. Variability of sizes differentiates colonic filling defects from lymphoid follicular pattern, which is commonly present in pediatric colon. Term "lymphoid hyperplasia" is reserved for larger lymphoid follicles, condition seen with inflammatory changes, such as IBD.

4. Functional megacolon.
   a. No anatomic obstructive abnormality is present; colonic ganglion cells are present.
   b. Presents with chronic constipation; symptoms are not present from birth.
   c. Often dietary or "habit" constipation. Occasionally, emotionally based (psychogenic).
   d. Need to differentiate from "ultrashort" Hirschsprung disease.
   e. Breast-fed children.
      *1.* Often not truly constipated.

2. Process breast milk so efficiently, that they can have remarkably few residue stools.

> **Imaging** Abdominal radiograph and enema examiantion reveal large, feces-filled, distended rectum, down to anus without transition zone. May be impossible to differentiate from Hirschsprung (fecal impaction can obscure transition zone).

5. Pseudomembranous colitis.
   a. Etiology.
      1. *Clostridium difficile.*
      2. Produces mucosal toxin that results in severe colitis (often appears after antibiotic therapy).
   b. Clinically presents as fever, diarrhea (bloody).
   c. Colonic mucosal yellow "plaques" are seen on colonoscopy.
   d. Treated with vancomycin.

> **Imaging** Abdominal radiographs can demonstrate bowel wall thickening or thumbprinting. Contrast study is contraindicated.

6. IBD.
   a. Ulcerative colitis.
   b. Seen in patients greater than 10 years of age.
   c. Presents with abdominal pain and diarrhea (often bloody).
   d. Disease confined to mucosa; almost always involves rectum, with contiguous proximal colonic involvment (unlike Crohn disease, no skip lesions).
   e. Increased risk of colon carcinoma.
   f. Crohn colitis.
      1. Although usually small bowel abnormality, Crohn disease can involve colon (up to 50% of cases).
      2. Can be difficult to differentiate radiographically from ulcerative colitis.

> **Imaging** Contrast enema reveals mucosal irregularity or granularity, often with punctate ulcerations (collar button). Colon may have tubular and featureless appearance (lead pipe). Sometimes, terminal ileum can be involved ("backwash ileitis"). Contrast enema is contraindicated in cases of toxic megacolon.

7. Hemolytic uremia.
   a. Clinical triad.
      1. Hemolytic anemia.
      2. Acute renal failure.

3. Thrombocytopenia.
   b. Clinical diagnosis with bloody diarrhea and anemia.
   c. Most common cause of pediatric acute renal failure.
   d. Usually have prodromal illness, raising question of infectious etiology (*Shigella dysenteriae* and *Escherichia coli* have been implicated). Pathophysiology, however, is of microangiopathy.
   e. Dangerous entity; high morbidity and mortality (30% to 40%).

**Imaging** Abdominal radiograph is often normal; may show featureless colon with thumbprinting owing to bowel wall thickening and dilatation. Ascites is usually present. On US, kidneys often demonstrate markedly echogenic renal cortex, with high resistive indices; also look for bowel wall thickening on US.

8. Neutropenic colitis (typhlitis).
   a. Necrotizing inflammation; almost always occurs in right lower quadrant of abdomen; usually involving cecum and right colon.
   b. Seen in oncology patients, neutropenia is usually caused by chemotherapy, including bone marrow transplantation.
   c. Can progress to pancolitis or toxic megacolon.
   d. Clinical presentation is abdominal pain and diarrhea.
   e. Prognosis is guarded.

**Imaging** Cecal colitis (bowel edema with thumprinting), thickened bowel wall, and adjacent mesenteric stranding or edema can be seen on US and CT. Focal ileus can also be present. Contrast study is contraindicated, due to increased risk of perforation.

9. Graft-versus-host disease.
   a. Presents 2 to 7 weeks after bone marrow transplant or organ transplant.
   b. Presents with watery diarrhea and skin rash.

**Imaging** Abdominal radiographs demonstrate bowel wall thickening, ascites, air-fluid levels, and often gasless abdomen. Contrast study can show loss of small bowel folds, with appearance of featureless, distended bowel loops ("sausage bowel").

10. Colonic tumors.
    a. Benign (rare).
       *1.* Lipomas (especially of ileocecal region).
       *2.* Hemangiomas.
       *3.* Polyps (see previous discussion of polyposis).

b. Malignant.
   1. Lymphoma (usually involves small bowel).
   2. Carcinoma.
      a. Extremely rare.
      b. Look for predisposing factor.
         1) Polyposis syndrome.
         2) Ulcerative colitis.
   3. Carcinoid (especially near appendix).

**Imaging** Contrast study may show filling defect. Benign lesions are usually smooth and nonobstructive, versus irregular, invading appearance of malignancy. Lymphoma can encase and invade bowel wall (see Chapter 10).

**SUGGESTED READINGS**

Abramson SJ, Berdon WE, Baker DH: Childhood typhlitis: Its increasing association with acute myelogenous leukemia. *Radiology* 1983; 146:61-64.

Bartram CI, Thornton A: Colonic polyp patterns in familial polyposis. *AJR* 1984; 142:305-308.

Berger LA, Wilkinson D: The investigation of colitis in infancy. *Pediatr Radiol* 1974; 2:145-154.

Bolandi L, Ferrentina M, Treviani, F, Bernard M, Gasbarrini G: Sonographic appearance of pseudomembranous colitis. *J Ultrasound Med* 1985; 4:489-492.

Brunner D, Feifarek C, McNeely D, Haney P: CT of pseudomembranous colitis. *Gastrointest Radiol* 1984; 9:73-74.

Dodds WJ: Clinical and roentgen features of the intestinal polyposis syndromes. *Gastrointest Radiol* 1976; 1:127-142.

Gore RM, Marn CS, Kirby DF, Vogelzang RL, Neiman HL: CT findings in ulcerative, granulomatous and indeterminate colitis. *AJR* 1984; 143:279-284.

Kawanami T, Bowen A, Girdany BR: Enterocolitis: Prodrome of the hemolytic-uremic syndrome. *Radiology* 1984; 151:91-92.

Kelvin FM, Oddson TA, Rice RP, Garbutt JT, Bradenham BP: Double contrast barium enema in Crohn disease and ulcerative colitis. *AJR* 1978; 131:207-213.

Kirks DR: Radiology of enteritis due to hemolytic-uremic syndrome. *Pediatr Radiol* 1982; 12:179-183.

McNamara MJ, Chalmers AG, Morgan M, Smith SEW: Typhlitis in acute childhood leukemia: Radiological features. *Clin Radiol* 1986; 37:83-86.

Miller M, Stringer DA, Chui-Mei T: Lymphoid follicular pattern in the colon: An indicator of barium coating. *J Can Assoc Radiol* 1987; 38:256-258.

Pasto ME, Deiling JM, O'Hara AE, Rifkin MD, Goldberg BB: Neonatal colonic atresia: Ultrasound findings. *Pediatr Radiol* 1984; 14:346-348.

Siegel MJ, Shackelford GD, McAllister WH: The rectosigmoid ratio. *Radiology* 1981; 139:497-499.

Winters WD, Weinberger W, Hatch EI: Atresia of the colon in neonates: Radiographic findings. *AJR* 1992; 159:1273-1276.

# 12
# Acute Abdomen

> **Key Concepts**
>
> 1. The two most frequent and acute abdominal emergencies in normal children are appendicitis and intussusception.
> 2. Intussusception is commonly seen in infants and children less than 2 years of age. The exact etiology is unknown; may be due to enlarged lymph nodes near the ileocecal valve, which can act as a lead point.
> 3. In older children (older than 2 years of age) with intussusception, look for lead points such as polyps, duplication cysts, Meckel diverticulum, and lymphoma.
> 4. Appendicitis is a clinical diagnosis (leukocytosis, fever, and pain). Ultrasound has been used to image the inflamed appendix.
> 5. A helpful mneumonic for pediatric bowel obstruction is: $(AIM)^2$ or *AAIIMM*.
>    a. *A*ppendicitis and *a*dhesions.
>    b. *I*ntussusception and *i*ncarcerated hernia.
>    c. *M*idgut volvulus and *m*iscellaneous causes (such as Meckel diverticulum, duplication cysts, Crohn disease, inflammatory bowel disease [IBD], or lymphoma).

A. Pneumoperitoneum ("free air").
   1. Entities associated with pneumoperitoneum.
      a. Necrotizing enterocolitis (NEC).
      b. Intestinal obstruction.
      c. Pneumothorax.
      d. Iatrogenic.
         *1.* Nasogastric tubes perforating gastroesophageal junction or stomach.
         *2.* Rectal thermometers.
   2. Free air is usually surgical emergency.

   > **Imaging** On supine abdominal radiographs, pneumoperitoneum can be subtle with vague, ill-defined lucencies. Look for "football sign" (large, central, rounded collection of air in peritoneum, and air outlining falciform ligament of liver). Cross-table supine film or left-lateral decubitus film (left side down) can demonstrate free air. Look for air to accumulate around liver edge on left decubitus film, and along anterior abdominal wall on cross-table radiograph.

B. NEC.
   1. Usually disease found in premature infants.
      a. Incidence of NEC is 13% for infants weighing between 500 and 700 grams.
      b. Incidence of NEC decreases to 3% in infants weighing between 1500 and 1700 grams.
   2. Etiology unknown; current hypothesis related to hypoxia.
      a. Hypoxia induces shunting of blood away from gut to brain.
      b. Resulting intestinal hypoxia leads to loss of mucosal integrity with bacterial invasion into bowel wall, causing pneumatosis (air in bowel wall).
      c. Predisposition to NEC.
         *1.* Patent ductus arteriosus (PDA).
         *2.* Left-to-right shunt of PDA decreases vascular supply to gut.
   3. Complications of NEC.
      a. Bowel ulceration.
      b. Transmural necrosis.
      c. Pneumatosis (air in bowel wall).
      d. Portal venous gas.
         *1.* Ominous finding (suggestive of transmural necrosis).
         *2.* Caused by gas forming bacteria, or intramural air that has entered portal system.
         *3.* Can be confirmed on ultrasound (US).

*4.* Associated with 80% to 90% fatality rate.
   e. Perforation (pneumoperitoneum).
   f. Death.
4. Clinical triad (typically presents between day 3 and 8).
   a. Abdominal distention.
   b. Gastric retention (gastric aspirates increase).
   c. Bloody stools.
5. Management.
   a. Conservative and supportive (no feeds, antibiotics).
   b. Surgical when extraluminal gas is suspected.
6. Complications following NEC.
   a. Stricture formation.
      *1.* As high as 25% of cases.
      *2.* Yet only half of these are actually symptomatic.
   b. Strictures usually occur in colon (70%), especially in left colon.
   c. Enterocolonic fistula can also be present.
7. "Epidemic" NEC.
   a. Etiology is probably bacterial (*Escherichia coli* or *Enterobacter*).
   b. Hallmark is sudden, rapid rise in NEC incidence in neonatal intensive care unit.
   c. Since it is not caused by ischemia, this form of NEC has lower complication and fatality rate than regular NEC.
   d. "Epidemic" NEC is also seen in higher birth weight babies, and earlier in life.

**Imaging** Abdominal radiograph reveals bulging flanks, bowel distension, bowel wall thickening, and unfolding of bowel loops. Look for hallmark pneumatosis intestinalis (lucencies within bowel wall, often linear; seen particularly in right colon ileocecal area, which has "water-shed" vascular supply). More ominous signs include portal venous gas (linear lucencies overlying liver) and pneumoperitoneum.

C. Appendicitis.
   1. Appendicitis is most common condition requiring acute abdominal surgery in children.
   2. Occurs in older child or adolesecent; only 2% of cases are found in children less than 2 years of age.
   3. Caused by blockage of appendiceal lumen by inspissated feces (appendicolith), lymphoid hyperplasia, worms, and so forth.
   4. Clinical diagnosis; imaging is only required in equivocal cases.
      a. Right lower quadrant (RLQ) pain.
      b. Fever.

c. Leukocytosis.
5. Yet up to 30% of operative cases have different postoperative diagnosis (gastroenteritis, IBD, or female pelvic pathology can all often mimic appendicitis).
6. Consequences of delayed diagnosis of appendicitis.
   a. Perforation (25% of all acute cases), abscess formation, and peritonitis.
   b. Late manifesation: infertility in females resulting from adhesions or scarring.

**Imaging** Abdominal radiographs are often normal or nonspecific.
- Appendicolith (calcified inspissated feces can be seen in RLQ). Appendicolith in presence of pain has 90% incidence of acute appendicitis.
- Localized ileus (sentinel loop); blurring or loss of properitoneal fat in RLQ suggests inflammation or abscess.
- Air-fluid levels (suggesting small bowel obstruction); pneumoperitoneum.

Barium enema.
- Unreliable and rarely indicated today.
- Nonfilling of appendix (however, appendix does not fill 10% of time in normal children); look for mass effect upon cecum.
- Enema can be useful in patient with cystic fibrosis (where differential diagnosis is appendicitis versus meconium ileus equivalent). In these patients, water-soluble enema can therapeutic.

US.
- Probably best modality available today for imaging of appendicitis.
- RLQ hypoechoic tubular structure measuring greater than 6 mm (in adolescents and adults); does not compress (90% sensitive and 95% specific).
- Occasionally, shadowing appendicolith can be seen.
- RLQ or pelvic free fluid.
- Periappendiceal abscess may be present, which is usually hypoechoic.

D. Intussusception.
1. Intussusception is prolapse of one portion of bowel into adjoining segment, resulting in bowel obstruction (Fig. 12-1).
2. Most are ileocolic (75% to 95%).
3. Most common abdominal emergency in early childhood (less than 2 years of age).

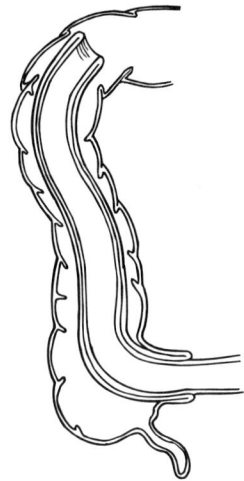

**Fig. 12-1** Ileal-cecal intussusception.

4. Up to 75% present before 2 years of age; 50% before 1 year of age (peak age range is 6 to 9 months); found more commonly in males than in females.
5. Idiopathic, with no known lead point (90%), presumed due to lymphoid hyperplasia, secondary to viral infection.
6. If older than 3 years of age, consider lead point as etiology.
   a. Meckel diverticulum.
   b. Duplication cysts.
   c. Polyps.
   d. Lymph nodes (Kawaski syndrome).
   e. Foreign body.
   f. Lipoma.
   g. Lymphoma.
7. Clinical presentation.
   a. Abdominal pain (legs drawn up to abdomen).
   b. Palpable abdominal mass.
   c. "Currant jelly" stools (bloody).
   d. Lethargic, listless child.
8. Intussusception is often intermittant process.
   a. Persistent, untreated intussusception can lead to serious complications, such as obstructed, ischemic, infarcted, or perforated bowel.
   b. Delay in treatment can lead to irreducible intussusception and increased risk of bowel perforation (resulting from ongoing and worsening bowel edema).

**Imaging** Abdominal radiograph.
- Can be normal in up to 25% of cases.
- Look for right-sided paucity of gas or right-sided mass effect (50% to 60%).
- "Colon cut-off" sign (midtransverse colon).
- Dilated loops of small bowel are suggestive of obstruction (25%).
- Abdominal radiograph can also exclude free air.

US.
- Can demonstrate "doughnut" sign (on transverse images) with hypoechoic edematous bowel surrounding central area of increased echogenicity ("pseudokidney").
- Examination can be technically difficult, because of surrounding bowel gas.

Enema.
- Can be both diagnostic and therapeutic (reduction of intussusception).
- Contraindications to enema are hypovolemic shock, peritonitis, or pneumoperitoneum. In addition, surgical staff should be notified prior to enema reduction, in event of bowel perforation or failed reduction.
- There are two enema techniques: hydrostatic (barium or water-soluble) versus pneumatic (air) reduction.
  - Hydrostatic.
    - Three reduction attempts at 3 feet height of barium or water-soluble contrast bag is traditional method of intussusception reduction.
    - Classic finding is "coiled spring" appearance of intussuscepted bowel. Free flow of barium or water-soluble contrast into small bowel signals successful intussusception reduction.
    - Main complication is bowel perforation, with risk of free barium in abdomen (peritonitis and scarring).
  - Air.
    - Air reduction of intussusception has been gaining acceptance in United States; is considered by its advocates to be safer and more effective.
    - Use insufflated air to reduce intussusception, maintaining pressure at less than 120 mm Hg in nonsedated child. With Valsalva maneuver

(crying), higher pressure is allowed, because of increased intraabdominal pressures.
- Small bowel obstruction is not contraindication for air enema, although risk of perforation does increase from less than 1% up to 10% to 12% when bowel obstruction is present (because of possible compromise or necrosis of obstructed bowel).
- Reduction is complete when there is free reflux of air into distal small bowel and absence of cecal mass. Residual density is often present at ileocecal valve (because of edema versus residual intussusception versus lead point).
 - In uncomplicated idiopathic intussusception, reduction can be achieved in up to 90% of cases. If intussusception will not reduce, or recurrs, or is seen in older child (greater than 2 years of age), suspect lead point (further imaging would include barium study, US, or even nuclear medicine, if bleeding Meckel diverticulum is suspected).
 - Between 5% and 10% of intussusceptions can recur, usually within 24 to 48 hours; therefore, most children are hospitalized following reduction for at least 24 hours.

E. Other causes of bowel obstruction.
   1. Inguinal hernia.
      a. Bowel herniation through patent processus vaginalis.
      b. Clinical diagnosis; common in infants (especially premature) and small children.
      c. Found more commonly in males than in females; on left side more commonly than on right.
      d. Can cause small bowel obstruction; often intermittant.

   **Imaging** Abdominal radiographs can demonstrate air-filled bowel loops, extending below symphysis pubis; if obstructed, can see dilated proximal bowel loops. On US, peristalsis of bowel loops within scrotum can be seen, often with associated hydrocele.

   2. Adhesions.
      a. Fibrotic bands that can narrow, incarcerate, and obstruct bowel.
      b. Predisposition.
         *1.* Previous history of surgery.

2. NEC.
3. Any inflammatory condition of abdomen.
3. Midgut volvulus (see Chapter 10).
   a. Twisting of bowel (malrotated bowel has short mesenteric base, predisposing to volvulus).
   b. Radiographs can be normal, although double bubble sign may be present in upper abdomen, due to distention or obstruction of stomach and proximal duodenum. Upper gastrointestinal examination is performed for diagnosis.
4. Miscellaneous (see Chapter 10).
   a. Meckel diverticulum.
   b. Duplication cysts (commonly found near ileocecal area).
   c. Inflammatory bowel disease (IBD).
   d. Lymphoma.

## SUGGESTED READINGS

Bissett GS, Kirks DR: Intussusception in infants and children: Diagnosis and therapy. *Radiology* 1988; 168:141-145.

Currarino G: Incarcerated inguinal hernia in infants: Plain films and barium enema. *Pediatr Radiol* 1974; 2:247-252.

Johnson JF, Woisard KK: Ileocolic intussusception: New sign on the supine cross table lateral radiograph. *Radiology* 1989; 170:483-486.

Kogutt MS: Necrotizing enterocolitis of infancy: Early roentgenologic patterns as a guide to prompt diagnosis. *Radiology* 1979; 130:367-370.

Oestreich AE, Adelstein EH: Appendicitis as the presenting complaint in cystic fibrosis. *J Pediatr Surg* 1982; 17:191-194.

Puylaert JB: Acute appendicitis: US evaluation using graded compression. *Radiology* 1986; 158:355-360.

Quillin SP, Siegel MJ: Appendicitis in children: Color Doppler sonography. *Radiology* 1992; 184:745-747.

Rabinowitz JG, Siegle RL: Changing clinical and roentgenologic patterns of necrotizing entercolitis. *AJR* 1976; 126:560-566.

Shiels WE, Maves CK, Hedlund GL, Kirks DR: Air enema for diagnosis and reduction of intussusception: Clinical experience and pressure correlates. *Radiology* 1991; 181:169-172.

Shiels WE, Bisset GS, Kirks DR: Simple device for air reduction of intussusception. *Pediatr Radiol* 1990; 20:472-474.

Shimkin PM: Radiology of acute appendicitis. *AJR* 1978; 130:1001-1004.

Sivit CJ: Diagnosis of acute appendicitis in children: Spectrum of sonographic findings. *AJR* 1993; 161:147-152.

Sivit CJ, Newman KD, Boenning DA, Nussbaum-Blask AR, Bulas DI, Bond SJ, Attorri R, Rebolo LC, Brown-Jones C, Garin DB: Appendicitis: Usefulness of US in the diagnosis in a pediatric population. *Radiology* 1992; 185:549-552.

Virjee JP, Gill GJ, Desa D, Somers S, Stevenson GW: Strictures and other late complications of neonatal necrotizing enterocolitis. *Clin Radiol* 1979; 30:25-31.

Weinberger E, Winters WD: Intussusception in children: The role of sonography. *Radiology* 1992; 184:601-602.

White SJ, Blane CE: Intussusception: Additional observations on the plain radiograph. *AJR* 1983; 139:511-513.

# 13
# Hepatobiliary System

### Key Concepts

1. In the infant with persistent neonatal jaundice, the major differential is neonatal hepatitis versus biliary atresia. Nuclear medicine scan can help differentiate the two, but sometimes liver biopsy is needed.
2. Hemangioma is the most common benign liver tumor in children, accounting for 50% of pediatric benign hepatic lesions.
3. Hepatoblastoma is the most common primary malignant liver tumor in children. Hepatoma or hepatocellular carcinoma is rare in children.
4. Cholelithiasis is uncommon in children; look for predisposing factors such as hemolytic anemias, administration of total parenteral nutrition (TPN), or cystic fibrosis.
5. In the neonate with a cystic mass, the following are common possibilities to consider: choledochal cyst, ovarian cyst, duplication cyst, omental or mesenteric cyst, or renal cystic pathology.

A. Neonatal jaundice.
   1. Physiologic.
      a. Common in neonates, especially breast-fed babies.
      b. No imaging required.
   2. Neonatal hepatitis.
      a. Etiology.
         *1.* Viral (hepatitis B or cytomegalovirus).
         *2.* Idiopathic.
      b. Liver functions poorly, but biliary excretion is still present.
      c. Major differential is biliary atresia.

> **Imaging** Ultrasound (US).
> - Hepatic US may demonstrate "starry-sky" appearance (prominent periportal fat in hypoechoic liver).
> - Can document gallbladder contraction and emptying (differentiating feature with biliary atresia).
> 
> Nuclear medicine.
> - Limited uptake of radiopharmaceutical Tc-99m diisopropyl iminodiacetic acid (Tc-99m [DISIDA] or mebrofenin); gallbladder or biliary activity and excretion are still present.
> - Persistent lack of bowel activity is strong evidence for biliary atresia.
> - Pretreatment with phenobarbitol for few days prior to nuclear medicine liver scan is recommended for infants (optimizes liver uptake of radiopharmaceutical).

   3. Biliary atresia (Fig. 13-1).
      a. Portions of biliary tree are not patent; unknown etiology.
      b. Present with jaundice, often with clay-colored stool (no bile reaches bowel).
      c. Associated with polysplenia.
      d. Initial treatment is portoenterostomy (Kasai procedure).
         *1.* Attempt to dissect out patent biliary radicals in hepatic portal area and directly anastomose to bowel.
         *2.* Preferably done in infants less than 2 months of age, reduces or delays long-term complications such as cirrhosis and liver failure.
         *3.* Most of patients with biliary atresia eventually require liver transplant.

> **Imaging** US may document an absent gallbladder. Usually, small gallbladder is seen. Lack of gallbladder filling and
> 
> *Continued*

> *Continued from previous page*
> subsequent emptying suggests biliary atresia. Nuclear medicine scan demonstrates hepatic uptake of radiopharmaceutical, but no excretion into biliary system or bowel. Definitive diagnosis is liver biopsy or cholangiogram (often operative at time of portoenterostomy).

4. Choledochal cyst.
   a. Focal cystic dilation of biliary system.
   b. Clinical presentation.
      1. Neonate.
         a. Jaundice.
         b. Palpable abdominal mass.
      2. Older child (classic clinical triad).
         a. Right upper quadrant (RUQ) pain.
         b. Jaundice.
         c. Fever.
   c. Complications.
      1. Ascending cholangitis.
      2. Stasis (stones).
   d. Types (Fig. 13-2).
      1. Type I.
         a. Fusiform dilatation of common bile duct (CBD).

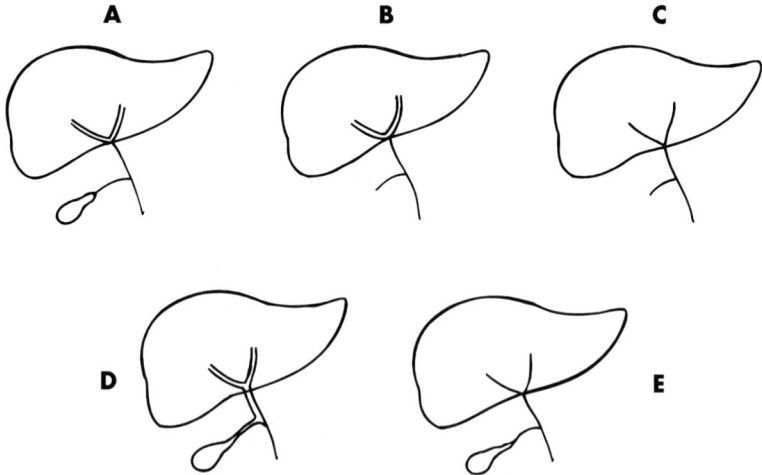

**Fig. 13-1** Types of biliary atresia. **A-E,** Different types of biliary atresia (single line denotes portions of atretic biliary tree).

b. Most common type (80% to 90%).
c. Considered to result from abnormal insertion of CBD and pancreatic duct with resulting reflux of pancreatic enzymes, which can weaken CBD wall, causing CBD dilatation.
2. Type II.
   a. Diverticulum of CBD.
   b. Not common (2%).
3. Type III.
   a. Choledococele (1% to 5%).
   b. Dilatation of intraduodenal portion of CBD.

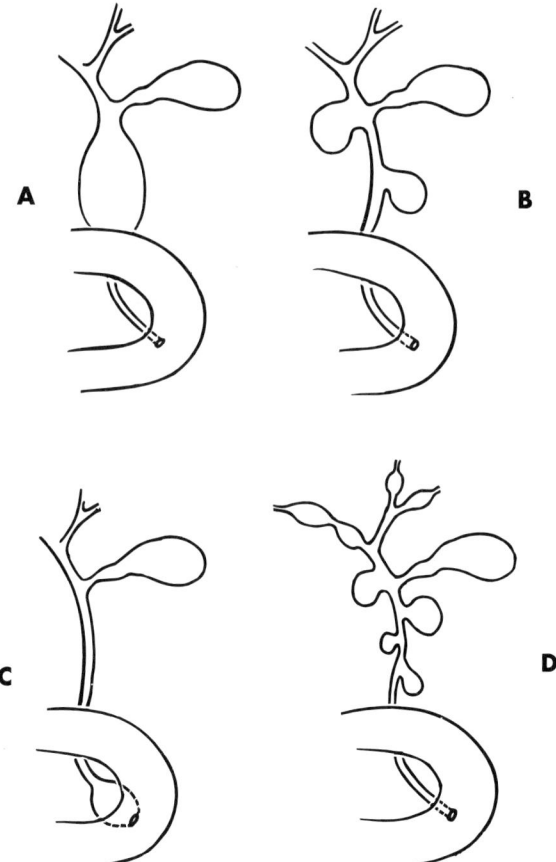

**Fig. 13-2** Types of choledochal cyst. **A,** Type I. **B,** Type II. **C,** Type III (choledococele). **D,** Type IV (some classify Caroli disease within this category).

c. Receives ostia of both CBD and main pancreatic duct.
  4. Type IV.
     a. Cystic dilatation of intrahepatic ducts.
     b. Second most common type (15% to 20%).
     c. Caroli disease has been included in this category.
        1) Diffuse ectasia of biliary tree.
        2) Associations with Caroli disease.
           a) Polycystic kidney disease (autosomal recessive, juvenile type).
           b) Hepatic fibrosis.

> **Imaging** RUQ abdominal mass, that often displaces bowel loops, can be seen on abdominal radiograph. US demonstrates cystic mass adjacent to gallbladder; try to establish connection between cystic mass and biliary tree. Nuclear medicine scan will show persistent uptake within choledochal cyst, because of stasis and delayed emptying.

B. Benign hepatic masses.
  1. Hemangioma.
     a. Common benign liver tumor.
     b. Accounts for 50% of pediatric benign hepatic lesions.

> **Imaging** Smooth, round, echogenic, hepatic lesion is seen on US; computed tomography (CT) demonstrates enhancement (peripheral to central).

  2. Hemangioendothelioma.
     a. Multiple, enlarged vascular spaces can be seen in these (often very large) liver lesions.
     b. Clinical presentation.
        1. RUQ mass in neonate.
        2. Cardiomegaly and pulmonary edema from high-output cardiac failure because of arteriovenous shunting through lesion.
     c. Associated with cutaneous hemangiomas (50%).

> **Imaging** Speckled calcifications are often present on abdominal radiographs (50%). US demonstrates lesion of mixed echogenicity, often with hypoechoic (vascular) spaces. Color and duplex Doppler can document blood flow through lesion. CT shows hypodense hepatic lesion that demonstrates vascular blush following contrast injection. Nuclear medicine (Tc-99m RBC scan) can demonstrate intense radiopharmaceutical pooling in this hepatic lesion.

3. Mesenchymal hamartoma.
   a. Cystic liver lesion; presents as asymptomatic mass.
   b. Constitutes 22% of benign pediatric liver masses.
   c. Etiology.
      1. Failure of fetal liver development.
      2. Cystic degeneration and fluid accumulation.
   d. More commonly seen in males than in females, presents in children less than 2 years of age.

> **Imaging** Large, cystic (often multicystic) lesion that can be seen anywhere in liver. Can be diagnosed on US, CT, or magnetic resonance imaging (MRI). Lack of internal vascular component differentiates from hemangioma.

4. Hepatic adenoma.
   a. Uncommon in children.
   b. Associations.
      1. Oral contraceptives.
      2. Glycogen storage disease.
      3. Fanconi anemia.
   c. Can acutely hemorrhage.

> **Imaging** Usually hypodense lesion on CT. Because of lack of Kupffer cells, lesion does not uptake radiopharmaceutical (99m Tc-sulphur colloid) leading to "cold spots."

5. Peliosis hepatis.
   a. Blood-filled cavities in liver; cavities can also be seen in spleen.
   b. Unknown etiology; associated with anabolic steroids.

> **Imaging** CT and US reveal large fluid-filled spaces in liver. MRI may demonstrate various stages of hemorrhage.

6. Other benign hepatic masses (uncommon in children).
   a. Focal nodular hyperplasia.
   b. Focal fatty infiltration (nodular).
   c. Regenerative nodules (in cirrhosis).

C. Malignant hepatic masses.
   1. Hepatoblastoma.
      a. Most common malignant primary neoplasm (67% of all pediatric hepatic tumors).
      b. Most occur in children less than 3 years of age; usually located in right lobe of liver.
      c. Elevated alpha-fetoprotein (AFP) is usually present.
      d. Associated with Beckwith-Wiedemann syndrome, hemihypertrophy, and biliary atresia.

> **Imaging** Often see calcifications on abdominal radiographs. US shows focal mass of mixed echogenicity within liver. Hypodense lesions are seen on CT with variable enhancement.

2. Hepatocellular carcinoma.
   a. Uncommon; seen in children greater than 4 years of age.
   b. Preexisting liver disease (such as cirrhosis) is often present (50%).
   c. Elevated serum AFP.
   d. Invasive tumor; often multicentric.

> **Imaging** Variable sonographic and CT appearance of this infiltrating lesion (often mixed echogenicity or density is seen). Calcifications are less common. Hyperintense lesion on MRI ($T_2$-weighted images).

3. Undifferentiated embryonal sarcoma.
   a. Rare, mesenchymal tumor (some consider it malignant "counterpart" to benign mesenchymal hamartoma).
   b. Seen in adolescents, young adults.

> **Imaging** Large, often echogenic (US) or hypodense (CT) lesion. Cystic (necrotic) spaces and calcifications may be present.

4. Metastasis.
   a. Less commonly seen in pediatric carcinomas than in adult carcinomas.
   b. Neoplasms that can have hepatic metastasis.
      *1.* Wilms tumor.
      *2.* Neuroblastoma.
      *3.* Lymphoma (Non-Hodgkins, often Burkitt type).

> **Imaging** Usually hypodense, round, scattered lesions on CT. Often hyperintense $T_2$ signal on MRI.

D. Hepatic cirrhosis.
   1. Diffuse liver parenchymal destruction with fibrotic replacement.
   2. Many etiologies.
      a. Hepatitis.
      b. Biliary atresia.
      c. Alagille syndrome (arteriohepatic dysplasia).
      d. Cystic fibrosis.
      e. Congenital hepatic fibrosis.
      f. Metabolic.

1. Alpha$_1$-antitrypsin deficiency.
    a. Also characterized by pulmonary destruction or fibrosis.
    b. Emphysema.
2. Glycogen storage diseases.
3. Tyrosinemia.
4. Galactosemia.
5. Wilson disease (copper storage abnormality).
6. Hemochromatosis.
    a. Iron deposition.
    b. Look for increased attenuation of liver on CT (also seen in hemolytic anemias, hemosiderosis).
  g. Budd-Chiari syndrome.
   1. Rare.
   2. Obstruction of hepatic veins, intrahepatic inferior vena cava (IVC), or extrahepatic IVC.
   3. Possible etiologies.
      a. Hypercoagulable states (such as sickle cell anemia).
      b. Neoplasms.
      c. Congenital IVC webs.
      d. Trauma.
      e. Liver transplantation.
   4. Doppler can demonstrate absence, reduction, or reversal of hepatic venous flow.
   5. Hepatic venoocclusive disease.
      a. Hepatic venous obstruction at central and lobular hepatic venous level, as opposed to major hepatic veins or IVC obstruction from Budd-Chiari syndrome.
      b. Associations.
         1) Chemotherapy toxicity.
         2) Graft-versus-host disease.
         3) Immunodeficiencies.

**Imaging** Early cirrhosis usually has normal imaging studies. Later, small, often nodular liver can be present. Fatty infiltration of liver can be seen as decreased attenuation of liver on CT, with increased sonographic echogenicity. Findings of portal hypertension can also be present: ascites, reversal of flow within portal system, varices (opening of umbilical vein, splenic, and esophageal varices), and splenomegaly.

E. Acquired biliary disease.
  1. Enlarged gallbladder (normal in fasting patient).

2. Gallbladder hydrops (acute noncalculous distension of gallbladder).
   a. Sepsis.
   b. Acalculous cholecystitis.
   c. Kawasaki syndrome (mucocutaneous lymph node syndrome).
      1. Caused by immune related vasculitis; probably postinfectious.
      2. Clinical presentation.
         *a.* Fever.
         *b.* Rash.
         *c.* Conjunctivitis.
         *d.* Cervical adenopathy.
      3. Associated with coronary artery aneurysms (20%).
3. Cholelithiasis (gallstones).
   a. Uncommon in children; look for predisposing factor.
      1. Bilirubinate stones are seen in various anemias, particularly hemolytic.
         *a.* Sickle cell anemia.
         *b.* Glucose-6-phosphate-dehydrogenase (G6PD)
         *c.* Spherocytosis.
      2. TPN.
      3. Cystic fibrosis.
         *a.* Ispissated secretions.
         *b.* Causes cystic duct obstruction or stasis.
   b. Can be seen in neonates; often idiopathic.
      1. Dehydration.
      2. Following diuretic therapy.
      3. Usually spontaneously resolves without intervention.
   c. Cholecystitis is rare in children.

**Imaging** US shows echogenic, shadowing foci within gallbladder. Amorphous, irregular, echogenic, but nonshadowing "sludge" can also be seen within gallbaldder (commonly seen in long-term fasting patients, like those receiving TPN). Sludge usually resolves with resumption of enteral feeding, although some believe that sludge is precursor to gallstones. Gallstones can be seen incidentally on abdominal radiographs or CT.

4. Gallbladder polyps.
   a. Extremely rare in children; usually adenomas.
   b. Nonshadowing, fixed echogenic foci within gallbladder can be seen on US.
5. Sclerosing cholangitis.

a. Inflammatory and destructive (fibrotic) process involving biliary tree.
b. Strong association with inflammatory bowel disease.
c. Cholelithiasis often present.

**Imaging** Dilatation of biliary tree can be seen on US and CT. Cholangiography (direct contrast injection into biliary system) reveals irregular dilatations and strictures. Usually involves entire intrahepatic biliary tree.

## SUGGESTED READINGS

Alwaidh MH, Woodhall CR, Carty HT: Mesenchymal hamartoma of the liver: A care report. *Pediatr Radiol* 1997; 27:247-249.

Barzilai M, Lerner A: Gallbladder polyps in children: A rare condition. *Pediatr Radiol* 1997; 27:54-56.

Boechat MI, Kangerloo H, Gilsanz V: Hepatic masses in children. *Semin Roentgenol* 1988; 3:185-193.

Boechat MI, Kangerloo H, Ortega J, Hall T, Feig S, Stanley P, Gilsanz, V: Primary liver tumors in children: Comparison of CT and MR imaging. *Radiology* 1988; 169:727-732.

Boon LM, Burrows PE, Mulliken JB: Hepatic vascular anomalies in infancy: A 27 year experience. *J Pediatr* 1996; 129:346-354.

Callahan J, Haller JO, Cacciarelli AA, Slovis TL, Friedman AP: Cholelithiasis in infants: Association with total parenteral nutrition (TPN) and furosemide. *Radiology* 1982; 143:437-439.

Dachman AH, Lichtenstein JE, Friedman AC, Hartman DS: Infantile hemangioendothelioma of the liver: Radiographic-pathologic-clinical correlation. *AJR* 1983; 140:1091-1096.

Dachman AH, Pakter RL, Ros PR, Fishman EK, Goodman ZD, Lichtenstein JE: Hepatoblastoma: Radiologic-pathologic correlation in 50 cases. *Radiology* 1987; 164:15-19.

Keller MS, Markle BM, Laffey PA, Chawla HS, Jacir N, Frank JL: Spontaneous resolution of cholelithiasis in infants. *Radiology* 1985; 157:345-348.

Kim OH, Chung HJ, Choi BG: Imaging of the choledochal cyst. *Radiographics* 1995; 15:69-88.

Maves CK, Caron KH, Bisset GS, Agarwal R: Splenic and hepatic peliosis: MR findings. *AJR* 1992; 158:75-76.

McCain AH, Bernardino ME, Sones PJ, Berkman WA, Casarella WJ: Varices from portal hypertension: Correlation of CT and angiography. *Radiology* 1985; 154: 63-69.

Miller JH, Greenspan BS: Integrated imaging of hepatic tumors in childhood. *Radiology* 1985; 154:83-90.

Neu J, Arvin A, Ariagno RL: Hydrops of the gallbladder. *Am J Dis Child* 1980; 134:891-893.

Pobiel RS, Bisset GS: Pictorial essay: Imaging of liver tumors in the infant and child. *Pediatr Radiol* 1995; 25:495-506.

Stanley P: Budd-Chiari syndrome. *Radiology* 1989; 170:625-627.

Weinreb JC, Cohen JM, Armstrong E, Smith T: Imaging of the pediatric liver. *AJR* 1986; 147:785-790.

# 14
# Pancreas and Spleen

> **Key Concepts**
> 1. Pancreatitis is uncommon in children. Etiologies include: trauma, congenital anomaly, sepsis, or idiopathic.
> 2. Mucus inspissation of the pancreatic ducts in children with cystic fibrosis can lead to obstruction and eventual destruction, fatty replacement, and fibrosis of the pancreas.
> 3. Splenomegaly in children is most commonly an infectious etiology, such as infectious mononucleosis. Hemolytic anemias and lymphoma or leukemia can also be considered.
> 4. Evaluation of the spleen is an important aspect in the work-up for ambiguous situs (asplenia or polysplenia).

## PANCREAS DEVELOPMENT

The pancreas develops from the two portions (dorsal and ventral). The dorsal portion is derived from the embryologic duodenum, and forms most of the head, body, and tail of the pancreas. The ventral portion arises from the primitive bile duct to form the uncinate process and part of the pancreatic head. The portions and their draining ducts fuse at about the sixth week of gestation. Although developing pancreatic ducts have several patterns of fusion, most commonly the main pancreatic duct is formed by fusion of the ventral duct (duct of Wirsung) and the proximal portion of the dorsal duct; the accessory pancreatic duct forms from the remainder of the dorsal duct (duct of Santorini) (Fig. 14-1).

A. Pancreas (congenital malformations).
   1. Annular pancreas.
      a. Circumferential pancreas surrounding duodenum.
      b. Unknown etiology; possibilities include bifid ventral portion or rotational problem with ventral portion.

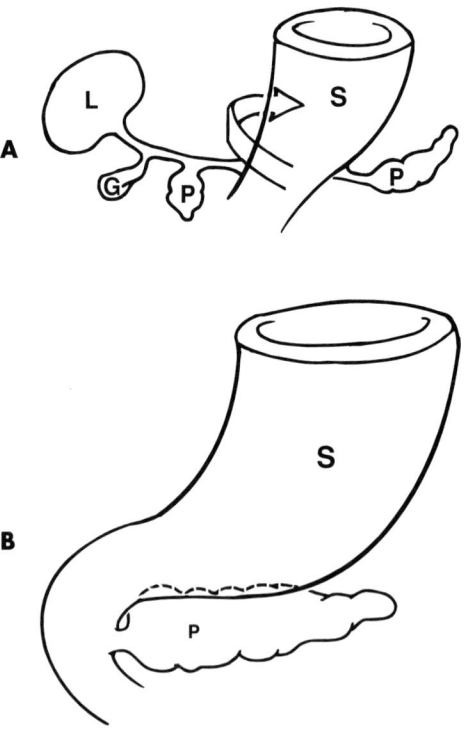

**Fig. 14-1** Pancreas development. **A,** Two portions of pancreas *(P)* rotate and eventually fuse forming normal pancreas. **B,** Normally developed pancreas. Liver *(L)*; gallbladder *(G)*; stomach *(S)*.

c. Partial duodenal obstruction (40% of cases).
d. Other associations.
   1. Malrotation.
   2. Down syndrome.
   3. Tracheoesophageal fistula.
   4. Anal atresia.
   5. Duodenal malformations.

**Imaging** Abdominal radiograph in infant can show double bubble pattern of bowel obstruction, if narrowing is too tight. It is difficult to ascertain annular pancreas on ultrasound (US); computed tomography (CT) might demonstrate circumferential nature of pancreas around duodenum.

2. Pancreas divisum.
   a. Failure of fusion between dorsal and ventral pancreatic ducts. Result is duct of Santorini drains superior pancreatic head, body, and tail, while duct of Wirsung drains inferior head and uncinate process.
   b. Incidence is unknown; may be as high as 10%.
   c. Possible increased incidence of pancreatitis.
      1. Up to 20% of patients with idiopathic pancreatitis have this anomaly.
      2. Perhaps due to inability of smaller duct of Santorini to handle normal pancreatic secretions.

**Imaging** Pancreas itself appears normal, or may have mild pancreatic head enlargement on cross-sectional imaging. However, endoscopic retrograde cholangiopancreatography (ERCP) can diagnose anomalous ducts.

3. Ectopic pancreas.
   a. Pancreatic tissue can be found in heterotopic locations apart from main gland.
      1. Antrum of stomach (70%).
      2. Duodenum.
      3. Appendix.
      4. Meckel diverticulum.
   b. Usually asymptomatic; often found incidentally in pathologic samples.

**Imaging** Gastric and duodenal lesions are occasionally detected during contrast upper gastrointestinal examinations or endoscopy; these lesions are polypoid; about half have central pit or umbilication (from rudimentary duct formation).

4. Schwachman syndrome (also known as Schwachman-Diamond syndrome).
   a. Exocrine pancreatic insufficiency.
   b. Charactertistics of syndrome.
      *1.* Bony dysplasia (metaphyseal chondrodysplasia).
      *2.* Short stature.
      *3.* Bone marrow dysfunction (neutropenia).
   c. Autosomal recessive.
   d. Often initially mistaken for cystic fibrosis because of multiple pneumonias and failure to thrive appearance of these children.

> **Imaging** Hypoplastic pancreas that may be echogenic (fatty-replaced) on US.

5. Von Hippel-Lindau disease.
   a. Autosomal dominant.
   b. Hallmarks.
      *1.* Hemangioblastoma of central nervous system.
         *a.* Retina.
         *b.* Cerebellum.
         *c.* Spinal cord.
      *2.* Cysts.
         *a.* Pancreatic.
         *b.* Renal.
   c. Increased risk of malignancy.
      *1.* Renal.
      *2.* Adrenal.
      *3.* Pancreatic.

> **Imaging** US and CT can demonstrate multiple pancreatic cysts, which can be quite large; pancreatic calcifications may be present. Look also for pancreatic masses (adults have increased risk of malignant masses of pancreas).

6. Hereditary pancreatitis.
   a. Autosomal dominant.
   b. Recurrent bouts of abdominal pain are usual presentation in child; recurrent pancreatitis is seen in adult (usually when diagnosis is made).

> **Imaging** Pancreatitis appearance (see following discussion); Pseudocyst formation can also occur. Over time, findings of chronic pancreatitis may develop (pancreatic atrophy, calcifications, and ductal dilatation).

B. Pancreas (acquired).
   1. Pancreatitis.

a. Uncommon in children; more diverse etiologies than seen in adults.
b. Most common etiologies.
   1. Trauma, including child abuse.
   2. Congenital anomaly.
      a. Pancreas divisum.
      b. Hereditary pancreatitis.
      c. Choledochal cyst.
   3. Sepsis.
   4. Viral infection (mumps).
   5. Idiopathic.
c. Clinical presentation.
   1. Abdominal pain.
   2. Pancreatic enzymes (amylase and lipase) are often elevated.
d. Treatment is usually conservative.
   1. Bowel rest.
   2. Analgesics.
   3. Supportive therapy.
e. Complications.
   1. Abscess.
   2. Pseudocyst formation.

**Imaging** Abdominal radiograph may demonstrate focal ileus anterior to pancreas ("sentinel loop"). US is frequently normal, but can show hypoechoic, enlarged edematous pancreas. Often pancreatic duct is dilated. Adjacent ascites, pseudocyst, and phlegmon (hypoechoic inflammatory mass or abscess) may also be identified. Similar findings can be seen on CT.

2. Cystic fibrosis (see Chapter 6).
   a. Mucus inspissation of pancreatic ducts.
      1. Leads to obstruction.
      2. Eventual destruction, fatty replacement, and fibrosis of pancreas.
   b. Pancreatic function.
      1. These patients have exocrine insufficiency, and often require pancreatic enzyme replacement.
      2. Endocrine dysfunction (diabetes) is uncommon, but has been seen in older survivors of cystic fibrosis.

**Imaging** US and CT demonstrate shrunken, fatty-replaced pancreas.

3. Nesidioblastosis.
   a. Islet cell hyperplasia (primitive remnant fetal cells).

b. Often presents in infants with persistent hypoglycemia (increased insulin production).
c. Can be associated with Beckwith-Wiedemann syndrome.
d. No discrete pancreatic mass is present; therefore, near total pancreatectomy may need to be performed to control condition.

**Imaging** US of pancreas is often normal, but can have enlarged appearance.

4. Pancreatic neoplasms.
   a. Extremely rare in children.
   b. Functional.
      *1.* Insulinoma.
         *a.* Clinically presents with hypoglycemia.
         *b.* Islet cell tumors can be associated with multiple endocrine neoplasia syndromes.
      *2.* "VIPoma."
         *a.* Vasoactive intestinal peptide.
         *b.* Presents with intractable diarrhea.
   c. Malignant neoplasms.
      *1.* Lymphoma.
      *2.* Pancreatoblastoma (remnant fetal cells).
      *3.* Adenocarcinoma in children (extremely rare).

**Imaging** Enlarged pancreas (often head) may be seen on US. However, definitive mass (usually hypoechoic) of functional tumors may not be seen. Contrast CT or even angiography may delineate this often hypervascular mass. Intraoperative US has been used to locate these small, often elusive pancreatic lesions. Malignant masses of pancreas, on other hand, are usually big and bulky, and can be diagnosed on CT or US.

C. Spleen (congenital).
   1. Ambiguous situs (see Chapter 19).
      a. Asplenia.
      b. Polysplenia.
   2. Accessory spleens or splenules.
      a. Common; incidence is approximately 10% to 20%.
      b. Often found near splenic hilum or surrounding spleen.

**Imaging** Can be seen on US or CT as small (less than 2 cm) homogenous nodules that match echogenicity or density of spleen. Although usually found near spleen, can be seen anywhere in abdomen.

3. Ectopic spleen ("wandering spleen").
   a. Etiology is believed to result from lack of fusion of dorsal mesogastrium with posterior peritoneum (which normally restricts spleen to left upper quadrant [LUQ] position).
   b. Spleen can be located anywhere in abdomen, but is usually found in lower left quadrant (LLQ).
   c. Complications.
      1. Intermittant torsion of splenic pedicle; can produce abdominal pain.
      2. Volvulus of pedicle with frank, splenic infarction.

> **Imaging** CT or US reveal homogenous, incidental abdominal mass that matches splenic echogenicity or density, with no spleen seen in normal LUQ position.

4. Benign splenic lesions.
   a. Cysts.
      1. Congenital.
         a. Epidermoid.
         b. Dermoid.
      2. Acquired.
         a. Traumatic.
         b. Infectious *(Echinococcus)*.
         c. Sequelae of ischemia or infarction.
      3. Congenital cyst has epithelial lining (unlike acquired).
   b. Hemangiomas.
      1. Kasabach-Merritt syndrome.
         a. Large splenic hemangiomas.
         b. Liver hemangiomas or hemangioendothelioma.
      2. Associated with thrombocytopenia and coagulopathy.
   c. Lymphangiomas.
   d. Hamartomas.

> **Imaging** Smooth, anechoic, well-circumscribed lesions can be seen on US. Multiple, septated cysts may suggest lymphangioma.

D. Spleen (acquired).
   1. Normal splenic sizes.
      a. Sonographic splenic size varies by age.
      b. General guidelines.
         1. 6 cm by 3 months of age.
         2. 7 cm by 1 year.
         3. 8 cm by 2 years.
         4. 9 cm by 4 years.

    5. 10 cm by 8 years.
    6. 11 cm by 10 years.
    7. 13 cm by 15 years of age.
 2. Splenomegaly.
    a. Infectious (most common).
       1. Infectious mononucleosis.
       2. Fungal (such as *Candida albicans* in immunocompromised host).
    b. Hemolytic anemias (such as spherocytosis or glucose-6-phosphate dehydrogenase).
    c. Storage diseases (Gaucher disease).
    d. Lymphoma or leukemia.
    e. Langerhans cell histiocytosis.
       1. Histiocytic infiltration of liver and spleen.
       2. Letterer-Siwe (rapidly fatal disorder, usually by age 3 years).
    f. Portal hypertension.
       1. Hepatic cirrhosis.
       2. Biliary atresia.
       3. Splenic vein thrombosis.
       4. Cavernous transformation of portal vein.

> **Imaging** In addition to enlarged spleen, large varices can also be present around spleen, often involving splenic hilar vessels. Look for abdominal ascites.

## SUGGESTED READINGS

Baggott BB, Long WB: Annular pancreas as a cause of extrahepatic biliary obstruction. *Am J Gastroenterol* 1991; 86:224-226.

Berrocal T, Simon MJ, Al-Assir I: Schwachman-Diamond syndrome: Clinical radiographic and sonographic aspects. *Pediatr Radiol* 1995; 25:289-292.

Choyke PL, Filling-Katz MR, Shawker TH, Gorin MB, Travis WD, Chang R, Seizinger BR, Dwyer AJ, Linehan WM: Von Hippel-Lindau disease: Radiologic screening for visceral manifestations. *Radiology* 1990; 174:815-820.

Daneman A, Gaskin K, Martin DJ, Cutz E: Pancreatic changes in cystic fibrosis: CT and sonographic appearances. *AJR* 1983; 141:653-655.

Dodds WJ, Taylor AJ, Erickson SJ, Lawson TL: Radiologic imaging of splenic anomalies. *AJR* 1990; 155:805-810.

Fleischer AC, Parker P, Kirchner SG: Sonographic findings of pancreatitis in children. *Radiology* 1983; 146:151-155.

Goerg C, Schwerk WB, Goerg K: Sonographic of focal lesions of the spleen. *AJR* 1991; 156:949-953.

Goerg C, Schwerk WB, Goerg K, Havemann K: Sonographic patterns of the affected spleen in malignant lymphoma. *J Clin Ultrasound* 1990; 18:569-574.

Grosfeld JL, Vane DW, Rescorla FJ, McQuire W, West KM: Pancreatic tumors in childhood: Analysis of 13 cases. *J Pediatr Surg* 1990; 25:1057-1062.

Herman TE, Siegel MJ: CT of acute splenic torsion in children with wandering spleen. *AJR* 1991; 156:151-153.

Herman TE, Siegel MJ: CT of the pancreas in children. *AJR* 1991; 157:375-379.

Miller JH, Greenfield LD, Wald BR: Candidiasis of the liver and spleen in childhood. *Radiology* 1982; 142:375-380.

Rosenberg HK, Markowitz RI, Kolberg H, Park C, Hubbard A, Bellah RD: Normal splenic size in infants and children: Sonographic measurements. *AJR* 1991; 157:119-121.

Siegel MJ, Martin KW, Worthington JL: Normal and abnormal pancreas in children: Ultrasound studies. *Radiology* 1987; 165:15-18.

Spencer NJB, Arthur RJ, Stringer MD: Ruptured splenic epidermoid cyst: Case report and imaging appearances. *Pediatr Radiol* 1996; 12:871-873.

Zeman RK, McVay LV, Silverman PM, Cattall EL, Benjamin SB, Fleischer DF, Garra BS, Jaffe MH: Pancreas divisum: Thin section CT. *Radiology* 1988; 169:395-398.

# SECTION III
## Cardiac and Great Vessels

# 15
# Congenital Heart Disease: Radiographic Approach

### Key Concepts

1. Congenital heart disease (CHD) occurs in approximately 1% of all live births.
2. Radiographic description of CHD involves the following mnemonic: "HAPS."
   a. *H*eart (size, configuration, and chamber enlargement).
   b. *A*ortic arch (right versus left arch).
   c. *P*ulmonary blood flow (increased versus decreased flow).
   d. *S*itus.
   e. *S*oft tissues or bones.
3. CHD can be divided into four main categories:
   a. Left-to-right shunts.
   b. Cyanotic heart disease with decreased pulmonary blood flow.
   c. Cyanotic heart disease with increased pulmonary blood flow.
   d. Left heart lesions.

A. Radiographic approach.
   1. Diagnosis of CHD can be made using variety of methods; there are many different approaches to interpretation of CHD (see Suggested Readings).
      a. Physical examination.
      b. Chest radiograph.
      c. Cardiac ultrasound (echocardiography).
      d. Cardiac catheterization.
      e. Magnetic resonance imaging (MRI).
   2. One such systematic approach to chest radiographic evaluation of CHD involves following steps (HAPS).
      a. Heart (size, configuration, chamber enlargement).
      b. Aortic arch (right versus left arch).
      c. Pulmonary blood flow (increased versus decreased flow).
      d. Situs.
      e. Soft tissues or bones.
   3. Heart size.
      a. Can be difficult to assess in neonates, because of thymus.
         *1.* Cardiothymic silhouette should be approximately 60% of neonatal hemithorax.
         *2.* In older children, 50% of thorax.
      b. If cardiomegaly is present, try to determine which specific cardiac chambers are involved.
         *1.* This information will help narrow differential.
         *2.* If available, don't forget to use lateral film. Specific chamber enlargement is often easier to discern on lateral radiograph than on anteroposterior (AP).
         *3.* Specific chambers.
            *a.* Right atrium.
               *1)* Look for bulging of right cardiac border on AP film.
               *2)* Right atrium can massively dilate (as can be seen in entities such as Ebstein anomaly or pulmonary atresia with intact septum).
            *b.* Right ventricle.
               *1)* Rotation of heart occurs with right ventricular enlargement. Result: right ventricular hypertrophy manifests as upward displacement of cardiac apex on AP film, such as is commonly seen in tetralogy of Fallot (TOF).
               *2)* On lateral film, normal right ventricular chamber should only be one third of distance of length of sternum to angle of Louis.
            *c.* Left atrium.

1) AP film may demonstrate uplifting of left main stem bronchus (resulting from left artial enlargement). Also, look for "double density" of left atrial enlargement beneath carina.
2) Lateral film is particularly helpful in assessment of left atrium; look for posterior displacement of left bronchus, such as is seen in mitral stenosis or ventricular septal defect (VSD).
3) Another hint: drop line as continuation of trachea on lateral film. In normal situation, that line should not "touch" heart. If it does, then left atrial or left ventricular enlargement is suspected.
   d. Left ventricle.
   1) Left ventricular enlargement rotates heart producing downward displacement to left cardiac apex on AP view. Again, lateral view is helpful.
   2) In left ventricular hypertrophy, left ventricle projects into retrocardiac space, posterior to inferior vena cava (IVC).
c. Pathognomonic heart configurations (Fig. 15-1).
   1. Occasionally, cardiac configuration is highly suggestive or pathognomonic for certain type of CHD.
   2. "Egg-shaped" or "egg-on-string."
      a. Oval shaped heart (egg).
      b. Thin mediastinum (string), because of small thymus and AP configuration of great vessels, as opposed to normal lateral orientation.
      c. Suggestive of transposition of great vessels (TGV).
   3. "Boot-shaped."
      a. This heart configuration has upturned cardiac apex with concave left hilum.
      b. Often associated with TOF, although any CHD with right ventricular hypertrophy can have this appearance.
   4. "Box-shaped."
      a. Right-sided enlargement (especially right atrial) that causes boxlike appearance of heart.
      b. Configuration is usually seen in Ebstein anomaly; can also occur with pulmonary or tricuspid atresia.
4. Aortic arch.
   a. Identification of right arch is important because of strong association with CHD.
      1. Truncus arteriosis (30% to 40% have right arch).
      2. TOF (25%).

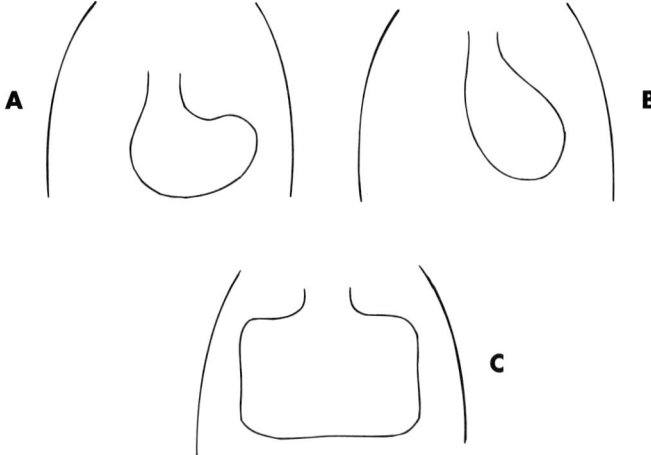

**Fig. 15-1** Schematic drawings of pathognomonic heart shapes. **A,** Upturned or boot-shaped heart; most often associated with TOF. **B,** Oval or egg-on-string heart; seen with TGV. **C,** Box-shaped heart; seen with enlargement of right atrium, as with Ebstein anomaly.

      3. TGV (5%).
      4. Vascular rings.
   b. Can be very difficult to evaluate in neonate because of thymus.
      1. Use trachea instead.
      2. Position of arch can be inferred by position of trachea.
      3. Left arch.
         *a.* Trachea positioned over right pedicles of spine.
         *b.* Also, rightward buckling of trachea can be seen with expiration.
         *c.* Can sometimes see left-sided indentation upon trachea.
      4. Right arch.
         *a.* Trachea centrally positioned over spine or over left pedicles.
         *b.* Leftward buckling of trachea is seen with expiration.
         *c.* Right-sided indentation in trachea may be present.
   c. In older children, actual aortic knob and descending aorta can usually be identified directly.
5. Pulmonary blood flow.
   a. Be careful during assessment of pulmonary blood flow; can be misleading and difficult to discern.
   b. Normal pulmonary flow does not rule out CHD.

1. Normal pulmonary flow can be seen in children with small left-to-right shunts, mild aortic or pulmonic stenosis, and mild coarctation of aorta.
2. Neonates have mild pulmonary hypertension, and radiographs will have normal to decreased flow, even with presence of shunt lesion; however, pulmonary flow will increase as soon as physiologic drop in pulmonary pressures occurs.

c. Increased pulmonary blood flow.
1. Large central pulmonary vessels (arterial).
   a. Usually due to left-to-right shunts.
   b. Shunts include VSD, atrial septal defect (ASD), and patent ductus arteriosus (PDA).
2. Vertical orientation to pulmonary vessels (venous).
   a. Suggestive of pulmonary venous congestion.
   b. Can be seen with left heart obstructive lesions.

d. Decreased pulmonary blood flow.
1. Associated with cyanotic CHD.
2. Seen in neonate with persistent pulmonary hypertension of the newborn (PPHN) (see Chapter 2).

e. Symmetry of pulmonary blood flow may also be significant.
1. Pulmonary stenosis can result in larger left-sided pulmonary artery, as opposed to right-sided, because of "jet effect" of stenosis.
2. Placement of corrective shunt to temporarily increase pulmonary flow in "blue baby" such as Blalock-Taussig shunt (subclavian artery to pulmonary artery); can result in asymmetric flow to one lung (see Chapter 18).

6. Situs (see Chapter 19).
   a. Need to locate cardiac apex and gastric bubble.
   b. If cardiac apex and gastric bubble are on opposite sides, there is CHD until proven otherwise.
   c. Situs indeterminus.
      1. Polysplenia.
         a. Left-sided.
         b. Interrupted IVC.
         c. Biliary atresia.
      2. Asplenia.
         a. "Right-sided."
         b. Midline liver.
         c. Severe, complicated CHD.

7. Soft tissues and bones.
   a. Look for bony anomalies.
      1. Segmentation often present; vertebral abnormalities like hemivertebrae or butterfly vertebrae are present.

2. Limb malformations.
    a. Holt-Oram syndrome.
    b. Radial ray malformation associated with CHD, often ASD.
  b. Cardiac problems can be part of syndrome like vertebral anomalies, anal atresia, CHD, tracheoesophageal fistula, renal and limb malformations (VACTERL).
  c. Often small child (failure to thrive).
  d. Look for rib notching.
    1. Associated with collateral flow from postductal coarctation of aorta.
    2. Rib notching often not apparent until at least 6 years of age.
    3. Can also be seen with Blalock-Taussig surgical shunts.
  e. Rib deformities can be due to prior thoracotomy.
    1. From coarctation repair.
    2. PDA ligation.
    3. Palliative shunt placement, such as Blalock-Taussig shunt.
8. Questions to ask.
  a. Once "HAPS" radiographic interpretation is complete, clinical information obtained from answering following questions is important.
    1. "Is there cyanosis?"
    2. "Is there a murmur?"
B. Differential diagnosis of CHD.
  1. CHD can be divided into four basic categories.
    a. Left-to-right shunts.
      1. VSD.
      2. ASD.
      3. PDA.
      4. Atrioventricular canal (AVC).
    b. Cyanotic heart disease with decreased flow.
      1. TOF.
      2. TGV (small shunt).
      3. Tricuspid atresia.
      4. Pulmonary atresia or critical pulmonic stenosis.
      5. Ebstein anomaly.
    c. Cyanotic heart disease with increased flow.
      1. TGV (large shunt).
      2. Total anomalous pulmonary venous return (TAPVR).
      3. Truncus arteriosus.
    d. Left-heart lesions.
      1. Aortic stenosis.
      2. Coarctation of aorta.
      3. Hypoplastic left heart.
      4. Anomalous left coronary artery.

        5. Endocardial fibroelastosis.
        6. Cor triatriatum.
    2. Method of generating differential diagnosis in evaluation of CHD.
        a. Gather information.
            1. Radiographic evaluation (HAPS).
            2. Clinical questions.
        b. Choose category of CHD (four basic categories as previously listed).
            1. Left-to-right shunt.
                a. Cardiomegaly.
                b. Increased pulmonary flow (central).
                c. Presence of murmur.
            2. Cyanotic heart disease (decreased pulmonary flow).
                a. Cardiomegaly.
                b. Decreased pulmonary flow.
                c. Cyanosis.
            3. Cyanotic heart disease (increased pulmonary flow).
                a. Cardiomegaly.
                b. Increased pulmonary flow.
                c. Cyanosis.
            4. Left-heart lesions.
                a. Cardiomegaly.
                b. Pulmonary congestion.
                c. Acyanotic.
        c. Once category is chosen, try to decide and evaluate which specific type of CHD within chosen category most fits your information. Remember: it is often difficult to distinguish one entity from another within single category.
        d. If uncertain, one can always "play statistics."
            1. Ten lesions make up 90% of CHD.
                a. VSD.
                b. TOF.
                c. PDA.
                d. Pulmonary stenosis.
                e. TGV.
                f. Hypoplastic left heart.
                g. ASD.
                h. Aortic stenosis.
                i. Coarctation of aorta.
                j. Endocardial cushion defects, AVC.
            2. Overall most common cyanotic heart disease is TOF.
            3. Most common cyanotic heart disease in newborn (first week of life) is TGV.

4. Most common shunt lesion is VSD, followed by PDA unless child has Down syndrome, then AVC is more common. PDA is more common in premature infants.
5. ASD is most common CHD discovered in older child or adult (especially in females).
6. Bicuspid aortic valve is most common congenital heart anomaly; frequently asymptomatic.

**SUGGESTED READINGS**

Choe YH, Kin YM, Han BK, Park KG, Lee HJ: MR imaging in the morphologic diagnosis of congenital heart disease. *Radiographics* 1997; 17:403-422.

Elliot LP (ed): *Cardiac Imaging in infants, children and adults,* Philadelphia, 1991, JB Lippincott.

Freedom RM, Culham JAG, Moes CAF (eds): *Angiocardiography of congenital heart disease,* New York, 1984, Macmillan.

Friedman WF, Higgins CB (eds): *Pediatric cardiac imaging,* Philadelphia, 1984, WB Saunders Company.

Gedgaudas E, Moller JH, Castaneda-Zuniga WR, Amplatz K: *Cardiovascular radiology,* Philadelphia, 1985, WB Saunders Company.

Jefferson K, Rees S: *Clinical cardiac radiology,* London, 1980, Butterworth.

Keith JD, Rowe RD, Vlad P (eds): *Heart disease in infancy and childhood,* New York, 1978, Macmillan.

Kelley MJ, Jaffe CC, Kleinman CS: *Cardiac imaging in infants and children,* Philadelphia, 1982, WB Saunders Company.

Silverman FN, Kuhn JP (eds): *Caffey's pediatric xray diagnosis* (cardiovascular section), Philadelphia, 1993, Mosby-Year Book.

Soto B, Kassner EG, Baxley WA: *Imaging of cardiac disorders* (vol 1 Congenital disorders), Philadelphia, 1992, JB Lippincott.

Swischuk LE: *Plain film interpretation in congenital heart disease,* Baltimore, 1979, Williams and Wilkins.

Swischuk LE: *Imaging of the newborn, infant and young child* (cardiovascular section), Baltimore, 1989, Williams and Wilkins.

Tonkin IND: *Pediatric cardiovascular imaging,* Philadelphia, 1992, WB Saunders Company.

# 16
## Congenital Heart Disease—Acyanotic

---

**Key Concepts**

1. Acyanotic heart disease can be broken down into two basic categories:
   a. Left-to-right shunts.
   b. Left heart lesions (often obstructive).
2. Left-to-right shunts account for nearly 50% of all forms of congenital heart disease (CHD), especially the patent ductus arteriosus (PDA) and ventricular septal defect (VSD).
3. Atrial septal defect (ASD) is the most common CHD to present later in life in the older child or adult, especially in females.
4. The three most common types of left heart lesions are hypoplastic left heart, aortic stenosis, and aortic coarctation.
5. In the infant presenting with findings of myocardial infarction, consider an aberrant left coronary artery.

A. Left-to-right shunts: account for 45% of all CHD.
  1. VSD.
     a. Very common; 20% to 25% of all CHD.
     b. Hole in ventricular septum allows blood flow to shunt from high-pressure left ventricle into right ventricle. Extra flow in right ventricle then floods lungs.
     c. Usually presents around 6 to 12 weeks of age (detection can be delayed because of physiologic high neonatal pulmonary artery pressures).
     d. Types of VSD.
        *1.* Membranous.
           *a.* High defect.
           *b.* Most common (80%).
        *2.* Supracristal or conal (outlet).
        *3.* Endocardial cushion or atrioventricular canal (inlet).
        *4.* Muscular.
           *a.* Low septal defect.
           *b.* Often multiple or Swiss cheese appearance.
     e. Majority of VSDs (50% to 70%) will close spontaneously by age 3.
     f. Treatment.
        *1.* In children with failure to thrive, or in whom shunt has not spontaneously closed, surgical correction should be done prior to age 3, in order to prevent irreversible pulmonary hypertension or Eisenmenger complex.
        *2.* Palliative pulmonary artery (PA) banding can be done in high-risk cases prior to definitive surgical closure; rare.

  **Imaging** On chest radiograph, heart is enlarged; look for right ventricular and left atrial enlargement (uplifting of left mainstem bronchus). Pulmonary blood flow is increased (large central vessels). Aortic knob is often small.

  2. PDA.
     a. Fifteen percent of CHD; more common in premature infant (25% to 30%).
     b. Normal ductus arteriosus (connects pulmonary artery to aorta) usually closes by one week of age as increasing $O_2$ levels constrict ductus. Calcifications can be seen of fibrotic remnant (ligamentum arteriosum).
     c. Pharmacologic therapy.
        *1.* Indomethacin accelerates closure of ductus (in premature infant); if pharmocologic therapy fails, surgical closure may be needed.

2. Prostaglandins (PGE1) keep ductus open.
   d. If PDA persists, listen for continuous machinelike murmur.

> **Imaging** In neonate, patent PDA usually manifests on chest radiograph as pulmonary edema with loss of sharp heart border and elevation of left main stem bronchus (resulting from left atrium enlargement). In older children, aortic knob may be enlarged and seen as density in aorticopulmonary (AP) window. Cardiomegaly and increased pulmonary blood flow is also present.

3. ASD.
   a. Between 8% and 10% of CHD.
   b. Most common CHD to present late in adult, because atrial shunting is low pressure.
   c. Females are more commonly affected than males (2:1).
   d. Classification.
      1. Ostium secundum.
         a. Most common (70%).
         b. Central defect near fossa ovalis.
      2. Ostium primum.
         a. Low ASD (20%).
         b. Part of endocardial cushion spectrum; associated with cleft mitral valve.
      3. Sinus venosus.
         a. High defect near superior vena cava (5% to 10%).
         b. Associated with partial anomalous pulmonary venous return, from right upper lung to right atrium.
   e. Large atrial shunts should be surgically closed; small ones are often monitored (possible complication of untreated ASD is late pulmonary hypertension).

> **Imaging** On chest radiograph, look for enlarged right ventricle but no left atrial enlargement. Increased pulmonary flow is also present with large central vessels (often more subtle finding than in other shunt lesions).

4. Endocardial cushion defect (ECD) or atrioventricular canal (AVC).
   a. Four percent of all CHD.
   b. Strong association with Down syndrome.
      1. Between 25% and 30% of Down children have ECD.
      2. Also look for characteristic double manubrial ossification centers and 11 pairs of ribs, both commonly seen in children with Down syndrome.

c. Caused by abnormal development of lower atrial and upper ventricular septum (endocardial cushion) with defects in tricuspid and mitral valves.
d. Types.
  1. Complete AVC.
    a. All four cardiac chambers communicate.
    b. ASD and VSD (left-to-right shunt) and common AV valve.
  2. Partial AVC.
    a. Primum ASD with cleft mitral valve.
    b. Classic angiographic finding is "gooseneck" deformity of left ventricular outflow tract, due to abnormal cleft mitral valve.
e. Surgical correction should be performed prior to onset of pulmonary hypertension (before 3 to 5 years of age). Common complication is AV valve dysfunction.

**Imaging** Chest radiograph shows cardiomegaly with increased pulmonary flow. Left atrium may be large, due to mitral insufficiency.

5. AP window.
  a. Opening between ascending aorta and pulmonary artery just above aortic valve; results in high-pressure left-to-right shunt.
  b. Uncommon; can be mistaken for truncus arteriosus (lack of separation between aorta and pulmonary artery [see Chapter 20]).

**Imaging** Chest radiograph demonstrates right ventricular and left atrial hypertrophy, and increased pulmonary flow of left-to-right shunt.

B. Left heart lesions: obstructive.
  1. Hypoplastic left heart.
    a. Presents early with congestive heart failure (CHF) and edema in neonate.
    b. Found more commonly in males than in females.
    c. Seven percent of all CHD; accounts for 25% of all cardiac deaths in first week of life.
      1. Premature foramen ovale closure.
      2. Pulmonary venous congestion.
    d. Components usually present.
      1. Rudimentary left ventricle.
      2. Hypoplastic ascending aorta.
      3. Atretic aortic valve.

e. Systemic blood flow is right-to-left shunt at PDA. There is also left-to-right shunt of oxygenated blood at atrial level.
f. Prognosis is poor even with surgery.
 1. Cardiac transplant.
 2. Norwood procedure.

> **Imaging** Chest radiograph shows cardiomegaly (often "globular" heart) with pulmonary venous congestion.

2. Aortic stenosis (AS).
  a. Between 6% and 8% of all CHD; found more commonly in males than in females.
  b. Bicuspid aortic valve is commonly present (50%), finding also seen in coarctation.
  c. Clinical presentation.
   1. Critical AS presents early in infancy with CHF from left heart obstruction.
   2. Syncope (in older children).
  d. Types.
   1. Valvular.
    a. Most common (70%); also more likely to calcify.
    b. Surgical correction.
     1) Valvotomy.
     2) Valve prosthesis.
   2. Supravalvular.
    a. Williams syndrome.
     1) Supravalvar aortic and pulmonary stenosis.
     2) Renal stenosis.
     3) Coronary artery stenosis.
     4) Hypercalcemia.
     5) Mental retardation.
     6) "Elfin faces."
    b. Poor prognosis.
   3. Subvalvular.
    a. Idiopathic hypertrophic subaortic stenosis.
     1) Asymmetric hypertrophy of left ventricular outflow tract.
     2) Strong familial connection, associated with Noonan syndrome and Turner syndrome.
     3) Can be cause of sudden cardiac failure, especially in active or athletic adolescent.
     4) Poor prognosis in symptomatic patients.

> **Imaging** In clinical AS, cardiomegaly (particularly left ventricular) is seen on chest radiograph with CHF present in

more severe cases (critical AS). In older child, look for ascending aortic bulge owing to "jet effect" from stenosis at valvular level.

3. Coarctation of aorta.
   a. Five percent of CHD.
   b. Marked narrowing of aorta resulting in impeded blood flow; no distal pulses.
   c. Strong association with bicuspid aortic valve (greater than 75%) and shunt lesions (PDA or VSD).
   d. Commonly seen in Turner syndrome.
   e. Types.
      1. Preductal (also known as "ductal dependent").
         *a.* Diffuse narrowing of isthmus prior to ductus.
         *b.* In utero collateral formation does not develop.
         *c.* Presents in neonatal period with CHF and cardiomegaly.
         *d.* More difficult surgical repair because of long segment of narrowing usually present.
      2. Postductal.
         *a.* Coarctation occurs past ductus; therefore, in utero collateral flow forms via internal mammary and intercostal vessels.
         *b.* Presents in older child or adolescent.
   f. Pseudocoarctation.
      1. Aortic buckling or narrowing.
      2. No pressure gradient over area of narrowing.
   g. Interrupted aortic arch.
      1. Retrograde flow from PDA maintains systemic circulation.
      2. Classified by site of aortic interruption.
         *a.* Between left common carotid artery and left subclavian artery (53%).
         *b.* Distal-to-left subclavian (42%).
         *c.* Between innominate artery and left common carotid artery (5%).

**Imaging** Left ventricular hypertrophy and congestive failure are present, depending on extent of aortic narrowing. Coarctation can be demonstrated on angiography, sonography (adjacent lung may interfere), or magnetic resonance imaging. On chest radiograph, rib notching may be present (apparent by age 3 to 6); forms as result of collateral flow in children with postductal coarctation.

4. Endocardial fibroelastosis.
   a. One percent of CHD.

b. Increased elastic and fibrotic tissue in left ventricular wall results in stiff ventricle with decreased cardiac output.
   c. Poor prognosis, especially when patient is symptomatic early in life.

> **Imaging** Chest radiograph demonstrates cardiomegaly with CHF.

5. Aberrant left coronary artery.
   a. Left coronary artery arises from PA.
   b. Blood flow progresses from aorta to right coronary artery, to left coronary artery, to PA (left-to-right shunt).
   c. Left ventricular ischemia and/or infarction can result. Severity depends on coronary artery dominance and presence of collateral flow.
   d. Usually presents in infancy with findings of myocardial infarction; electrocardiogram findings are helpful.

> **Imaging** Cardiomegaly and CHF may be present on chest radiograph because of myocardial infarction. Angiography is conclusive with no left coronary origin from aorta. Instead, there is retrograde filling of left coronary artery and PA from right coronary artery.

6. Cor triatriatum.
   a. Pulmonary veins combine into accessory chamber prior to reaching left atrium ("triatriatum" means three atria).
   b. Separating this chamber from left atrium is perforated membrane that impedes blood flow, resulting in obstruction with pulmonary venous congestion.

> **Imaging** Pulmonary venous congestion is seen on chest radiograph. Angiography can demonstrate accessory chamber and pulmonary veins.

7. Other lesions that can affect left heart.
   a. Myocarditis or cardiomyopathy.
      1. Viral (Coxsackievirus).
      2. Storage disorder (Pompe disorder).
   b. Kawasaki syndrome.
      1. Coronary artery aneurysm or stenosis.
      2. Myocardial infarction.
   c. Rheumatic fever.
      1. Myocarditis.
      2. Mitral stenosis or insufficiency (less likely to affect aortic valve).
   d. Pericardial effusion (viral, renal dysfunction).

> **Imaging** Chest radiograph demonstrates nonspecific cardiomegaly with congestive failure depending on degree of cardiac dysfunction.

C. Pulmonary artery abnormalities.
  1. Pulmonary artery stenosis.
     a. Twelve percent of CHD.
     b. Right ventricular hypertrophy with increased RV trabeculation.
     c. Classification.
        *1.* Ventricular (infundibular).
        *2.* Valvular.
        *3.* Peripheral.

> **Imaging** On chest radiograph, look for characteristic poststenotic bulge of main PA or left PA. Rest of pulmonary flow is usually normal.

  2. Idiopathic primary pulmonary hypertension.
     a. Rare; found more commonly in females than in males.
     b. No treatment; ultimately fatal.

> **Imaging** Characterized by large central pulmonary arteries on chest radiograph, often with peripheral "pruning" of pulmonary tree.

  3. Eisenmenger complex.
     a. Pulmonary hypertension secondary to pulmonary vascular changes from left-to-right shunt.
     b. Eventually, reversal of shunt occurs with subsequent cyanosis.

> **Imaging** Findings same as are seen in idiopathic pulmonary hypertension.

  4. Chronic lung disease.
     a. Chronic destruction of lungs leads to increased pulmonary resistence and eventual cor pulmonale (right heart failure).
     b. Common causes of end-stage lung disease.
        *1.* Cystic fibrosis.
        *2.* Chronic destructive pulmonary disease (adults).
        *3.* Chronic pulmonary emboli (sickle cell anemia).
        *4.* Bronchopulmonary dysplasia.

> **Imaging** Same as is seen in primary pulmonary hypertension; however, severe lung damage is also evident on chest radiograph (honeycomb lung with hyperaeration and fibrotic or cystic changes).

**SUGGESTED READINGS**

Bisset GS, Kirks DS, Strife JL, Schwartz DC: Cortriatriatum: Diagnosis by MR imaging. *AJR* 1987; 149:567-568.

Bisset GS, Meyer RS: Obstructive left heart lesions. *Semin Roentgenol* 1985; 20:247-253.

Broderick TW, Higgins CB, Guthaner DF, Friedman WF, Stevenson JG, French JW: Critical aortic stenosis in neonates. *Radiology* 1978; 129:393-399.

Burrows PE: Magnetic resonance imaging of the aorta in children. *Semin Ultrasound CT MR* 1990; 11:221-233.

Green CE, Gottdiener JS, Goldstein HA: Atrial septal defect. *Semin Roentgenol* 1985; 20:214-225.

Greenberg MA, Fish BG, Spindola-Franco H: Congenital abnormalities of the coronary arteries. *Radiol Clin North Am* 1989; 23:1127-1146.

Jaffe RB: Radiographic manifestations of congenital anomalies of the aortic arch. *Radiol Clin North Am* 1991; 29:319-334.

Martin EC, Strafford MA, Gersony W: Initial detection of coarctation of the aorta. *AJR* 1981; 137:1015-1017.

Norwood WI, Kirkin JK, Sanders SP: Hypoplastic left heart syndrome: Experience with palliative surgery. *Am J Cardiol* 1980; 45:87-91.

Soto B, Bargeron LM, Diethelm E: Ventricular septal defect. *Semin Roentgenol* 1985; 20:200-213.

Swischuk LE: Patent ductus arteriosus. *Semin Roentgenol* 1985; 20:236-243.

Towbin RB, Schwartz DC: Endocardial cushion defects: Embryology, anatomy and angiography. *AJR* 1981; 136:157-162.

# 17
# Congenital Heart Disease—Cyanotic

> **Key Concepts**
>
> 1. Cyanotic heart disease can be grouped into two categories: cyanosis with decreased pulmonary flow and cyanosis with increased pulmonary flow.
> 2. Inverse relationship between pulmonary flow and cyanosis: the more flow, the less cyanosis and vice versa.
> 3. The most common form of cyanotic heart disease is tetralogy of Fallot (TOF). The four components of TOF are:
>    a. Pulmonary stenosis.
>    b. Right ventricular hypertrophy (RVH).
>    c. Overriding aorta.
>    d. Ventricular septal defect (VSD).
> 4. Transposition of great vessels (TGV) is the most common cyanotic congenital heart disease (CHD) in the neonate. It can present with either increased or decreased pulmonary blood flow (depending on the size of the coexisting left-to-right shunt).
> 5. Total anomalous pulmonary venous return (TAPVR) is cyanotic heart disease with increased pulmonary blood flow.

A. Cyanotic heart disease: decreased pulmonary flow.
   1. TOF.
      a. Most common of cyanotic CHD and 15% of all CHD.
      b. Components of TOF.
         1. Pulmonary stenosis.
            a. Right ventricular outflow obstruction.
               1) Infundibular.
               2) Valvar.
               3) Supravalvar.
            b. Determines severity of disease, time of presentation, and prognosis of child.
            c. Range of severity.
               1) Severe.
                  a) "Blue baby."
                  b) Presents as neonate.
               2) Mild.
                  a) "Pink Tet" (TOF).
                  b) Presents later in life with cyanosis upon exertion.
         2. RVH.
         3. VSD.
         4. Aorta that overrides right and left ventricles.
         5. If atrial septal defect (ASD) is present, called "pentalogy of Fallot."
      c. Associations.
         1. Right arch with "mirror-image" orientation is present in 25% of cases of TOF (see Chapter 20).
         2. Vertebral anomalies, anal atresia, cardiac abnormalities, tracheoesophageal fistula, renal and limb malformations (see Chapter 9); Down syndrome.
      d. Surgical options.
         1. Palliative surgery.
            a. Blalock-Taussig shunt.
            b. Subclavian artery shunt to pulmonary artery (PA).
         2. Definitive surgery.
            a. Right ventricular outflow reconstruction.
            b. Conduit (homograft).

> **Imaging** Chest radiograph can demonstrate "boot-shaped" heart (RVH) with decreased pulmonary blood flow, dependent on amount of pulmonary stenosis present (markedly decreased flow with severe stenosis and near normal flow in "pink Tet").

   2. TGV.

a. Most common cyanotic CHD to present in neonate.
b. Aorta and pulmonary artery positions are reversed.
   1. Anteriorly positioned aorta comes off of right ventricle.
   2. Posteriorly positioned pulmonary artery originates from left ventricle.
c. Left-to-right (L-to-R) shunt lesion required for survival.
   1. Type and amount of shunt will determime pulmonary blood flow.
   2. Therefore, TGV can be placed into both differential categories of cyanotic heart disease (decreased pulmonary flow with small shunts and increased pulmonary flow with large or multiple shunts).
   3. L-to-R shunt lesion is often VSD.
   4. If L-to-R shunt is inadequate (severe cyanosis), then emergent balloon septostomy (Rashkind procedure) can be performed to create shunt at atrial level.
d. Right arch occurs in 5% to 10% of cases.
e. Surgical repair.
   1. Jatene procedure.
      a. "Arterial switch."
      b. Done at birth, during neonatal period.
   2. Mustard procedure.
      a. Atrial switch.
      b. Poor prognosis due to eventual right ventricle (RV) failure, when faced with long-term systemic pressures.
      c. Arrthymias.
f. Corrected transposition of great vessels.
   1. Type of transposition with major cardiac anatomic abnormalities.
      a. Ventricular and atrial discordance with aorta arising from left-sided RV.
      b. Normal physiologic routing of blood results, hence name "corrected" transposition.
   2. Asymptomatic condition; however, high association with conduction abnormalities and atrioventricular (AV) block.
   3. Classic chest radiographic finding is "straightening" of left heart border, because of position of aorta.
g. Transposition complexes.
   1. Double outlet right ventricle (DORV) I.
      a. Both PA and aorta arise from RV.
      b. VSD is only left ventricular outlet.
   2. DORV II.
      a. Also known as Taussig-Bing syndrome.

        b. Aorta from RV with PA overriding high VSD.
    3. Single ventricle.
        a. Rare; less than 1% of CHD.
        b. Anterior aorta and posterior PA arise from one single chamber.
        c. Single ventricle is usually "left-type" (morphologically similar to left ventricle).

**Imaging** Chest radiograph may show oval or egg-shaped heart with narrow superior mediastinum (because of abnormal aortopulmonary relationship and lack of thymic tissue). Pulmonary flow depends on presence of shunt and degree of pulmonary stenosis. (Large shunt can result in increased flow, and small shunt can result in decreased flow).

3. Tricuspid atresia.
    a. Third most common cyanotic CHD after TOF and TGV.
    b. Agenesis of tricuspid valve.
        1. Blood flow reaches left heart via an intraatrial defect (patent foramen ovale or ASD).
        2. VSD then returns blood flow to right ventricle and PA.
    c. Extracardiac malformations, such as skeletal or gastrointestinal (20%).
    d. Treatment.
        1. Palliative surgery (Blalock-Taussig shunt).
        2. Definitive surgery; Fontan procedure (conduit connecting right atrium [RA] to PA).

**Imaging** Chest radiograph shows cardiomegaly (particularly right atrial enlargement) with decreased pulmonary flow.

4. Pulmonary atresia.
    a. No forward flow from right ventricle to PA because of valve atresia.
    b. When intact septum is present.
        1. Massive enlargement of RA.
        2. Pulmonary flow.
            a. Bronchial collateral flow to lungs.
                1) Also known as "pseudotruncus."
                2) When VSD is present, pulmonary atresia can be considered most severe form of TOF.
            b. In infants via patent ductus arteriosus (PDA).

**Imaging** Cardiomegaly with right heart enlargement and decreased pulmonary blood flow is seen on chest radiograph.

Occasionally, unusual "vascular branching patterns" are seen (owing to presence of bronchial collateral flow to lung). Marked concavity is seen in region of aorticopulmonary (AP) window (owing to missing pulmonary artery flow).

5. Ebstein malformation.
   a. Low insertion of tricuspid valve with resulting "atrialization" of RV and small distal RV pumping chamber.
   b. Right-to-Left atrial shunt with decreased pulmonary flow.
   c. Similar findings are seen in Uhl disease (hypoplasia of RV myocardium).

**Imaging** Chest radiograph shows massive right atrial enlargement with decreased pulmonary flow (sometimes described as boxlike heart).

B. Cyanotic heart disease: increased pulmonary flow.
   1. TAPVR.
      a. Two percent of all CHD.
      b. All pulmonary veins drain abnormally into right heart, instead of into left atrium (can also be partial anomalous pulmonary venous return, with some of pulmonary veins draining to correct position).
      c. Clinical presentation.
         *1.* Congestive heart failure.
         *2.* Tachypnea.
         *3.* Feeding difficulties.
      d. Classification.
         *1.* Type I.
            *a.* Nonobstructive supracardiac.
            *b.* Most common, 80% to 90%.
            *c.* Classic "snowman" appearance of heart due to pulmonary flow into left superior vena cava (appearance not usually present in infants).
         *2.* Type II.
            *a.* Cardiac.
            *b.* Pulmonary flow into coronary sinus or RA.
         *3.* Type III.
            *a.* Infradiaphragmatic.
            *b.* Pulmonary venous flow, via esophageal hiatus, into infradiaphragmatic vitelline vein system (inferior vena cava, portal vein, hepatic veins, or ductus venosis).
            *c.* Often obstructed, with pulmonary venous congestion (cyanosis with feeds).

> **Imaging** Increased pulmonary markings are present on chest radiograph; significant cardiomegaly is often not seen. With type I TAPVR, may have "snowman" appearance of heart with superior mediastinal widening (in older children).

2. Truncus arteriosus.
   a. Rare; has strong association with right arch, mirror-image configuration (30% to 40%).
   b. Failure of division of truncus arteriosus (fetal structure that forms aorta and PA).
   c. Common vessel results (truncus arteriosus) that supplies coronary, pulmonary, and systemic circulations.
   d. Classification.
      *1.* Type I.
         *a.* Single main PA originating from truncus.
         *b.* Splits into left and right PA.
      *2.* Type II.
         *a.* Right PA and Left PA arise from dorsal truncus.
      *3.* Type III.
         *a.* Right PA and Left PA arise from lateral truncus.
      *4.* Pseudotruncus.
         *a.* Pulmonary flow originates from descending aorta.
         *b.* Actually form of pulmonary atresia with bronchial collaterals.

> **Imaging** Chest radiograph demonstrates cardiomegaly with increased pulmonary blood flow (similar to a L-to-R shunt). Look for right arch and absent pulmonary segment (concavity at AP window).

3. TGV (see previous discussion).
   a. TGV can also present with increased pulmonary flow depending on size of shunt (usually PDA or VSD).

**SUGGESTED READINGS**

Becker S, Hoeffel JC, Worms AM, Pernot C: Angiographic appearance of tetraology of Fallot: 100 cases. *Ann Radiol* 1980; 23:23-31.

Budorick NE, McDonald V. Flisak ME, Moncada RM: The pulmonary veins. *Semin Roentgenol* 1989; 24:127-140.

Freedom RM, Moes CAF: Hypoplastic right heart complex. *Semin Roentgenol* 1980; 20:169-183.

Hernanz-Schulman M, Fellows KE: Persistent truncus arteriosus: Pathologic, diagnostic, and therapeutic considerations. *Semin Roentgenol* 1985; 20:121-129.

Mirowitz SA, Gutierrez FR, Canter CE, Vannier MW: Tetraology of Fallot: MR findings. *Radiology* 1989; 171:207-212.

Moes CAF, Freedom RM, Burrows PE: Anomalous pulmonary venous connections. *Semin Roentgenol* 1985; 20:134-150.

Shapiro SR, Potter BM: Transposition of the great arteries. *Semin Roentgenol* 1985; 20:110-120.

Soto B, Pacifico A, Cebellos R, Bargeron LM: Tetraology of Fallot: Angiographic-pathologic correlative study. *Circulation* 1981; 64:558-566.

Strife JL: Tetraology of Fallot. *Semin Roentgenol* 1985; 20:160-168.

Tao MS, Partridge J, Radford D: Plain chest radiograph in uncomplicated Ebstein's disease. *Clin Radiol* 1986; 37:551-553.

Turley K, Tucker WY, Ullyot DJ, Ebert PA: Total anomalous pulmonary venous connection in infancy: Influence of age and type of lesion. *Am J Cardiol* 1980; 45:92-97.

Unger FM, Cavanaugh DJ, Johnson GF, Tuuri DT, Berkman R: Radiologic real-time echocardiographic evaluation of the cyanotic newborn. *Radiographics* 1986; 6:603-660.

# 18
## Surgical Repair of Congenital Heart Disease

---

**Key Concepts**

1. Most left-to-right shunts (ventricular septal defect [VSD] or atrial septal defect [ASD]) close on their own and do not require surgical intervention.
2. Pharmacologic therapy (indomethacin) can close a patent ductus arteriosus (PDA). If unsuccessful, surgical ligation can be done.
3. The Blalock-Taussig procedure (subclavian artery to pulmonary artery) is the most common surgical shunt used for palliative measures in children with cyanotic heart disease.
4. The Fontan procedure (a conduit between the right atrium [RA] and pulmonary artery [PA]) is a common surgical procedure for right heart lesions or complex congenital heart disease (CHD) cases.
5. Mediastinal widening in the immediate postoperative radiograph is an indication of hematoma. If the mediastinum is progressively widening, consider ongoing hemorrhage (an emergency).

A. Surgical corrections and palliative procedures.
   1. VSD or ASD repair.
      a. Most will close spontaneously, from 50% to 70% of VSD by age 3.
      b. Surgical repair.
         *1.* Performed when catheterization data indicates high pulmonary pressures (impending pulmonary hypertension).
         *2.* Failure to thrive.
         *3.* Surgical repair: dacron "patch" over defect.
   2. PDA.
      a. Medical or pharmacologic therapy (indomethacin to close ductus).
      b. Surgical ligation.
      c. Coil embolization.
   3. Blalock-Taussig (BT shunt).
      a. Original "blue-baby operation," first described in 1945.
      b. Subclavian artery to PA, preferably on side opposite aortic arch.
      c. Modifed BT shunt: graft from subclavian artery to PA.
      d. Palliative procedure prior to surgical correction. Used to allow time for child to grow prior to final surgical intervention.
      e. Often see asymmetric pulmonary flow on chest radiograph.
   4. Fontan procedure.
      a. Establishes flow between RA and PA.
      b. Right atrial tunnel connects systemic venous return to PA.
      c. Definitive repair for right heart lesions (such as tricuspid atresia).
      d. Often used in complex cardiac cases.
         *1.* Single ventricle.
         *2.* Double outlet right ventricle.
   5. Jatene operation.
      a. Arterial switch for transposition of the great vessels (TGV).
      b. Potential complication is coronary artery occlusion or disruption during arterial "switch."
      c. Must be done in neonatal period.
   6. Glenn operation.
      a. Superior vena cava to right pulmonary artery.
      b. Can be bidirectional.
      c. Low pressure venous flow to lung.
         *1.* Relies on changing intrathoracic pressure to generate forward flow through anastomosis.
         *2.* Positive pressure ventilation is contraindicated in these children, because it can impair venous return and prevent forward flow through anastomosis.
      d. Can be used prior to definitive Fontan procedure.
         *1.* Tricuspid atresia.

2. Single ventricle.
7. Rashkind procedure.
   a. Balloon atrial septostomy.
   b. Used for TGV when small, inadequate shunt is present (atrial septostomy allows for greater mixing of flow, therefore decreasing severe cyanosis).
   c. Can also perform operative atrial septectomy (Blalock-Hanlon operation).
8. Rastelli operation.
   a. Valved conduit from right ventricle (RV) to PA.
   b. Pulmonary outflow reconstruction for truncus arteriosus and pulmonary atresia.
9. Norwood procedure.
   a. Used for hypoplastic left ventricle repair.
   b. Two stage procedure.
      1. Single "pumping chamber" is created (RV) with connection from PA to descending aorta.
      2. Fontan procedure.
10. Mustard-Senning technique.
    a. Original TGV repair.
    b. Intraatrial baffle, resulting in "atrial switch."
    c. Long-term.
       1. This procedure retains RV as systemic ventricle (attached to aorta).
       2. Results in eventual right heart failure, arrythmias, and complete heart block; seen later in life (adolescence and early adulthood).
11. Aortic shunts to PA.
    a. Types.
       1. Potts operation (descending aorta to left pulmonary artery).
       2. Waterston operation (ascending aorta to right pulmonary artery [RPA]).
       3. Cooley operation (ascending aorta to main PA; also known as "aortopulmonary graft").
    b. These shunts are rarely used today because of complication of pulmonary hypertension (caused by long-term systemic or aortic flow into lungs).
12. Subclavian artery patch.
    a. Severe coarctation (often preductal coarctation because of long segment that is usually involved).
    b. Interrupted arch.
B. Radiographic findings of CHD repair.
   1. Sternotomy.

a. Look for midline sutures or wires.
   b. Used for definitive repair for the following CHD.
      *1.* VSD or ASD.
      *2.* Aortic and pulmonary stenosis (unless treated with balloon valvotomy).
      *3.* Tetralogy of Fallot.
      *4.* TGV.
      *5.* Aberrant coronary artery surgery.
2. Thoracotomy.
   a. Look for lateral deformity of fourth or fifth ribs.
   b. Left-sided thoracotomy.
      *1.* PDA ligation.
      *2.* Coarctation repair.
      *3.* Pulmonary artery banding.
      *4.* Vascular ring division.
   c. Right-sided thoracotomy.
      *1.* Systemic to PA shunts.
         *a.* Palliative procedure done on opposite side of aortic arch.
         *b.* Look for surgical clips in superior mediastinum.
      *2.* Esophageal atresia or tracheoesophageal fistula repair.
         *a.* Thoracotomy is preferably performed on opposite side of aorta.
3. Postoperative chest radiographic findings.
   a. Mediastinal widening.
      *1.* Immediately postoperative.
         *a.* Hemorrhage.
         *b.* If progressively widening, consider vascular leak (emergency).
      *2.* Thymic rebound in recovering child may occur several months later.
   b. Pleural effusions.
      *1.* Especially right-sided initially; can progress to involve left side.
      *2.* If pleural effusion is large and persistent, consider chylothorax secondary to damage to thoracic duct.

**SUGGESTED READINGS**

Cleveland DC, Kirklin JK, Naftel DC, Kirklin JW, Blackstone EH, Pacifico AD: Surgical treatment of tricuspid atresia. *Ann Thorac Surg* 1984; 38:447-457.

Jatene AD, Fontes VF, Souza LC, Paulista PP, Neto CA, Sousa JE: Anatomic correction of transposition of the great arteries. *J Thorac Cardiovasc Surg* 1982; 83:20-26.

Kirklin JW, Blacksone EH, Kirklin JK, Pacifico AD, Aramendi J, Bargeron LM: Surgical results and protocols in the spectrum of tetralogy of Fallot. *Ann Surg* 1983; 198:251-265.

Mazzucco A, Rizzoli G, Fracasso A, Stellin G, Valfre C, Pellegrino P, Bartolotti U, Gallucci V: Experience with operation for total anomalous pulmonary venous connection in infancy. *J Thorac Cardiovasc Surg* 1983; 85:686-690.

Norwood WI, Lang P, Hansen D: Physiologic repair of aortic atresia-hypoplastic left heart syndrome. *N Engl J Med* 1983; 308:23-26.

Soulen RL, Donner R, Capitanio M: Postoperative evaluation of complex congenital heart disease by magnetic resonance imaging. *Radiographics* 1987; 7:975-1000.

Weinberg PM: Anatomy of tricuspid atresia and its relevance to current forms of surgical therapy. *Ann Thorac Surg* 1980; 29:306-311.

# 19
# Situs Abnormalities

### Key Concepts

1. Situs abnormalities are rare (0.01% of population).
2. The association with congenital heart disease (CHD) merits evaluation for situs abnormalities whenever considering CHD and vice versa.
3. Anytime the cardiac apex is on the opposite side of the gastric air bubble, CHD is present until proven otherwise.
4. Situs ambiguous (also called situs indeterminus or the heterotaxy syndromes) involves two types: asplenia (bilateral "right-sidedness") or polysplenia (bilateral "left-sidedness").
5. Situs ambiguous is strongly associated with CHD (often complex CHD), especially asplenia.

A. Evaluation for situs abnormalities ("Three A's").
   1. Aortic arch.
   2. Air bubble (stomach).
   3. Cardiac Apex.
   4. Anytime the cardiac apex is on opposite side of gastric air bubble, CHD is present until proven otherwise.
   5. If possible, also look for hepatic position and branching pattern of bronchi, in order to determine presence of asplenia or polysplenia (Fig. 19-1).
B. Types of situs abnormalities.
   1. Situs solitus and levocardia (normal orientation).
      a. Less than 1% incidence of CHD.

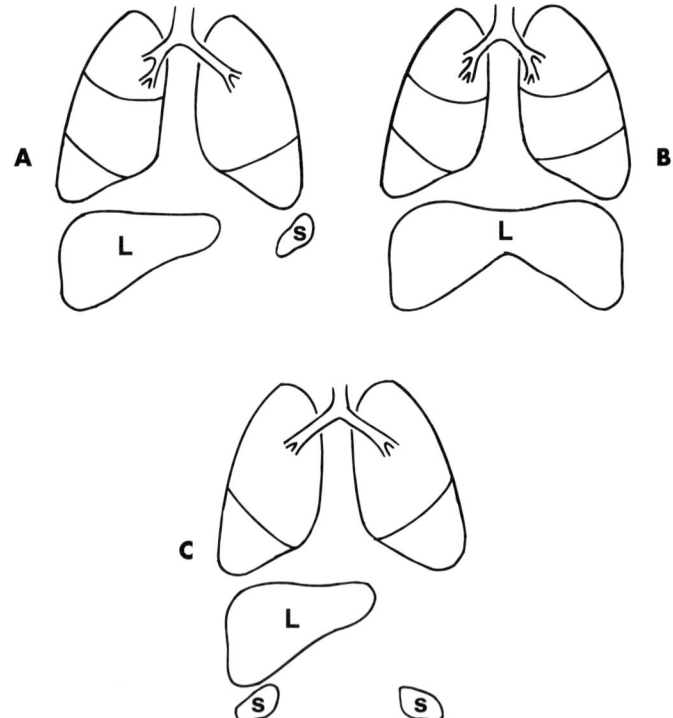

**Fig. 19-1** Branching patterns of ambiguous situs. **A,** Normal situs with trilobed right lung and bilobed left lung (note normal tracheal branching pattern); liver *(L);* spleen *(s).* **B,** Asplenia with bilateral, trilobed lungs and midline liver *(L);* spleen is absent. **C,** Polysplenia with bilateral, bilobed lungs and multiple spleens *(s),* often on both sides; liver can be on either side *(L).*

b. Gastric bubble on left.
  c. Spleen on left, liver on right.
  d. Bilobed left lung with hyparterial bronchus (left mainstem bronchus passes above left pulmonary artery [PA]).
  e. Trilobed right lung with eparterial bronchus (right mainstem bronchus passes below right PA).
  f. Left cardiac apex.
2. Situs solitus and dextrocardia.
  a. Greater than 95% incidence of CHD.
  b. Normal abdominal situs with right cardiac apex.
  c. Note: cardiac apex and gastric bubble are on opposite sides; therefore, incidence of CHD is high.
3. Situs inversus and levocardia.
  a. Incidence of CHD (100%).
  b. Left-to-right reversal of abdominal viscera.
  c. Left cardiac apex.
  d. Again note cardiac apex and gastric bubble are on opposite sides; therefore, incidence of CHD is high.
4. Situs inversus and dextrocardia.
  a. Between 3% and 5% incidence of CHD (lower incidence of CHD because cardiac apex and gastric bubble are on same side).
  b. Left-to-right reversal of abdominal viscera.
  c. Right cardiac apex.
  d. Associated with Kartagener syndrome.
    *1.* Sinusitus.
    *2.* Bronchiectasis.
    *3.* Situs inversus.
    *4.* Dextrocardia.
5. Situs ambiguous or indeterminus (Fig. 19-1).
  a. Also known as asplenia, polysplenia, or heterotaxy syndromes.
  b. Asplenia (also known as Ivemark syndrome).
    *1.* Strong association with CHD (often complex, severe CHD).
    *2.* Found more commonly in males than in females.
    *3.* Bilateral right-sidedness.
    *4.* Absent spleen.
    *5.* Centrally located liver.
    *6.* Stomach can be on either side.
    *7.* Bilateral, trilobed lungs (right-sided) with eparterial bronchi (pulmonary artery crosses above bronchi).
    *8.* Anomalies of systemic and pulmonary venous return, such as total anomalous pulmonary venous return (especially type III or infradiaphragmatic).

c. Polysplenia.
   1. Associated with biliary atresia; found more commonly in females than in males.
   2. Bilateral left-sidedness.
   3. Two or more spleens, located bilaterally.
   4. Varied hepatic and gastric position.
   5. Often have malrotation of bowel.
   6. Bilateral, bilobed lungs (left-sided) with hyparterial bronchi (pulmonary artery crosses beneath bronchi).
   7. Interrupted inferior vena cava (70%) with azygous or hemiazygous continuation.

**SUGGESTED READINGS**

Rose V, Izukawa T, Moes CAF: Syndromes of asplenia and polysplenia: A review of the cardiac and noncardiac malformations with special reference to diagnosis and prognosis. *Br Heart J* 1975; 37:840-852.

Tonkin IL, Tonkin AK: Visceroatrial situs abnormalities: Sonographic and computed tomographic appearance. *AJR* 1982; 138:509-515.

Van Mierop LHS, Eisen S, Scheibler GL: The radiographic appearance of the tracheobronchial tree as an indicator of visceral situs. *Am J Cardiol* 1970; 26:432-435.

Van Praagh R: Diagnosis of complex congenital heart disease: Morphologic anatomic method and terminology. *Cardiovasc Intervent Radiol* 1984; 7:115-120.

Van Praagh R: Importance of segmental situs in the diagnosis of congenital heart disease. *Semin Roentgenol* 1985; 20:254-271.

Winer-Muran HT, Tonkin IL: The spectrum of heterotaxy syndromes. *Radiol Clin North Am* 1989; 27:1147-1170.

# 20
# Congenital Abnormalities of the Aortic Arch

### Key Concepts

1. Left aortic arch, aberrant right subclavian artery is the most common congenital aortic anomaly (1:200).
2. Right aortic arch (mirror-image branching) is almost always associated with congenital heart disease (CHD).
3. If a healthy patient has a right arch, expect an aberrant left subclavian artery.
4. The most common vascular ring is the double aortic arch (compresses the trachea and the esophagus).
5. Coarctation of the aorta has two forms: preductal (also known as "ductal dependent") and postductal. Preductal type presents immediately at birth with "coarctation syndrome." Postductal coarctation presents later in life, because of the presence of collateral flow.

## EMBRYOLOGY OF THE AORTIC ARCH

The aortic arch develops between the sixth and eighth week of development. Six pairs of aortic arches form (Fig. 20-1). The first and second pairs involute early; the third pair forms the common carotid arteries; the fourth pair forms the aortic arch; the fifth pair regresses; the sixth pair forms the pulmonary arteries and ductus arteriosus. The subclavian arteries develop from the seventh intersegmental arteries that arise from the proximal dorsal aorta.
A. Aortic patterns.
   1. Left aortic arch.
      a. Left aortic arch, normal great vessel branching.
         *1.* Three great vessels.
            *a.* Right innominate.
            *b.* Left common carotid.
            *c.* Left subclavian.
         2. Normal variants.
            *a.* Common origin of innominate and left common carotid (also known as bovine arch).
            *b.* Vertebral artery origin from aortic arch.
         *3.* On chest radiograph, normal trachea is slightly deviated to right (more pronounced on expiration), and indented by aortic knob on left.

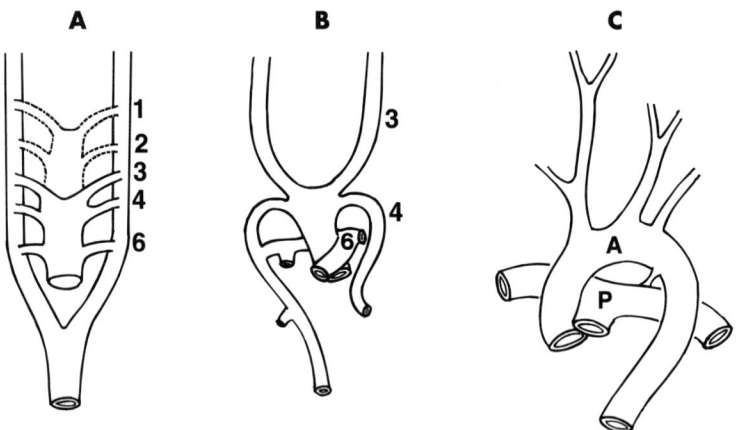

**Fig. 20-1** Aortic arch development. **A,** Early development of aortic arch with six paired aortic arches (first, second, and fifth arches are rudimentary and disappear). **B,** Continuing development of aortic arches with third arches forming carotid arteries, fourth arches becoming aorta (usually left fourth arch), and sixth arches forming pulmonary artery and ductus arteriosus. **C,** Normal left aortic arch *(A)*, pulmonary artery *(P)*, and great vessels.

b. Left aortic arch, aberrant right subclavian artery (Fig. 20-2).
   1. Four great vessels.
      a. Right and left common carotid (CC).
      b. Left subclavian.
      c. Aberrant right subclavian.
   2. Most common congenital aortic anomaly (1:200).
   3. Asymptomatic.
      a. Often incidental finding on computed tomography (CT), magnetic resonance imaging (MRI), or barium swallow.
      b. Barium swallow can show posterior impression upon esophagus, extending from lower left to upper right.
c. Left aortic arch, isolated right subclavian artery.
   1. Very rare.
   2. Three great vessels off of arch.
      a. Right and left common carotid.
      b. Left subclavian.
   3. Isolated right subclavian artery.
      a. Fills via right vertebral artery.
      b. Also known as congenital "subclavian steal syndrome."
2. Right aortic arch (1% to 2% of general population).
   a. Right aortic arch, aberrant left subclavian artery (Fig. 20-3).
      1. Four great vessels.
         a. Right and left common carotid.
         b. Right subclavian.
         c. Aberrant left subclavian.
      2. Most common type of right arch; CHD incidence is 5% to 10%.
      3. Often incidental finding on barium swallow with posterior impression extending from lower right to upper left.

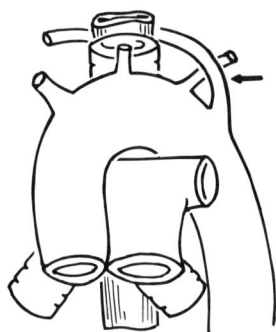

**Fig. 20-2** Left arch, aberrant right subclavian artery *(arrow)*.

4. Can form vascular ring.
    a. Right arch.
    b. Left subclavian or aortic diverticulum (persistent rudimentary distal left arch).
    c. Left pulmonary artery (PA).
    d. Ductus arteriosus.
  b. Right aortic arch, mirror-image branching (Fig. 20-4).
    1. Three great vessels.
      a. Left innominate.
      b. Right common carotid.
      c. Right subclavian.
    2. "Good news, bad news" situation.
      a. Good news: no vascular ring.
      b. Bad news: 98% are associated with CHD.

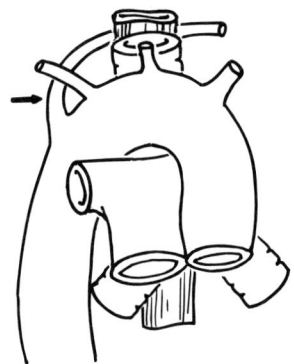

**Fig. 20-3** Right arch, aberrant left subclavian artery *(arrow)*.

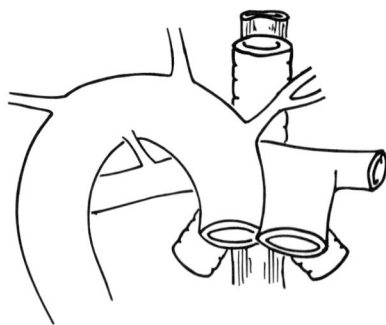

**Fig. 20-4** Right arch, mirror-image branching.

3. CHD types.
    a. Tetralogy of Fallot (TOF); 25% have right arch.
    b. Truncus arteriosus; 35% to 45% have right arch.
    c. Transposition of great vessels (TGV); 5% have right arch.
  c. Right aortic arch, isolated left subclavian artery.
    1. Very rare.
    2. Three great vessels.
       a. Left and right common carotid.
       b. Right subclavian.
    3. Left subclavian artery fills via left vertebral artery (congenital subclavian steal syndrome).
  d. Pertinent facts about right arch.
    1. Mirror image and aberrant left subclavian comprise 98% of all right arch configurations.
    2. Mirror-image branching is almost always associated with CHD.
    3. If healthy adult has right arch, expect aberrant left subclavian.
    4. If aberrant or isolated subclavian is present, it is opposite arch orientation. (For example, right arch can only have aberrant left subclavian and vice versa.)
B. Vascular rings.
  1. Definition: Anomaly in which there is encircling of trachea and esophagus by aortic arch and/or its various vascular derivatives.
    a. Asymptomatic (incomplete vascular rings).
    b. Symptomatic.
       1. Tracheal compression: cough, stridor, wheezing.
       2. Esophageal compression: dysphagia, regurgitation, aspiration.
  2. Double aortic arch (Fig. 20-5).

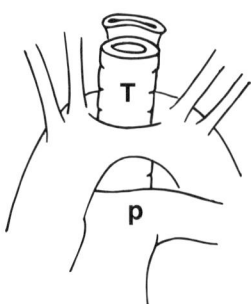

**Fig. 20-5** Double aortic arch. Aortic arch encircles trachea *(T)* and esophagus, forming vascular ring. Four great vessels are present: left and right subclavian and carotid arteries, respectively; pulmonary artery *(p)*.

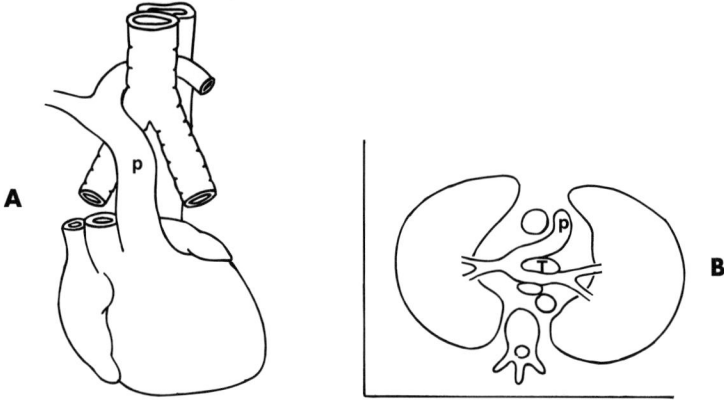

**Fig. 20-6** Pulmonary sling. **A,** Aberrant left pulmonary artery (comes off of right pulmonary artery) passes between trachea and esophagus, forming pulmonary sling. **B,** Axial view of pulmonary sling; pulmonary artery *(p)*; trachea *(T)*.

    a. "True" vascular ring.
    b. Most common vascular ring; rarely associated with CHD.
    c. Can be highly symptomatic early on in life; presents later in life, if vascular ring is "loose."

> **Imaging** On chest radiograph and angiography, right arch is usually higher, larger, and more posterior than left arch. Posterior impression upon esophagus (seen on barium swallow) varies depending on which arch is larger.

3. Pulmonary sling (Fig. 20-6).
    a. Aberrant origin of left pulmonary artery from right PA.
    b. Course of aberrant left PA.
        *1.* Left PA courses between trachea and esophagus.
        *2.* Only vascular ring to pass between trachea and esophagus (bronchogenic cyst can also occur in location).

> **Imaging** Lateral chest radiograph may show anterior bowing of tracheal air column. Anomalous course of left PA can also be seen on cross-sectional imaging (CT and MRI).

4. Right arch with aberrant left subclavian (see previous discussion).
5. Anomalous innominate artery (Fig. 20-7).
    a. More distal innominate artery origin on arch than is normally seen; can result in anterior tracheal compression as it crosses over trachea.

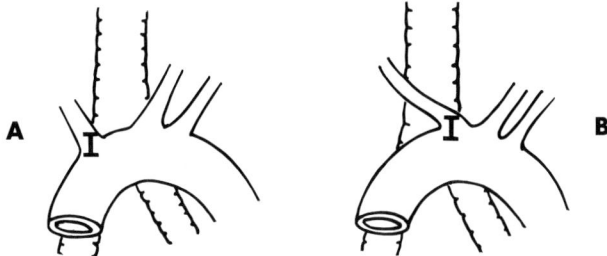

**Fig. 20-7** Anomalous innominate artery. **A,** Normal appearance of great vessels (note position of normal innominate artery *[Il]*). **B,** Origin of innominate artery *(I)* is more distal than normal, causing vessel to cross over trachea. This anomalous innominate artery position can be symptomatic.

   b. Usually asymptomatic, but can present with stridor or apneic episodes.
   c. Bronchoscopy can confirm symptomatic pulsatile narrowing of trachea.
   d. Treatment.
      *1.* Aortopexy that lifts and attaches aorta to sternum.
      *2.* Relieves compression upon trachea.

> **Imaging** Anterior compression upon trachea can be seen on lateral chest radiograph. MRI can demonstrate innominate course as it compresses trachea. (Remember, however, that anterior tracheal compression can be normal finding in young asymptomatic children.)

C. Other congenital aortic arch abnormalities.
   1. Cervical aortic arch.
      a. Rare; usually asymptomatic.
      b. Can present as pulsating mass in right or left supraclavicular fossa.
      c. Great vessel anomalies.
         *1.* Separate origin of carotid contralateral to arch.
         *2.* Varied origin of ipsilateral carotid and subclavian arteries.
      d. Aorta descends on opposite side of arch.

> **Imaging** Chest radiograph shows mediastinal mass that extends superiorly. Angiography can show cervical position of aortic arch apex.

   2. Coarctation of aorta (Fig. 20-8).

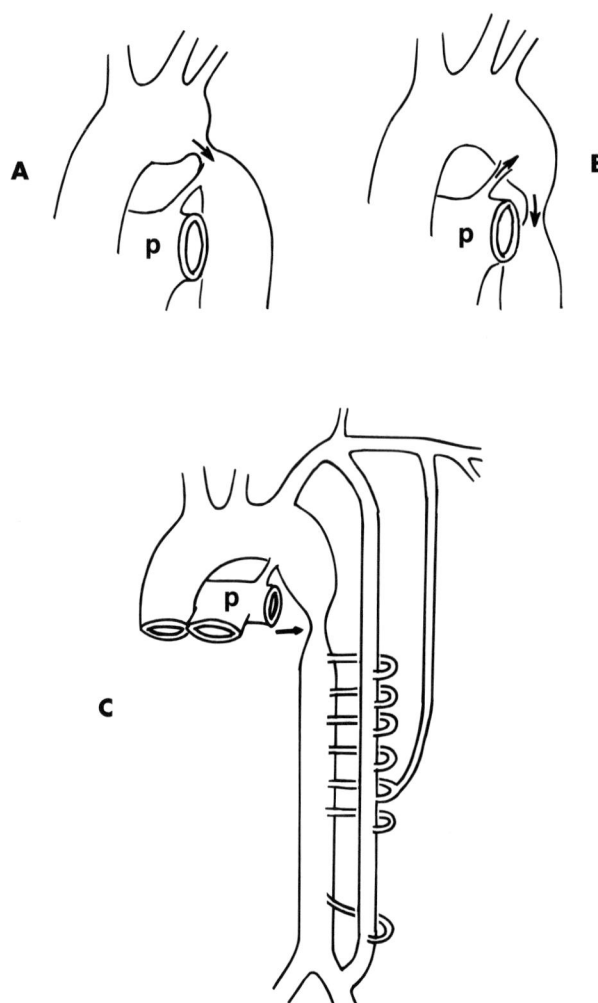

**Fig. 20-8** Coarctation of aorta. **A,** Preductal (ductal-dependent) coarctation of aorta with narrowing of aorta prior to ductus arteriosus; pulmonary artery *(p)*. **B,** Postductal coarctation of aorta; occurs distal to ductus arteriosus; pulmonary artery *(p)*. **C,** Postductal coarctation *(arrow)* with demonstration of collateral flow; forms in utero, via mammary and intercostal vessels, to supply adequate blood flow to aorta, beyond coarctation; pulmonary artery *(p)*.

a. Congenital malformation with constriction of aorta; can vary from mild stenosis to complete atresia.
b. Strong association with bicuspid aortic valve (80%), Turner syndrome, and DiGeorge syndrome.
c. Almost never associated with right heart obstructive lesions, such as TOF or pulmonary atresia.
d. Types.
   1. Postductal coarctation.
      a. Constriction at or distal to ductus arteriosus.
      b. Most common.
      c. Collateral circulation forms in utero; presents later in life.

**Imaging** Small indentation can be visible on chest radiograph just below aortic knob (coarctation) followed by convexity (poststenotic dilatation). Also look for rib notching.

   2. Preductal coarctation (also known as ductal dependent).
      a. Constriction proximal to ductus.
      b. Coarcted segment is usually longer.
      c. Associated with other CHD defects.
         1) Left-to-right shunt such as patent ductus arteriosus (PDA) or ventricular septal defect (VSD).
         2) Aortic stenosis.
      d. No collateral circulation formation in utero; results in immediate clinical presentation ("infantile coarctation syndrome").

**Imaging** Chest radiograph will show grossly enlarged heart with pulmonary congestion.

   e. Interrupted arch.
      1. Atresia of arch; clinically presents like severe coarctation.
      2. Types.
         a. Interruption distal to left subclavian (42%).
         b. Interruption between left CC and left subclavian (52%).
         c. Interruption between innominate artery and left CC (5%).
      3. Associated with PDA (95%) that supplies flow to descending aorta past interruption.
   f. Pseudocoarctation.
      1. Elongated, kinked aorta.
      2. Associated with bicuspid aortic valve.
      3. No focal stricture with mild or no pressure gradient present; therefore, is asymptomatic.
3. Truncus arteriosus.

a. Failure of division of primitive common truncus arteriosus into aorta and PA. Result is single large vessel overriding ventricular septum; supplies systemic, pulmonary, and coronary circulations.
b. Associated with VSD, cyanosis, and increased pulmonary vasculature.
c. Uncommon anomaly (0.5% of all CHD).
d. Strong association with right arch (35% to 45%).
e. Types.
  1. Type I.
     a. Most common (50%).
     b. PA that arises as single branch off of lateral wall of main trunk.
  2. Type II.
     a. Thirty percent.
     b. Separate origin of left and right PAs from dorsal wall of truncus.
  3. Type III.
     a. Ten percent.
     b. Separate origin of left and right PAs from side of truncus.
  4. Type IV.
     a. Pseudotruncus (10%).
     b. Absence of PA (atresia).
     c. Arterial supply to lungs via bronchial arteries or other collaterals.
  5. Hemitruncus.
     a. Very rare.
     b. Acyanotic; associated with PDA (80%).
     c. Only one PA (usually right) that arises from truncus; other PA arises from right ventricle or systemic collaterals.
4. TGV.
  a. Ten percent of all CHD.
  b. Second only to TOF as cause of cyanotic heart disease.
  c. Most common cause of cyanosis in neonate.
  d. Relative positions of PA and aorta are reversed. Result is two closed systems (incompatible with life). Therefore, must have intracardiac shunt or extracardiac shunt to allow communication between two systems, such as PDA, VSD, or atrial septal defect.

**Imaging** Heart size is often normal at birth, although it may have "egg-on-a-string" (oval) appearance on chest radiograph. Pulmonary flow is variable depending on associated lesions (left-to-right shunt).

5. Corrected TGV.
   a. Physiologic correction of blood flow despite major abnormalities in overall structure of heart and great vessels.
      *1.* Transposition (reversal of aorta and PA origins).
      *2.* Inversion.
         *a.* Abnormal left and right relationship of ventricles and valves.
         *b.* L loop (anatomic right ventricle is on left and vice versa).
   b. Blood route.
      *1.* Systemic venous blood to right atrium (via bicuspid mitral valve), to right-sided (but anatomic left) ventricle, into posteriorly placed PA, into lungs.
      *2.* Blood flow from lungs goes into left atrium (via tricuspid valve) into left-sided (but anatomic right) ventricle; then finally, blood flows into anteriorly placed aorta.
      *3.* If no other lesions exist, no symptoms are present.
   c. However, majority of cases have associated cardiovascular abnormalities.
      *1.* VSD (50%).
      *2.* Pulmonic stenosis.
      *3.* Conduction abnormalities (atrioventricular [AV] block).
      *4.* Left AV valve problems.

**Imaging** Chest radiograph can show abnormal convexity along left upper cardiac border (due to ascending aorta, which forms left cardiac border).

## SUGGESTED READINGS

Berdon WE, Baker DH: Vascular anomalies and the infant lung: Rings, slings and other things. *Semin Roentgenol* 1972; 7:39-64.

Bisset GS: Cardiovascular system. In *Magnetic resonance imaging in children.* Philadelphia, B.C. Decker, 1990.

Bisset GS, Meyer RA: Obstructive left heart lesions. *Semin Roentgenol* 1985; 20:244-253.

Bisset GS, Strife JL, Kirks DR, Bailey WW: Vascular rings: MR imaging. *AJR* 1987; 149:251-256.

Felson B, Strife JL: Cervical aortic arch: A commentary. *Semin Roentgenol* 1989; 24:114-120.

Hopkins KL, Patrick LE, Simoneaux MD, Bank ER, Parks WJ, Smith SS: Pediatric great vessel anomalies: Initial clinical experience with spiral CT angiography. *Radiology* 1996; 200:811-815.

Lowe GM, Donaldson JS, Backer CL: Vascular rings: 10 year review of imaging. *Radiographics* 1991; 11:637-646.

McLoughlin MJ, Weisbrod G, Wise DJ, Yeung HPH: Computed tomography in congenital anomalies of the aortic arch and great vessels. *Radiology* 1981; 138:399-403.

Predey TA, McDonald V, Demos T, Moncada R: CT of congenital anomalies of the aortic arch. *Semin Roentgenol* 1989; 24:96-113.

Schulman M, Fellows K: Persistant truncus arteriosus. *Semin Roentgenol* 1985; 20:121-129.

Shapiro SR, Potter BM: Transposition of the great arteries. *Semin Roentgenol* 1985; 20:110-120.

Shuford WH, Sybers G, Edwards FK: The three types of right aortic arch. *AJR* 1970; 109:67-74.

Stewart JR, Kincaid OW, Titus JL: Right aortic arch: Plain film diagnosis and significance. *AJR* 1966; 97:377-384.

Strife JL, Baumel S, Dunbar JS: Tracheal compression by the innominate artery in infancy and childhood. *Radiology* 1981; 139:73-75.

# SECTION IV
## Genitourinary System

# 21
# Congenital Renal Abnormalities

---

**Key Concepts**

1. Hydronephrosis is the most common cause of neonatal abdominal mass; congenital causes include ureteropelvic junction (UPJ) obstruction or ureterovesical junction (UVJ) obstruction.
2. Multicystic dysplastic kidney (MCDK) is the second most common cystic abdominal mass in the neonate.
3. Contralateral renal malformations are common, occurring in up to 30% or 40% of cases.
4. Ectopic ureter presents in the female with constant dribbling, because it inserts below the level of the sphincter or into the vagina.
5. Polycystic kidney disease is classified as autosomal recessive, polycystic kidney disease (four types: perinatal, neonatal, infantile, and juvenile) versus autosomal dominant, polycystic kidney disease (adult type).

A. Embryology: (Fig. 21-1).
   1. Pronephros.
      a. Forms by second week of gestation.
      b. Rudimentary excretory system that disappears by the fifth week of gestation.
   2. Mesonephros.
      a. Originates from mesoderm and consists of nephrons with primitive glomeruli.
      b. Drains into mesonephric (wolffian) duct, which opens into cloaca (Latin for "sewer").

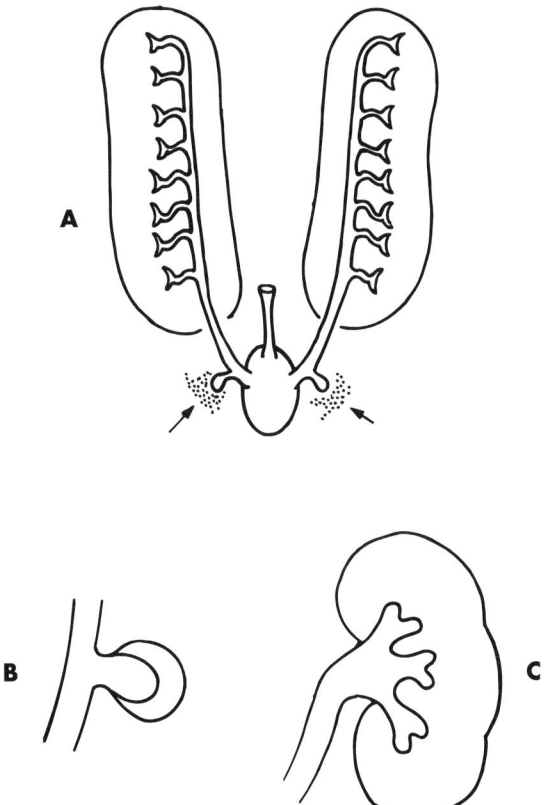

Fig. 21-1  Renal embryology. A, Ureteric bud induces adjacent mesonephric blastema *(arrows)*. Note mesonephric ducts of early primitive urinary system. B, Following ureteric induction of mesonephric blastema, kidney develops collecting system and cortical tissue (C).

c. This primitive system will regress by twelfth week of gestation.
d. Some portions of mesonephros become associated with male genital tract.
   1. Vas.
   2. Epididymis.
   3. Seminal vesicles.
   4. Ejaculatory ducts.
3. Metanephros.
   a. Forms by fifth week of gestation.
   b. Develops from ureteric bud (caudal aspect of mesonephric duct) and nephrogenic blastema (mesoderm located in lumbosacral region).
   c. Ureteric bud elongates and penetrates nephrogenic blastema during sixth week of gestation.
   d. Ureteric bud forms primitive ureter and renal pelvis, while nephrogenic blastema forms renal parenchyma.
   e. "Renal ascent" occurs during sixth and seventh weeks, as nephrogenic mass "ascends" posterior abdominal wall into renal fossa (actually, result of lumbosacral growth).
   f. Ninety degree medial rotation of developing kidney also occurs during renal ascent, brings kidney into normal position within renal fossa with anteromedial renal pelvis.
   g. Renal blood flow is supplied by splanchnic arteries off aorta and via supracardinal anastomoses (venous drainage).
4. Critical events in development of kidney.
   a. Ureteric bud appearance.
   b. Ureteric bud invagination of nephrogenic blastema.
   c. Renal ascent.
   d. Disruption of these events can lead to renal malformations.
      1. Failure at first two stages results in agenesis or hypoplasia of kidney.
      2. Ureteric bud can split resulting in duplication.
      3. Failure or arrest of renal ascent results in renal ectopia and malrotation.
B. Congenital urologic abnormalities.
   1. Renal agenesis.
      a. Bilateral.
         1. 1:8000; ratio of incidence in males to females is 3:1.
         2. Clinical presentation with bilateral agenesis.
            a. Oligohydramnios.
            b. Potter syndrome face (with low-set, floppy ears).
            c. Pulmonary hypoplasia.
               1) Associated with spontaneous pneumothorax.
               2) Often immediate cause of death.

b. Unilateral.
      1. Common (1:500).
      2. Due to ureteric bud failure.
      3. Usually ipsilateral ureter down to trigone is also absent.
      4. Can have contralateral renal malformation or dysplasia.
   c. Associated with genital malformations.
      1. Girls.
         a. Hydrometrocolpos.
         b. Unicornuate uterus.
         c. Vaginal atresia.
         d. Mayer-Rokitansky-Küster-Hauser syndrome.
            1) Renal agenesis.
            2) Müllerian abnormalities such as absent uterus.
      2. Boys.
         a. Cryptorchidism or absent testes.
         b. Seminal vesicle cysts.
         c. Hypospadias.

**Imaging** Renal fossa is absent on computed tomography, ultrasound, and intravenous pyelography (CT, US, and IVP); often bowel loops fall into empty space. Prominent adrenal can be seen on US.

2. Renal ectopia.
   a. Abnormally positioned kidney; greater incidence in boys than in girls.
   b. Kidney did not ascend completely.
      1. Final position somewhere between pelvis and renal fossa.
      2. Usually functions normally but pelvic kidney can be problematic during pregnancy.
   c. Ascends too far (thoracic kidney).
   d. Crossed-fused ectopia (Fig. 21-2).
      1. Crossing over of kidney with fusion to contralateral kidney.
      2. Ureter still enters bladder on its original side.
   e. If ectopic, kidney will not undergo normal rotation.
      1. Resulting anteriorly positioned renal pelvis can cause obstruction or stasis.
      2. There is also higher incidence of hypertension in renal ectopia.

**Imaging** When empty renal fossa is seen on CT or US, look elsewhere for potential ectopic kidney. Common locations are in pelvis behind bladder, or in lower abdomen.

3. Horseshoe kidney (Fig. 21-3).
   a. Renal fusion with lower poles fusing across midline; forms isthmus of renal tissue or fibrous band.

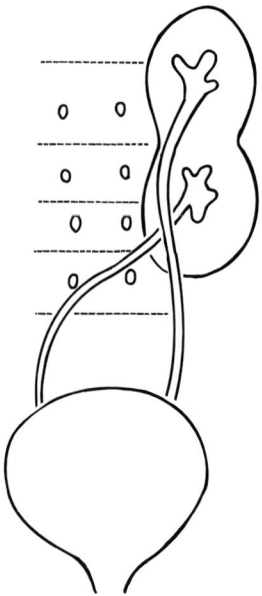

**Fig. 21-2** Crossed-fused ectopia.

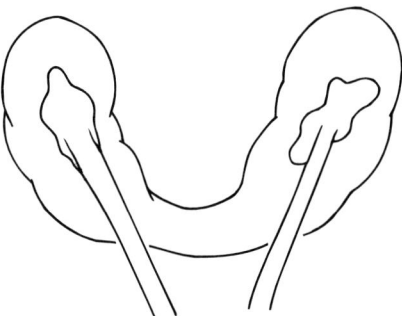

**Fig. 21-3** Horseshoe kidney. Note malrotated collecting system (anterior ureter rather than medially oriented ureter).

   b. Common (1:500).
   c. Etiology.
      1. Displaced ureteric bud with fusion of metanephric blastema.
      2. Because of fusion, normal rotation does not occur; results in anteriorly placed renal pelvis and ureters.
   d. Usually asymptomatic but can have complications.

1. UPJ obstruction.
2. Infections.
3. Stone formation.
e. Associated with Turner syndrome.

> **Imaging** On CT, US, or IVP, renal tissue can be seen crossing midline over spine uniting both kidneys.

4. Renal duplex.
   a. Sequela of premature branching of metanephric duct.
   b. Common; incidence in females is greater than in males (4:1).
   c. Usually unilateral and incomplete with distal joining of duplex ureters, and normal ureteral insertion at trigone.
   d. Complete duplex.
      1. Weigert-Meyer rule.
         a. When duplication is complete, lower pole moiety inserts in or near normal position, while upper pole ureter inserts medially and inferiorly to normal position.
         b. Therefore, upper pole moiety has longer submucosal tunnel, resulting in lower incidence of vesicoureteral reflux as compared to lower pole ureters.
      2. Upper pole ureter is more commonly obstructed (often by ureterocele), while lower pole ureter is associated with vesicoureteral reflux.

> **Imaging** US will show hypoechoic cortical band across medullary area, separating upper and lower poles of duplex. IVP will directly demonstrate duplicated collecting sytem and ureters.

   e. Ureterocele (obstructed upper pole) (Fig. 21-4).
      1. Congenital dilatation of intramucosal distal ureter.
         a. Simple.
            1) Located entirely within bladder with normal insertion position.
            2) Radiolucent filling defect known as "cobra head" or "spring onion."
         b. Ectopic.
            1) Ureter and resulting ureterocele insert in ectopic position on bladder.
            2) Often associated with upper pole moiety of duplex.
      2. Usually unilateral; found more commonly in females than in males (5:1).
      3. Complications.
         a. Can cause bladder outlet obstruction.

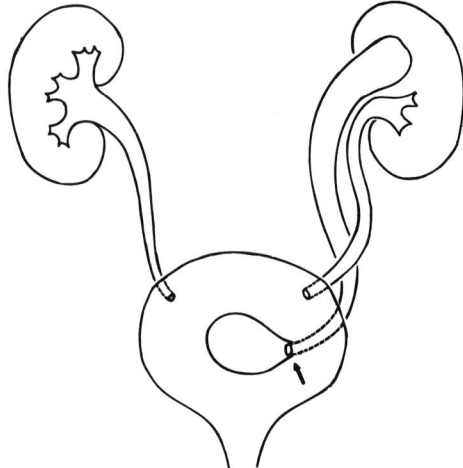

**Fig. 21-4** Left-sided duplex kidney with ureterocele. Upper pole ureter or ureterocele *(arrow)* inserts into bladder in more medial and inferior position as compared to lower pole ureter. Note drooping lily appearance of left lower pole collecting system, which is inferiorly displaced by obstructed upper pole.

        *b.* Can distort ureteral insertion causing reflux of lower pole ureter.
    4. Treatment of ureterocele, ectopic ureter, or obstructed nonfunctioning upper pole is heminephroureterectomy.

> **Imaging** US can demonstrate dilated upper pole with visualization of dilated, often tortuous distal ureter. Ureterocele can often be seen in bladder as thin-walled structure. On voiding cystourethrogram (VCUG), early filling of bladder will demonstrate filling defect (ureterocele) near UVJ; (if bladder is too full, ureterocele may be compressed and not visible). Corresponding obstructed upper pole (often poorly functioning) can be seen on IVP on delayed views. Also look for "drooping lily" sign (displacement of lower pole by either obstructed upper pole or suprarenal mass).

    *f.* Ectopic ureter; often upper pole of duplex (Fig. 21-5).
        *1.* Ureter that inserts in abnormal position on bladder or extravesicle insertion.
            *a.* Urethra.
            *b.* Vagina.
            *c.* Vas.

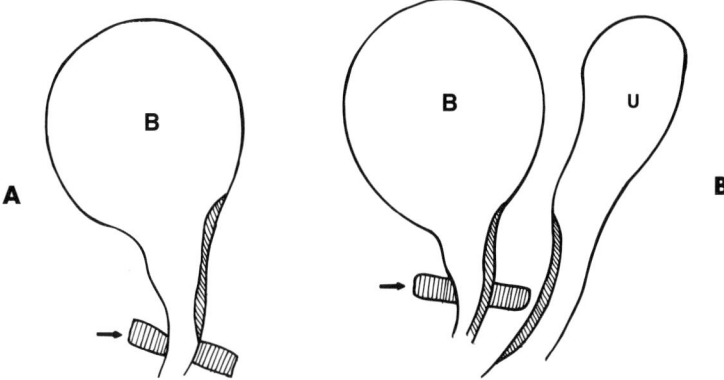

**Fig. 21-5** Ectopic ureteral insertions. Bladder *(B)*; Uterus *(U)*. **A,** Male ectopic ureteral insertion sites *(shaded regions)* are above sphincter *(arrow)*. **B,** Female ectopic ureteral insertion sites *(shaded regions)* can be below sphincter *(arrow)* leading to constant dribbling.

    2. In males.
        *a.* Ectopic ureter can present as epididymitis or hydronephrosis.
        *b.* Ectopic ureter always inserts above external sphincter; therefore, no incontinence in males.
    *3.* In females.
        *a.* Ureter can insert below external bladder sphincter.
        *b.* Result: ectopic ureter in female can present with urinary tract infection, constant wetting, or incontinence ("always wet, every day for as long as anyone can remember").

> **Imaging** One of few indications for IVP in child (with exception of obstructing renal calculi) is in search for ectopic ureter (classic history is female who is constantly wet), often associated with duplex system. Can be difficult to visualize actual ectopic ureter because of poorly functioning, obstructed system.

  5. Hydronephrosis.
    a. Most common cause of neonatal abdominal mass.
    b. Dilatation of renal collecting system can be due to obstruction versus more common reflux; therefore, VCUG examination to evaluate reflux is necessary component of subsequent imaging workup.
    c. UPJ obstruction.
        *1.* Possible etiologies.

a. Related to intrinsic abnormality (abnormal musculature).
b. Increased fibrosis (caused by external compression from aberrant vessel or kinks).
2. Large number of UPJ obstructions are left sided, 20% contralateral.
3. Wide range of severity.
4. Treatment depends on severity of obstruction.
   a. Mild obstruction can be followed with US.
   b. Severe obstruction requires surgical correction with excision and reanastomosis of narrowed site (pyeloplasty).

**Imaging** US can demonstrate dilated renal pelvis and often calyces. Nuclear renal scan diethylenetriaminepentaacetic acid (DTPA) can confirm obstruction at UPJ level: less than 10 minute emptying half-time is normal; greater than 20 minutes emptying half-time is abnormal. Between 10 and 20 minutes is intermediate; Whitaker test (pressure-flow study) may be done in these cases to determine presence of true obstruction.

d. UVJ obstruction.
   1. Functional obstruction or megaureter.
      a. Distal-most ureter is aperistaltic and often dilated.
      b. However, ganglion cells are present (therefore, it is not analogous to Hirschsprung disease).
      c. Fibrosis may be seen.
   2. Found more commonly in males than in females; incidence in left ureter is greater than in right, with 20% bilateral.
   3. Vesicoureteral reflux may also be present.
   4. Treatment depends on severity, possibly requiring surgical excision of distal aperistaltic segment with reimplantation of ureters.
   5. UVJ can be associated with congenital megacalyces.
      a. Hypoplastic medullary pyramids leading to calicectasis and increased calyceal numbers (often numbering over twenty) with no effect on renal function.
      b. Renal appearance may simulate hydronephrosis, but there is no obstruction.

**Imaging** US demonstrates dilated distal ureter in addition to dilated renal pelvis. Coexistant reflux as seen on VCUG examination is possible. Nuclear medicine (DTPA renal scan) or IVP shows obstruction at UVJ level with non-peristaltic distal ureteral segment.

e. Posterior urethral valves (see Chapter 22).
f. Prune-belly (Eagle-Barrett) syndrome (see Chapter 22).
6. MCDK.
   a. Second most common cystic abdominal mass in neonate (next to hydronephrosis).
   b. Bilateral MCDK is not compatible with life.
   c. Discovery of unilateral MCDK.
      *1.* On prenatal US.
      *2.* On first day of life as palpable mass.
      *3.* Incidental finding later in life.
   d. Etiology is probably due to atresia of ureteropelvic junction.
   e. Two forms.
      *1.* Pelvoinfundibular.
         *a.* Atresia of pelvis and ureter.
         *b.* Multiple noncommunicating cysts.
      *2.* Hydronephrotic.
         *a.* Less commonly seen.
         *b.* Dominant cyst is seen near renal pelvis.
   f. Both of these forms of MCDK are associated with hypoplastic renal artery and severely diminished or absent renal function.
   g. Contralateral abnormality (20% to 30%).
      *1.* Reflux.
      *2.* Especially UPJ obstruction.
   h. Historically, these dysplastic kidneys were removed for fear of hypertension, infection, or even malignancy. These fears are unfounded, and now MCDK is simply followed on US, usually demonstrating involution.
   i. Prognosis of unilateral MCDK depends on status of contralateral kidney.
      *1.* Often demonstrates compensatory hypertrophy.
      *2.* Most common contralateral abnormality is reflux.

**Imaging** US demonstrates little if any renal cortex with large cysts of varying sizes that do not communicate. (Remember to evaluate contralateral kidney.) Nuclear medicine (DTPA renal scan) shows little if any function of MCDK.

7. Polycystic kidney disease.
   a. No longer just simple infantile versus adult forms.
   b. Classification.
      *1.* Autosomal recessive, polycystic kidney disease: spectrum.
         *a.* Perinatal.
            *1)* Severe renal involvement.

2) Lethal.
   b. Neonatal.
      1) Moderate renal involvement to severe renal involvement with death usually by 1 year of age.
      2) Mild hepatic periportal fibrosis may be present.
   c. Infantile.
      1) Renal and/or hepatic failure not apparent until 5 to 10 years of age.
      2) Large kidneys, however, are noted much earlier.
   d. Juvenile.
      1) Hepatomegaly and periportal fibrosis diagnosed early on.
      2) Little renal involvement.

**Imaging** Perinatal, neonatal, infantile forms: US demonstrates nephromegaly with increased echogenicity of kidneys bilaterally; central renal fat-collecting system is not apparent. IVP may show delayed nephrographic phase, with brushlike tubules. Juvenile form: often normal appearance to kidneys, with hepatic findings of portal hypertension.

   2. Autosomal dominant, polycystic kidney disease.
      a. Adult form that can present (in rare cases) in late childhood.
      b. Cysts are located throughout enlarged kidney with hepatic cysts (30%) but little hepatic fibrosis.
      c. Intracranial berry aneurysms can occur (20%).
8. Medullary cystic disease.
   a. Medullary sponge disease.
      1. Tubular ectasia; possibly medullary dysplasia.
      2. Often incidental finding on radiographic studies.
      3. Associated with calculi and pyelonephritis.

**Imaging** US is often normal; can possibly see nephrocalcinosis or renal calculi. On IVP, radiating contrast from renal pyramids can be present ("paintbrush" appearance).

   b. Medullary cystic disease (juvenile nephronophthisis).
      1. Juvenile onset.
      2. Microscopic cysts with interstitial nephritis.
      3. Common cause for idiopathic renal failure in adolescents; no gender difference in incidence.

**Imaging** US may show small, scarred kidneys with cortical echogenicity and poor corticomedullary differentiation. Biopsy diagnosis.

## SUGGESTED READINGS

Avni EF, Thoug Y, Lalmand B, Didier F, Droulle P, Schulman CC: Multicystic dysplastic kidney: Natural history from in utero diagnosis and postnatal follow-up. *J Urol* 1987; 138:1420-1424.

Bisset GS, Strife JL: The duplex collecting system in girls with urinary tract infection: Prevalence and significance. *AJR* 1987; 148:497-500.

Churchill BM, Abara EO, Mc Lorie GA: Ureteral duplication, ectopy and ureteroceles. *Pediatr Clin North Am* 1987; 34:1273-1289.

Fernbach SK, Feinstein KA, Spencer K, Lindstrom CA: Ureteral duplication and its complications. *Radiographics* 1997; 17:109-127.

Grainger R, Murphy DM, Lane V: Horseshoe kidney: A review of presentation, associated congenital anomalies and complications in 73 patients. *Ir Med J* 1983; 76:315-317.

Hayden CK, Swischuk LE: Renal cystic disease. *Semin Ultrasound CT MR* 1991; 12:361-373.

Kaneko K, Suzuki Y, Fukado Y, Yabuta K, Miyano T: Abnormal contralateral kidney in unilateral MCDK. *Pediatr Radiol* 1995; 25:275-277.

Koff SA, McDowell GC, Bayard M: Diuretic radionuclide assessment of obstruction in the infant: Guidelines for successful interpretation. *J Urol* 1988; 140:1167-1168.

Mandell J, Peters CA, Retik AB: Current concepts in the prenatal diagnosis and management of hydronephrosis. *Urol Clin North Am* 1990; 17:247-262.

Nussbaum AR, Dorst JP, Jeffs RD, Gearhart JP, Sanders RC: Ectopic ureter and ureterocele: Their varied radiographic manifestations. *Radiology* 1986; 159:227-235.

Premkumar, Berdon WE, Levy J, Amodio J, Abramsons J, Newhouse JH: Emergence of hepatic fibrosis and portal hypertension in infants and children with autosomal recessive polycystic kidney disease: Initial and follow-up sonographic and radiographic findings. *Pediatr Radiol* 1988; 18:123-129.

Sanders RC, Hartman DS: Sonographic distinction between neonatal multicystic dysplastic kidney and hydronephrosis. *Radiology* 1984; 151:621-625.

Vargas B, Lebowitz RL: The coexistence of congenital megacalyces and primary megaureter. *AJR* 1986; 147:313-316.

Vincour L, Slovis TL, Perlmutter AD, Watts FB, Chung CH: Follow-up studies of multicystic dysplastic kidneys. *Radiology* 1988; 167:311-315.

Zerin JM: Hydronephrosis in the neonate and young infant: Current concepts. *Semin Ultrasound CT MR* 1994; 15:306-316.

# 22

# Lower Urinary (Bladder and Urethra) Development and Disorders

### Key Concepts

1. Neurogenic bladder is a dysfunction related to neurologic causes that, in children, is most commonly due to a congenital etiology such as myelomeningocele or spinal dysraphism.
2. Urachal anomalies occur because of failure of the embryonic urachus to completely involute. Types of urachal anomalies include patent urachus, urachal remnant or diverticulum, or urachal cyst.
3. Prune-belly (Eagle-Barrett) syndrome is found almost exclusively in males and has a classic triad of hypoplastic or absent abdominal musculature, cryptorchidism, and marked dilation of the urinary tract.
4. Obstruction from posterior urethral valves in males causes a hypertrophied and thick-walled bladder. The resulting altered vesicoureteral orifice predisposes to reflux, which can lead to bilateral hydroureteronephrosis.
5. Lower genitourinary (GU) tract tumors are uncommon in pediatrics, yet 10% of all rhabdomyosarcoma originates in the lower urinary tract, especially in the prostate. The most common type is embryonal, a lobulated tumor that fills the bladder viscus, often called "sarcoma botryoides" ("bunch of grapes").

## EMBRYOLOGY

The developing lower gastrointestinal tract, reproductive tract, and the lower urinary tract formations are closely related (see Figs. 11-1 and 22-1).

By the third week of gestation, the distal portion of the hindgut terminates in the cloaca (a cavity lined with endoderm). The distal-most portion of the cloaca is in contact with the ectoderm forming a cloacal membrane. By the fifth week of gestation, a wedge of mesoderm (urorectal septum) grows caudally to separate cloaca into ventral (urogenital) and dorsal (rectal) portions. This urorectal septum reaches the cloacal membrane by the seventh week of gestation, rupturing the membrane and dividing it into urogenital and anal membranes; this results in the formation of the perineum.

The ventral portion of the cloaca will eventually form the urethra, while rectum and anus form from dorsal part. In males, development is now complete, (since males have one opening for both genital functions and urinary functions). In females, however, GU portions must divide again (via the urogenital septum) to form separate genital (vaginal) and urinary (urethral) openings.

If the cloacal membrane fails to regress (that is, fails to make contact with urorectal septum), then there is interference with the normal fusion of the anterior abdominal and pelvic walls (malformation known as cloacal exstrophy).

A. Cloacal abnormalities.
  1. Abnormal formation of urorectal septum and cloacal membrane; can also have failure of fusion of anterior abdominal wall.
  2. Spectrum of abnormalities.
     a. Epispadias (mild).
     b. Exstrophy (severe).
  3. Common features that may be present.
     a. Widened pubic symphysis.
     b. Omphalocele.
     c. Spinal dysraphism.
  4. Epispadias (urethral meatus located anywhere along dorsum of penis).
  5. Hypospadias.
     a. Males.
        *1.* Termination of urethra along ventral aspect of penis.
        *2.* Common; 1:300 males.
        *3.* Associated with horseshoe kidney, inguinal hernia.
     b. Females.
        *1.* Form of hypospadias is seen in females and is called urogenital sinus defect.
        *2.* Common opening for both urinary and genital systems.
           *a.* Normal finding in early development.

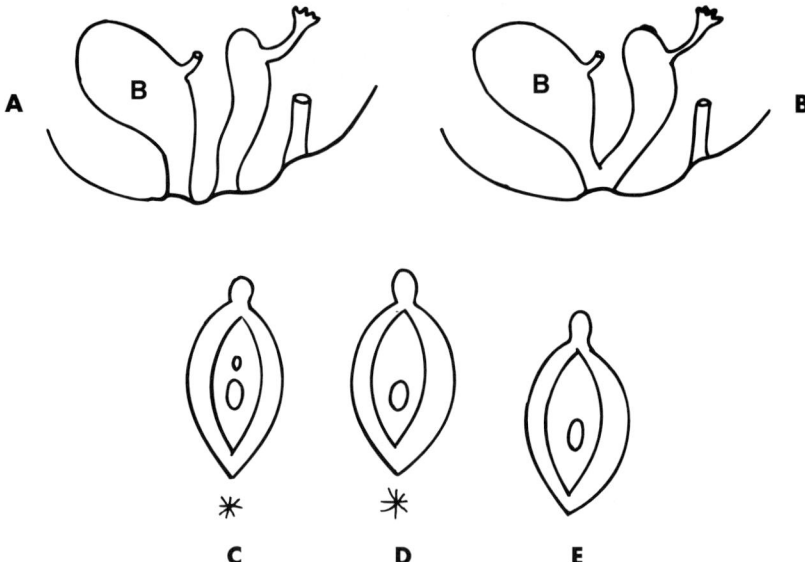

**Fig. 22-1** Female cloacal malformations. **A,** Normal female development with three divisions of cloaca: anal, vaginal, and urethral (bladder, *B*). **B,** Urogenital sinus defect with lack of separation of GU portion of cloaca (both vagina and urethra share perineal opening). **C,** Normal female perineal openings: urethral, vaginal, and anal *(\*)*. **D,** Urogenital sinus defect: only two openings, as urethra and vagina share GU tract opening; anus *(\*)*. **E,** Persistent cloacal malformation: only one opening for both GI and GU tracts.

   *b.* Obviously normal persistent finding in males, but abnormal in females.
3. Spectrum of abnormalities (Fig. 22-1).
4. Term female hypospadias has been used to describe these abnormalities, since urethra can enter anterior wall of vagina with no urethral meatus on perineum.
5. Can occur with virilization of female.
   *a.* Adrenal cortical hyperplasia.
   *b.* Adrenal genital syndrome with 21 hydroxylase deficiency.
6. Can be associated with vaginal atresia.
7. Although usually this disorder is asymptomatic, potential complications include:
   *a.* Urinary tract infection (UTI) or vaginal reflux.
   *b.* Urethral stenosis.
   *c.* Vaginal obstruction.

8. Labial adhesions can cause extensive vaginal reflux during voiding cystourethrogram (VCUG) examination; can mimic urogenital sinus abnormality.
6. Cloacal malformation.
   a. Only one common perineal opening for urinary, genital, and rectal tracts.
   b. Rare; 1:40,000.
   c. Females.
7. Bladder exstrophy.
   a. 1:30,000; found more commonly in males than in females.
   b. Bladder is not anteriorly fused.
   c. Urethral and trigonal areas are exposed, as everted bladder is continuous with anterior abdominal wall.
   d. Rarely have associated upper urinary tract abnormalities.
8. Cloacal exstrophy.
   a. Rare; 1:200,000.
   b. Primary defect in anterior abdominal wall mesoderm with resulting exstrophied (exposed) cloaca.
   c. Incidence of omphalocele or myelomeningocele (50%).

B. Bladder abnormalities.
1. Bladder formation.
   a. Around second week of gestation, ventral outgrowth of hindgut (known as allantois) appears.
   b. This allantoic stalk connection to cloaca is urachus (which becomes fibrous remnant known as medial umbilical ligament).
2. Bladder innervation.
   a. Complex, since it has both reflex control and voluntary control.
   b. Innervation.
      *1.* Sympathetic (thoracic vertebrae T11 and T12; lumbar vertebrae L1 and L2).
         *a.* Controls smooth muscle neck of bladder that maintains "tone" of bladder.
         *b.* This tone needs to be relaxed prior to voiding ("you can't urinate and run at the same time").
      2. Parasympathetic (S2, S3, S4 or pudenal).
         *a.* Controls striated voluntary sphincter which relaxes.
         *b.* Detrusor contracts to empty bladder.
      *3.* Two systems work in synergy, once conscious control is mastered.
   c. Infant voiding.
      *1.* Bladder contracts in response to stretch reflex.
      2. Afferent impulse to sacrum with efferent response; results in detrusor contraction and internal sphincter relaxation.

d. Child.
   1. Learns to inhibit detrusor (stretch reflex) response.
   2. Learns to voluntarily control external sphincter.
3. Urachal anomalies (Fig. 22-2).
   a. Patent urachus.
      1. Failure of embryonic urachus to involute.
      2. Persistent communication between bladder and umbilicus.
      3. Presents with urine leaking from umbilicus.

> **Imaging** Water-soluble contrast study can demonstrate connection between bladder and umbilicus (either following umbilicus or bladder catheterization).

   b. Urachal remnant or diverticulum.
      1. Continued bladder communication with urachus, but no umbilicus connection.

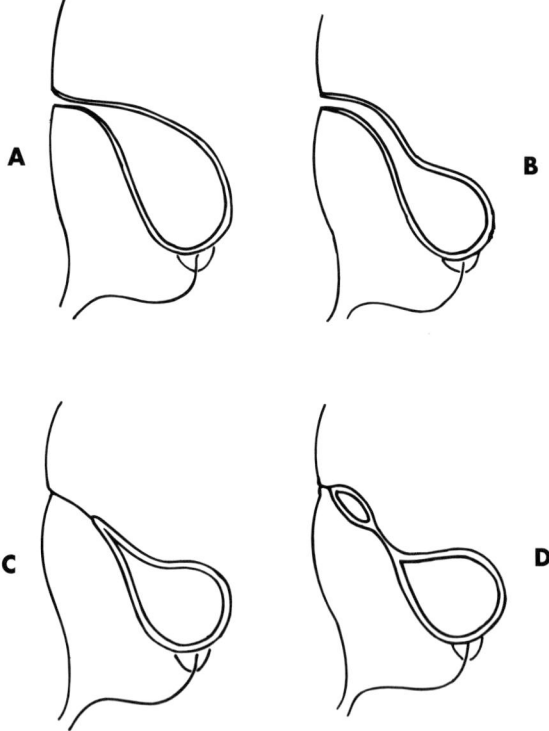

**Fig. 22-2** Urachal anomalies. **A,** Embryonic. **B,** Patent urachus. **C,** Urachal diverticulum. **D,** Urachal cyst.

2. Best seen on lateral film of VCUG examination.

**Imaging** On VCUG examination, appears as "outpouching" of superior aspect of bladder, pointing in direction of umbilicus.

    c. Urachal cyst.
        *1.* Fluid-filled remnant of urachus with no communication to either umbilicus or bladder.
        *2.* Can become infected.

**Imaging** Suspected when impression is seen upon superior aspect of bladder on VCUG examination. Ultrasound (US) and computed tomography can confirm urachal cyst by demonstrating fluid collection anywhere along course of urachus.

4. Neurogenic bladder.
    a. Bladder dysfunction related to neurologic causes.
    b. Sacral parasympathetic pathology.
        *1.* Unable to relax striated sphincter.
        *2.* Results in large, overflow-voiding bladder.
    c. Upper motor neuron injury (spastic, contracted bladder).
    d. Etiology in children is usually congenital (myelomeningocele or spinal dysraphism).
    e. Symptoms.
        *1.* Bladder.
            *a.* Failure to empty (flaccid with overflow-voiding bladder).
            *b.* Failure to retain (small, spastic bladder).
        *2.* Loss of bladder sensation.
        *3.* Incontinence.
        *4.* Frequency, dribbling.
        *5.* Reflux and UTI.
    f. Two main concerns.
        *1.* Renal damage (reflux from overloaded, obstructed bladder).
        *2.* Incontinence.
        *3.* Result: these children are often on routine catheterization regimen.

**Imaging** Look for posterior spinal defects on radiographs. On VCUG and US, trabeculated, irregular, thick-walled bladder is seen; can be large capacity or small capacity (Christmas-tree shaped), often with paraureteral diverticula or Hutch diverticulum near trigone, which can predispose to reflux.

5. Prune-belly (Eagle-Barrett) syndrome.
   a. Classic triad.
      1. Hypoplastic or absent abdominal musculature.
      2. Cryptorchidism.
      3. Marked dilation of urinary tract without obstruction.
   b. Found almost exclusively in males (1:40,000), but can have rare female "pseudoprune."
   c. Associations.
      1. Pulmonary hypoplasia.
      2. Dysplastic kidneys (can lead to renal failure).

**Imaging** On VCUG and US, hypertrophied bladder with urachal remnant may be seen. Reflux is often present in dilated, tortuous ureters, renal pelvis, or calyces.

6. Nocturnal enuresis or daytime frequency.
   a. Common, often frustrating problem.
   b. Found in males more commonly than in females; hereditary component.
   c. Probably related to delayed maturation of bladder control (detrusor inhibition).
   d. No increased incidence of UTI.
   e. Excellent prognosis with increasing age.

**Imaging** All imaging studies are normal.

7. Unstable bladder.
   a. Characterized by occasional uninhibited detrusor contractions; attempt at continence is maintained via external sphincter contraction, although "accidents" frequently occur.
   b. Can void spontaneously and normally on command.
   c. UTI is common.
   d. Found in females much more commonly than in males; average age is between 6 and 8 years.
   e. Disorder improves and resolves with age; may respond to anticholinergics such as oxybutinin (Ditropan), which decreases unexpected detrusor contraction.

**Imaging** Often no imaging findings; can have mildly thickened bladder wall seen on US examination.

8. Dyssynergia or Hinman syndrome.
   a. Also known as nonneurogenic, neurogenic bladder.
   b. Dyscoordination of voiding with unexpected simultaneous detrusor and external sphincter contraction, which prevent adequate emptying of bladder.

c. Difficulty initiating voiding; straining often required to empty bladder.
d. Chronically increased intravesical pressure results in obstructive changes in bladder.
e. UTIs and incontinence are common.
f. Very similar appearance to classic neurogenic bladder.
g. No gender difference in incidence.

**Imaging** On VCUG and US examination, thick, irregular bladder wall is often present. Reflux may be due to functional bladder obstruction. Difficulty in voiding is seen; posterior urethra may also be dilated.

9. Megacystis.
   a. Also known as "lazy" bladder.
   b. Dilated, smooth, hypotonic bladder with little detrusor activity.
   c. Usually related to infrequent voiding (lazy) or refluxing urine (megacystis-megaureter).
   d. Found in females more often than in males; 2 and 6 years of age.
   e. Syndromes with large, nonobstructive bladders (megacystis).
      1. Prune-belly (Eagle-Barrett) syndrome.
      2. Megacystis-microcolon syndrome.
         a. Large bladder with microcolon (dilated small bowel).
         b. Hypoperistalsis of bowel.
         c. Usually death ensues by age 1.

C. Urethra.
   1. Posterior urethral valves.
      a. 1:5000 to 8000 males.
      b. Often discovered on prenatal US, 75% present in first year of life, 50% in first 3 months.
      c. Formation of prominent "folds" (plicae colicularis) from verumontanum in posterior urethra that can cause obstruction to urinary flow through urethra.
      d. Types.
         1. Type I.
            a. Anterior margins of normal plicae colicularis fuse.
            b. Most common.
         2. Type II.
            a. Mucosal folds extend cranially from verumontanum up to bladder neck.
            b. Most rare.
         3. Type III.
            a. Obstructing disklike membrane is present distal to verumontanum.

                b. Uncommon.
            e. Posterior obstruction of urethral valves.
                1. Causes hypertrophied and thick-walled bladder.
                2. Resulting altered vesicoureteral orifice predisposes to reflux; can lead to bilateral hydroureteronephrosis.
                3. If pressure is great enough, collecting system of kidneys can rupture, causing urine ascites or urinoma.

> **Imaging** US can demonstrate thick-walled bladder and posterior urethra. Often dilated distal ureters that extend up to the hydronephrotic kidneys can be seen. On VCUG, thick, trabeculated bladder is present. Upon voiding, dilated posterior urethra is seen, and reflux is often present (30%). Valves themselves are often not visualized, but presence of dilated posterior urethra in male patient is presumptive for diagnosis.

    2. Urethral strictures.
        a. Found almost exclusively in males.
        b. Associations.
            1. History of previous instrumentation.
            2. Trauma to pelvis or urethra.
            3. Infectious *(Neisseria gonorrhea)*.

> **Imaging** On VCUG or retrograde urethrogram, contrast opacifies narrowed urethral segment.

D. Masses.
    1. Benign.
        a. Polyps.
            1. Fibroepithelial polyps can be seen in bladder (especially in bladder base or posterior urethra).
            2. Can present with obstruction.
        b. Hemangioma.
        c. Neurofibroma.

> **Imaging** Smooth filling defect noted on contrast study. Can often be seen on US.

    2. Malignant.
        a. Rhabdomyosarcoma.
            1. Ten percent of all rhabdomyosarcoma originate in lower urinary tract, especially in prostate.
            2. Tumor in infants or small children.
            3. Types.
                *a.* Embryonal.
                    *1)* Most common type.

2) Lobulated tumor filling bladder viscus, often called sarcoma botryoides (bunch of grapes).
   b. Alveolar.
   c. Polymorphic.

**Imaging** US may show irregular, lobulated mass at base of bladder. Similar finding can be seen as filling defect (within bladder) on VCUG examination.

## SUGGESTED READINGS

Agrons GA, Wagner BJ, Lonergan GJ, Dickey GE, Kaufman MS: Genitourinary rhabdomyosarcoma in children: Radiologic-Pathologic correlation. *Radiographics* 1997; 17:919-937.

Armis ES, Blaivas JG: The role of the radiologist in evaluating voiding dysfunction. *Radiology* 1990; 175:317-318.

Cacciarelli AA, Kass EJ, Yang SS: Urachal remnants: Demonstration in children. *Radiology* 1990; 174:473-475.

Cremin BJ: A review of ultrasonic appearance of posterior urethral valves and ureteroceles. *Pediatr Radiol* 1986; 16:357-364.

Fotter R, Kopp W, Klein E, Hollwarth M, Uray E: Unstable bladder in children: Functional evaluation by modified cystourethography. *Radiology* 1986; 161:811-813.

Friedland GW, Perkash I: Neuromuscular dysfunction of the bladder and urethra. *Semin Roentgen* 1983; 18:255-266.

Hernanz-Schulman M, Lebowitz RL: The elusiveness and importance of bladder diverticula in children. *Pediatr Radiol* 1985; 15:399-402.

Hinman F: Nonneurogenic neurogenic bladder (the Hinman syndrome) 15 years later. *J Urol* 1986; 135:769-777.

Jaramillo D, Lebowitz RL, Hendren WH: Cloacal malformation: Radiologic findings and imaging recommendations. *Radiology* 1990; 177:441-448.

Johnson JF, Hedden RJ, Piccolello ML, Wacksman J: Distension of the posterior urethra: Association with nonneurogenic neurogenic bladder (Hinman syndrome) *Radiology* 1992; 185:113-117.

Kindo A: Cystourethrogram characteristics of bladder instability in children. *Urology* 1990; 35:242-246.

Klimberg I: The development of voiding control. *Am Urol Assoc* (Update Series) 1988; 7:161.

Koff SA: The evaluation and management of voiding disorders in children. *Urol Clin North Am* 1988; 15:769-775.

Leicher-Duber A, Schumacher R: Urachal remnants in asymptomatic children: Sonographic morphology. *Pediatr Radiol* 1991; 21:200-202.

Macpherson RI, Leithiser RE, Gordon L, Turner WR: Posterior urethral valves: An update and review. *Radiographics* 1986; 6:753-792.

Musselman P, Kay R: The spectrum of urinary tract fibroepithelial polyps in children. *J Urol* 1986; 136:476-477.

# 23
# Urinary Tract Infection

### Key Concepts

1. Urinary tract infections (UTI) are very common. They are the second most common infection in children after upper respiratory infection (URI).
2. Vesicoureteral reflux is the retrograde passage of urine from the bladder up to the kidney. The most common etiology is a deficient submucosal "tunnel" at the level of the uretero-vesical junction (UVJ) that allows urine to reflux up the ureter, often following either volume or pressure (voiding) challenge.
3. The radiological workup in the child with suspected vesicoureteral reflux is a renal ultrasound (US) and voiding cystourethrogram (VCUG) examination.
4. Prophylactic antibiotic administration is the therapy used in children with reflux, because most cases will eventually resolve. Surgical intervention (reimplantation of the ureters) is reserved for select cases.
5. Persistent, recurrent UTIs in children with untreated reflux can lead to reflux nephropathy (permanent renal damage and scarring, poor renal function, and/or hypertension).

A. UTI.
  1. Very common; second most common infection in children after URI.
  2. Occurs much more frequently in females than in males; familial (mother/daughter/sister); uncommon in African-Americans.
  3. In neonates, occurs more frequently in males than in females (3:1); probably due to increased male incidence of urinary tract abnormalities.
  4. Associations.
     a. Vesicoureteral reflux.
     b. Obstructive abnormality (such as posterior urethral valves or ureteropelvic junction obstruction).
     c. Structural restriction.
        *1.* Females: labial adhesions.
           *a.* Membranous covering of urethral and vaginal opening.
           *b.* Varying degrees of labial adhesion is common disorder.
           *c.* Labia can be separated manually or via estrogen creme administration.
              *1)* However, labial adhesions often recur.
              *2)* Labia will open permanently at puberty with physiologic hormonal stimulation.
           *d.* If catheterization is difficult or impossible, consider labial adhesion as possible etiology.
        *2.* Males: tight foreskin (phimosis).
     d. Bladder dysfunction.
  5. Reflux nephropathy.
     a. Recurrent UTIs can cause permanent renal damage and scarring.
     b. Poor renal function.
     c. Hypertension.
  6. Indications for imaging.
     a. Males.
        *1.* After first urinary tract infection.
        *2.* Look for anatomic problems (posterior urethral valves).
     b. Females.
        *1.* With pyelonephritis, or in patients who do not respond to treatment.
        *2.* After recurrent UTIs. But how many constitute recurrent? (Some physicians advocate imaging after first UTI, especially in girls less than 5 years of age).
     c. UTI in first year of life (male or female).
  7. Imaging modalities.
     a. VCUG.
        *1.* Fluoroscopic examination.
           *a.* Evaluates for vesicoureteral reflux.

        b. Bladder appearance and emptying.
    2. Timing of VCUG examination: two theories.
        a. Waiting until acute infection subsides.
            *1)* Infection can itself "cause" reflux or worsen preexisting reflux (endotoxin from gram-negative bacteria such as *Escherichia coli* can eradicate tone of UVJ).
            *2)* Reflux of infected urine or contrast can further damage kidneys.
        b. Imaging during acute infection.
            *1)* "Immaturity" of distal ureter maldeveloped, resulting in shortened tunnel into bladder mucosa causes reflux. If transient reflux is in fact induced by infection, this would be important information to know.
            *2)* Since children are covered on antibiotics for UTI, chance of pyelonephritis from refluxing-infected contrast would be unlikely.
            *3)* Bladder cystitis may make examination (filling of bladder) very uncomfortable.
        c. Current practice.
            *1)* Perform VCUG in a convenient but timely fashion.
            *2)* However, remain cognizant of risks and discomfort.
    3. VCUG examination technique.
        a. Remember to fill bladder as much as possible.
            *1)* Reflux sometimes occurs only at high volumes.
            *2)* Repeat filling of infant that voids spontaneously may be needed ("cyclical VCUG").
            *3)* Bladder capacity (approximate).
                *a)* 30 to 50 cc for neonate.
                *b)* 100 cc at 1 year.
                *c)* 200 cc at 5 years.
                *d)* 300 to 400 cc for 10 years and up.
            *4)* Simple rule for bladder capacity.
                *a)* Child's age (in years) + 2 = bladder capacity (in ounces).
                *b)* Remember 1 ounce is equivalent to 30 cc.
        b. Need to look for reflux during voiding as well.
            *1)* Some children only reflux under high pressures.
            *2)* Have child void in oblique position to watch trigone region for potential reflux.
b. Renal US.
    *1.* Look for renal size (scarring), dilated pelvocalyceal system, and dilated distal ureters.

2. Do not forget to obtain bladder images.
3. Power Doppler has been helpful in evaluation of acute pyelonephritis.
   c. Nuclear medicine.
      1. Nuclear cystography.
         a. Imaging preference for follow-up of reflux.
            1) Less radiation than fluoroscopy.
            2) Drawback is poor anatomic detail.
         b. Some advocate nuclear cystography for first imaging evaluation of reflux in females. Unlike males, females rarely have anatomic urethral pathology that could be missed on nuclear cystography.
         c. Can be used for reflux screening (high-risk populations).
            1) Siblings or children of known refluxers.
            2) Child with unilateral multicystic dysplastic kidney, (because of increased incidence of reflux in contralateral kidney).
      2. Renal scan.
         a. Dimercaptosuccinic acid.
            1) Acute pyelonephritis.
            2) Renal scarring (reflux nephropathy).
B. Vesicoureteral reflux.
   1. Retrograde passage of urine from bladder up to kidney.
   2. Etiology.
      a. Most commonly due to deficient submucosal tunnel, allows urine to reflux up ureter, often following either volume or pressure (voiding) challenge.
      b. Weakening of UVJ musculature; usually caused by persistent high-pressure situation (as is encountered in posterior urethral valves or neurogenic bladder).
   3. More commonly seen in females than in males; commonly seen in duplicated collecting systems, especially lower pole.
   4. Grading of reflux (Fig. 23-1).
      a. Grade I: Reflux into distal ureter only (considered insignificant).
      b. Grade II: Reflux into nondilated collecting system.
      c. Grade III: Reflux into dilated collecting system.
      d. Grade IV: Reflux into dilated collecting system with tortuous ureters.
      e. Grade V: Worsening of IV; look for intrarenal reflux and increased tortuosity of ureters.
   5. Long-term outcome.

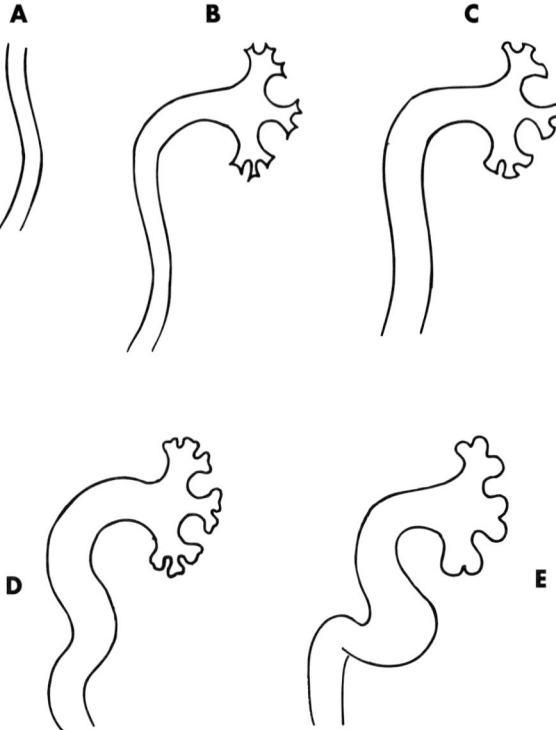

**Fig. 23-1** Types of vesicoureteral reflux. **A,** Type I. **B,** Type II. **C,** Type III. **D,** Type IV. **E,** Type V.

   a. Most reflux (grades I, II, and even III) resolve by school age, as distal ureteral "tunnel" lengthens to reach adult levels. Simple prophylactic antibiotics with yearly follow-up is usual course for this group of children.
   b. The worse the reflux, the greater the chance of renal scarring; ranges from 20% for grade II reflux to over 50% for grade IV reflux.
   c. Surgical intervention (reimplantation of ureters) is considered in:
      1. Massive refluxers (grade V).
      2. Older children that have not resolved reflux.
      3. Children with persistent pyelonephritis and scarring while on antibiotics ("break-through UTI").
      4. Children with ureters associated with Hutch diverticulum (diverticulum at ureteral insertion, resulting in persistent reflux that does not resolve with age).

d. Reflux nephropathy.
   1. Renal cortical atrophy.
   2. Often focal (preferentially upper pole).
   3. Blunted calyces.
   4. Hypertension.
   5. Can lead to end stage renal disease.

**SUGGESTED READINGS**

Andrich MP, Majk M: Diagnostic imaging in the evaluation of the first urinary tract infection in infants and young children. *Pediatrics* 1992; 90:436-441.

Ben-Ami T, Rozin M, Hertz M: Imaging of children with urinary tract infection: A tailored approach. *Clin Radiol* 1989; 40:64-68.

Bisset GS, Strife JL, Dunbar JS: Urography and voiding cystourethrography: Findings in girls with urinary tract infection. *AJR* 1987; 148:479-482.

Ginalski JM, Michaud A, Genton N: Renal growth retardation in children: Sign suggestive of vesicoureteral reflux. *AJR* 1985; 145:617-619.

Gore MD, Fernbach SK, Donaldson JS, Shkolnik A, Zaontz MR, Kaplan WE: Radiographic evaluation of subureteric injection of Teflon to correct vesicoureteric reflux. *AJR* 1989; 152:115-119.

Iskey G: Vesico-ureteric reflux, urinary tract infection and renal damage in children. *Lancet* 1995; 346:489-490.

Jequier S, Forbest PA, Nogrady MB: The value of ultrasonography as a screening procedure in a first documented urinary tract infection in children. *J Ultrasound Med* 1985; 4:393-400.

Kangerloo H, Gold RH, Fine RN, Diament MJ, Boechat MI: Urinary tract infection in infants and children evaluated by ultrasound. *Radiology* 1985; 154:367-373.

Kenney PJ: Imaging of chronic renal infections. *AJR* 1990; 155:485-494.

Lavocat MP, Granjon D, Allard D, Gay C, Freycon MT, Dubois F: Imaging of pyelonephritis. *Pediatr Radiol* 1997; 27:159-165.

Lebowitz RL, Mandell J: Urinary tract infection in children: Putting radiology in its place. *Radiology* 1987; 165:1-9.

Lebowitz RL, Olbing H, Parkkulainen KV, Smellie JM, Tamminen-Mobius TE: International system of radiographic grading of vesicoureteric reflux. *Pediatr Radiol* 1985; 15:105-109.

Mason WG: Urinary tract infections in children: Renal ultrasound evaluation. *Radiology* 1989; 153:109-111.

Paltiel HJ, Rupich RC, Kirulata HG: Enhanced detection of vesicoureteral reflux in infants and small children with use of cyclic voiding cystourethrography. *Radiology* 1992; 184:753-755.

Reid BS, Bender TM: Radiographic evaluation of children with urinary tract infections. *Radiol Clin North Am* 1988; 26:393-407.

Schneider K, Jablonski C, Wiessner M, Kohn M, Fendel H: Screening for vesicoureteral reflux in children using real-time sonography. *Pediatr Radiol* 1984; 14:400-403.

Strife JL, Bisset GS, Kirks DR, Schlueter FJ, Gelfand MJ, Babcock DS, Han BK: Nuclear cystography and renal sonography: Findings in girls with urinary tract infections. *AJR* 1989; 153:115-119.

Sty JR: Imaging in acute renal infection. *AJR* 1987; 148:471-477.

Winter WD: Power Doppler sonographic evaluation of acute pyelonephritis in children. *J Ultrasound Med* 1996; 15:91-96.

# 24
# Acquired Renal Disease

### Key Concepts

1. Acute renal failure in the neonate could be due to Tamm-Horsfall proteinuria (normal proteins in the infant urine that can precipitate out of solution). The resulting "clogging" of the tubules can cause a form of neonatal acute tubular necrosis (ATN).
2. The most common cause of new onset, previously undiagnosed pulmonary edema in the child, is renal dysfunction, such as poststreptoccocal glomerulonephritis.
3. The classic triad of hemolytic uremia is hemolytic anemia, thrombopcytopenia, and acute renal failure. Gastrointestinal complications, such as bowel wall hemorrhage can also occur.
4. Renal artery stenosis (RAS) causes hypertension because of increased renin production related to the decreased perfusion of the kidney. RAS is more commonly seen as a cause of pediatric hypertension than adult hypertension; it often presents with sudden onset of hypertension that has a poor response to medical therapy.
5. Endocrine cause for pediatric hypertension should also be considered, such as pheochromocytoma, located in the adrenal or anywhere along the sympathetic chain. The resulting catecholamine production can cause severe hypertension.

A. Acute renal failure.
   1. Neonatal.
      a. Tamm-Horsfall proteinuria.
         *1.* Normal proteins in infant urine that can precipitate out of solution, particularly with dehydration.
         *2.* Clogging of tubules can lead to form of neonatal ATN.
         *3.* Can also be incidental finding; usually resolves quickly.

   **Imaging** Renal ultrasound (US) reveals echogenic medullary pyramids; usually no hydronephrosis is present.

      b. Renal vein thrombosis.
         *1.* Usually unilateral.
         *2.* Predisposing factors.
            *a.* Dehydration.
            *b.* Indwelling catheters (also a factor in renal artery thrombosis; often with associated abnormal coagulable state).
            *c.* Infant of diabetic mother (hemoconcentration).

   **Imaging** Initially, renal US reveals enlarged kidney that becomes increasingly hypoechoic with poor corticomedullary differentiation within week or two of event. Doppler evaluation is helpful in confirming absent renal venous flow and/or clot, seen within renal vein or inferior vana cava. If kidney recovers, normal appearance will gradually return. Otherwise, kidney atrophies and becomes echogenic.

   2. Shock, hypoperfusion, or hypotension.
   3. Glomerulonephritis.
      a. Poststreptococcal.
         *1.* Usually seen in school age children.
         *2.* Etiology is probably immune-complex related.
         *3.* Most common cause of new onset is previously undiagnosed pulmonary edema in child.
         *4.* Vast majority will resolve.
      b. Other types (may require biopsy for diagnosis).
         *1.* Minimal change disease.
         *2.* Rapidly progressive.
         *3.* Henoch-Schönlein purpura.

   **Imaging** Renal US may demonstrate increased cortical echogenicity consistent with "medical renal disease" (nonspecific finding that may be due to any of types of glomerulonephritis listed above). However, kidneys may appear normal.

4. Hemolytic uremia.
   a. Usually occurs in children under 5 years of age.
   b. Infectious etiology that triggers microangiopathy.
      1. Gastrointestinal.
         a. *Escherichia coli* O157:H7.
         b. Produces "shigella-like" toxin that causes endothelium damage.
      2. Respiratory virus.
   c. Classic triad.
      1. Hemolytic anemia.
      2. Thrombopcytopenia.
      3. Acute renal failure.
   d. Gastrointestinal complications (common, up to 25%).
      1. Bowel wall hemorrhage and/or intussusception.
      2. Bowel perforation.
      3. Colitis.

**Imaging** Renal US reveals echogenic, often enlarged kidney. Abdominal radiograph may show thumbprinting of bowel due to hemorrhage in bowel wall; also be aware of high risk of bowel perforation (free air).

5. Nephrotoxic agents.
   a. Iodinated contrast material.
   b. Aminoglycoside antibiotics (gentamicin).
   c. Myoglobin.

B. Nephrocalcinosis.
   1. Hypercalcuria.
      a. Long-term diuretics (especially in preterm infants).
      b. Williams syndrome.
   2. Renal medical disease.
      a. Renal tubular acidosis, distal only.
      b. Medullary sponge kidney.
      c. Bartter syndrome (renal tubular transport defects).
   3. Lesch-Nyhan syndrome.
      a. Severe mental retardation and self-mutilation.
      b. Hypoxanthine guanine-phosphoribosyl transferase is missing enzyme; probably interfers with uric acid metabolism. Resulting hyperuricemia can cause oxypurine (xanthine and uric acid) crystal deposition.

> **Imaging** Renal US can show echogenic medullary pyramids; small echogenic (nonshadowing) foci at corticomedullary junction may also be present. Differential diagnosis of echogenic medullary pyramids includes Tamm-Horsfall proteinuria (see previous discussion), papillary necrosis (seen with sickle cell anemia), blood clot or debris, and fungal infection (fungal "balls").

C. Chronic renal failure.
  1. Chronic glomerulonephritis (30%).
     a. Rapidly progressive.
     b. Focal glomerulosclerosis.
     c. Membranoproliferative.
     d. Lupus nephritis.
     e. IgA nephropathy.

> **Imaging** Renal US is nonspecific; usually reveals echogenic, often small kidney.

  2. Reflux nephropathy (25%).
     a. Renal cortical atrophy caused by repeated infections (pyelonephritis); usually in children with vesicoureteral reflux (often undiagnosed and subsequently untreated).
     b. Scarring can be focal or global, upper pole predilection (35%).
     c. Complications are progressive renal failure and hypertension.

> **Imaging** US can show cortical thinning and renal scarring; US has replaced intravenous pyelogram examination in evaluation of renal scarring. Nuclear medicine (dimercaptosuccinic acid [DMSA] scan) effectively diagnoses renal cortical scarring. DMSA scan is also useful in diagnosis of acute pyelonephritis.

  3. Hereditary causes (15%).
     a. Alport syndrome.
     b. Nephronophthisis.
        1. Medullary cystic disease.
        2. Renal size may be preserved despite rising creatinine levels.
     c. Cystinosis or oxalosis.
  4. Congenital (13%).
     a. Obstructive nephropathy.
     b. Posterior urethral valves.
     c. Neurogenic bladder.
  5. Systemic complications.
     a. Cardiomegaly.
     b. Pleural or pericardial effusions.

c. Pulmonary edema or congestive heart failure.
d. Hypertension.
e. "Renal rickets" (renal osteodystophy).
6. Treatment.
a. Dialysis (peritoneal versus vascular).
b. Renal transplant.

> **Imaging** Renal US often reveals small, echogenic kidneys. Decreased blood flow with elevated resistive index may be present on Doppler evaluation (related to increased vascular resistance in kidney). Bony changes from renal failure (renal osteodystrophy) are also evident on radiographs (see Chapter 35). Delayed bone age and short stature can occur as well.

D. Hypertension.
1. Renal etiology (see previous discussion).
2. Renovascular.
   a. Renal artery stenosis.
      *1.* Causes hypertension resulting from increased renin production; both are related to decreased perfusion of kidney.
      *2.* More commonly seen as cause of pediatric hypertension than adult hypertension; often sudden onset of hypertension.
      *3.* Has poor response to medical therapy.
      *4.* Usually is isolated stenotic lesion of renal artery due to fibromuscular dysplasia.
      *5.* Can be seen in children with neurofibromatosis (often bilateral).
      *6.* Treatment.
         *a.* Angioplasty of stenotic lesion.
         *b.* Surgical correction.

> **Imaging** Renal US is not reliable indicator of renal artery stenosis; look for "pulsus tardus and parvis" (decreased arterial upstroke on Doppler). Nuclear medicine (captopril) scan has been helpful. In cases of renovascular hypertension, administration of captopril (angiotensin-converting enzyme inhibitor which reverses renin-induced hypertension) results in increased uptake of radiopharmaceutical. Decreased glomerular filtration rate can also be seen on stenotic side. The gold standard, however, remains angiography ($CO_2$ angiography in cases of rising creatinine with renal failure), can directly demonstrate stenotic renal artery lesion.

   b. Page kidney.

1. Posttraumatic hypertension.
2. Subcapsular hematoma squeezes kidney, resulting in increased renin production.
   c. Renal arteriovenous malformation or aneurysm.
      1. Complication after renal biopsy.
      2. Can occur following renal trauma or surgery.
      3. Kawasaki syndrome (usually causes coronary artery ancurysms).
3. Endocrine.
   a. Adrenal.
      1. Pheochromocytoma.
         a. Tumor of adrenal medulla.
         b. Can arise within adrenal medulla or anywhere along sympathetic chain.
         c. Catecholamine production causes hypertension.
         d. Associated with the multiple endocrine neoplasms type II.

**Imaging** US or computed tomography may show adrenal or sympathetic chain mass. Can be difficult to locate; may need to use nuclear medicine I-131 metaiodobenzylguanidine scan.

      2. Adrenocortical tumor or hyperplasia.
         a. Cushing syndrome.
         b. Increased glucocortical steroid production leads to increased aldosterone production.
         c. Congenital adrenal hyperplasia.
         d. Can have aldosterone-producing tumor.
            1) Often small, difficult-to-locate lesions.
            2) Low potassium.
      3. Neuroblastoma (see Chapter 7).
   b. Thyroid.

## SUGGESTED READINGS

Choyke PL, Grant EG, Hoffer FA, Tina L, Korec S: Cortical echogenicity in the hemolytic uremia syndrome: Clinical correlation. *J Ultrasound Med* 1988; 7:439-442.

Desberg AL, Paushter DM, Lammert GK, Hale JC, Troy RB, Novick AC, Nally JV, Weltevreden AM: Renal artery stenosis: Evaluation with color Doppler flow imaging. *Radiology* 1990; 177:749-753.

Farnsworth RH, Rossleigh MA, Leighton DM, Bass SJ, Rosenberg AR: The detection of reflux nephropathy in infants by Tc99m DMSA studies. *J Urol* 1991; 145:542-546.

Frankel DG, Narla D: Imaging of children with chronic renal failure. *J Pediatr* 1996; 129:S33-S38.

Glicklich D, Tellis VA, Quinn T, Mallis M, Greenstein SM, Schechner R, Heller S, Freeman LM, Kutcher R, Veith F: Comparison of captopril scan and Doppler ultrasonography as screening tests for renal artery stenosis. *Transplantation* 1990; 49:217-219.

Lalmand B, Avni EF, Nasr A, Ketelbant P, Struyven J: Perinatal renal vein thrombosis: Sonographic demonstration. *J Ultrasound Med* 1990; 9:437-442.

Patriquin HB: Doppler sonography in renal diseases. *Curr Opin Radiol* 1991; 3:663-668.

Riebel TW, Abraham K, Wartner R, Muller R: Transient renal medullary hyperechogenicity in ultrasound studies or neonates: Is it a normal phenomenon and what are the causes? *Clin Ultrasound* 1993; 21:25-31.

Rosenfeld DL, Preston MP, Salvaggi-Fadden: Serial renal sonographic evaluation of patients with Lesch-Nyhan syndrome. *Pediatr Radiol* 1994; 24:509-512.

Rosenfield AT, Siegel NJ: Renal parenchymal disease: Histopathologic-sonographic correlation. *AJR* 1981; 137:793-798.

Salisz JA, Kass EJ, Cacciarelli AA: Transient acute renal failure in the neonate. *Urology* 1993; 41:137-140.

Schultz PK, Strife JL, Strife CF, McDaniel JD: Hyperechoic renal medullary pyramids in infants and children. *Radiology* 1991; 181:163-167.

Starinsky R, Vardi O, Batasch, Goldberg M: Increased renal medullary echogenicity in neonates. *Pediatr Radiol* 1995; 25:S43-S45.

Westra SJ, Zaninovic AL, Hall TR, Kangarloo H, Boechat MI: Imaging of the adrenal gland in children. *Radiographics* 1994; 14:1323-1340.

# 25
# Renal Masses

---

### Key Concepts

1. Wilms tumor is the most common renal malignancy in children with most cases discovered in preschool-age children.
2. Mesoblastic nephroma (also known as a fetal renal hamartoma) is the most common solid renal tumor in the newborn period.
3. Leukemia or lymphoma can infiltrate the kidneys, appearing as diffusely enlarged kidneys or multifocal nodules.
4. Renal cell carcinoma is extremely rare in childhood.
5. Angiomyolipoma is a benign renal lesion composed of fat, smooth muscle, and vessels that has a strong association with tuberous sclerosis.

A. Wilms tumor.
   1. Most common childhood solid abdominal malignancy (10% of all childhood tumors).
   2. Majority of all cases are discovered from age 1 to 5 (75%); peak is 2 to 3 years of age.
   3. Clinical presentation.
      a. Most commonly presents with asymptomatic abdominal mass.
      b. Sudden hemorrhage into mass may cause more acute, painful presentation.
      c. Hypertension.
      d. Hematuria.
   4. Associated with congenital abnormalities.
      a. Beckwith-Wiedemann syndrome.
      b. Hemihypertrophy.
      c. Aniridia.
   5. Pathology (type of embryonal sarcoma).
      a. Favorable histology (no anaplasia or sarcomatous elements).
      b. Unfavorable histology.
         1. Anaplastic cells with sarcomatous elements.
         2. Less common (10%).
         3. Tends to be seen in older children.
         4. Worse prognosis and outcome.
   6. Nephroblastomatosis.
      a. Also known as renal blastema; precursor of Wilms tumor.
      b. Multifocal, embryonic, nephrogenic rests that retain potential for malignant induction into Wilms tumor.
      c. Bilateral Wilms tumor 5% to 10%; often related to nephroblastomatosis (tumor also tends to present at earlier age).

   **Imaging** Ultrasound (US) shows multiple, usually bilateral, hypoechoic, lobular lesions; on computed tomography (CT), renal lesions of nephroblastomatosis are low density.

   7. Staging.
      a. Stage I.
         1. Tumor limited to kidney.
         2. Complete resection.
         3. 5-year survival rate is 97%.
      b. Stage II.
         1. Tumor beyond kidney.
         2. Complete resection of tumor still possible.
         3. 5-year survival rate is 92%.
      c. Stage III.
         1. Residual tumor remains in abdomen.

2. No metastatic disease.
3. 5-year survival rate is 87%.
   d. Stage IV.
      1. Metastatic sites (such as lung, liver, or bone).
      2. May have renal vein or inferior vena cava (IVC) invasion.
      3. 5-year survival rate is 73%.
   e. Stage V.
      1. Bilateral renal involvement.
      2. 5-year survival rate is 50% to 70%.

**Imaging** US and CT demonstrate expansive, intrarenal mass, often inhomogeneous with calcifications uncommon (5%). Hemorrhage into tumor mass may be present. Mass usually does not cross midline (unlike neuroblastoma). Look for tumor thrombus in renal vein or IVC.

B. Mesoblastic nephroma.
   1. Also known as fetal renal hamartoma.
   2. Most common solid renal tumor in new-born period; usually presents in first 3 months of life.
   3. Benign, hamartomatous lesion composed mostly of spindle cells; no malignant potential or metastatic spread.
   4. Cured by surgical resection.

**Imaging** US reveals mixed echogenic, inhomogeneous lesion that distorts renal parenchyma. Cysts and calcifications are commonly present.

C. Multilocular cystic nephroma.
   1. Benign tumor, presenting between 3 months to 4 years of age.
   2. Consists of mass (often large) composed of multiple noncommunicating cysts with thin septations; cysts contain straw-colored fluid.
   3. Not invasive lesion; sharp borders are present, making lesion easily distinguished from surrounding normal renal parenchyma.
   4. Must differentiate from cystic Wilms tumor.
   5. Curative surgical resection.

**Imaging** US and CT can identify multicystic nature of this renal lesion. Presence of thick-walled septa is more suggestive of cystic Wilms tumor than of thin-walled multilocular cystic nephroma.

D. Leukemia or lymphoma.
   1. Usually infiltrates kidneys bilaterally.
   2. Can appear as diffusely enlarged kidneys versus multifocal nodules.
   3. Look for adjacent retroperitoneal adenopathy.

4. Renal function often remains normal, although cell lysis (following chemotherapy) may result in tubule obstruction (uric acid uropathy) and acute renal failure.

> **Imaging** Diffusely enlarged, inhomogeneous kidneys may be present on either CT or US. Hypechoic or hypodense nodules may also be seen.

E. Renal cell carcinoma.
   1. Rare in childhood, can be seen in adolescents.
   2. Can present with hematuria, palpable mass, or flank pain.
   3. Vascular tumor that can extend into renal vein or IVC, often with resulting metastatic disease.
   4. Associated with von Hippel-Lindau disease.
      a. Renal, pancreatic, or hepatic cysts.
      b. Central nervous system hemangioblastomas.

> **Imaging** US reveals inhomogeneous mass that distorts renal architecture; can cause hydronephrosis. Look for marked tumoral enhancement on CT.

F. Angiomyolipoma.
   1. Benign renal lesion composed of fat, smooth muscle, and vessels.
   2. Strong association with tuberous sclerosis.
      a. Present in 80% of children with tuberous sclerosis.
      b. Tuberous sclerosis present in 50% of patients with angiomyolipoma.
   3. Angiomyolipoma can be small; look for fat and calcifications in lesions.

> **Imaging** Often vascular, inhomogeneous renal lesion with characteristic fat density and calcifications on CT. US demonstrates echogenic lesion.

## SUGGESTED READINGS

Babyn P, Owens C, Gyepes M, D'angio G: Imaging patients with Wilms tumor. *Hematol Oncol Clin North Am* 1995; 9:1217-1252.

Beckwith JB: Wilms tumor and other renal tumors of childhood: An update. *J Urol* 1986; 136:320-324.

Beckwith JB, Kiviat NB, Bonadio JF: Nephrogenic rests, nephroblastomatosis and the pathogenesis of Wilms tumor. *Pediatr Pathol* 1990; 10:1-36.

Bell DG, King BF, Hattery RR, Charboneau JW, Hoffman AD, Houser OW: Imaging characteristics of tuberous sclerosis. *AJR* 1991; 156:1081-1086.

Cohen MD: Imaging and staging of Wilms tumors: Problems and controversies. *Pediatr Radiol* 1996; 26:307-311.

Decampo JF: Ultrasound of Wilms tumor. *Pediatr Radiol* 1986; 16:21-24.

Fernbach SK, Feinstein KA, Donaldson JS, Blaum ES: Nephroblastomatosis: Comparison of CT with US and urography. *Radiology* 1988; 166:153-156.

Hartman DS, Davis CJ, Sanders RC, Johns TT, Smirniotopoulous J, Goldman SM: The multilocular renal mass: Considerations and differential features. *Radiographics* 1987; 7:29-52.

Hartman DS, Lesar MSL, Madewell JE, Lichtenstein JE, Davis CJ: Mesoblastic nephroma: Radiologic-pathologic correlation of 20 cases. *AJR* 1981; 136:69-74.

Narla LD, Slovis TL, Watts FB, Nigro M: Renal lesions of tuberosclerosis (cysts and angiomyolipoma): Screening with sonography and computerized tomography. *Pediatr Radiol* 1988; 18:205-209.

Navoy JF, Royal SA, Vaid YN, Mroczek-Musulman EC: Wilms tumor: Unusual manifestations. *Pediatr Radiol* 1995; 25:76-86.

Reiman TAH, Siegel MJ, Shackelford GD: Wilms tumor in children: Abdominal CT and US evaluation. *Radiology* 1986; 160:501-505.

Slasky BS, Bar-Ziv J, Freeman AI, Peylan-Ramu N: CT appearances of involvement of the peritoneum, mesentery, and omentum in Wilms tumor. *Pediatr Radiol* 1997; 27:14-17.

Weinberger E, Rosenbaum DM, Pendergrass TM: Renal involvement in children with lymphoma: Comparison of CT with sonography. *AJR* 1990; 155:347-349.

White KS, Kirks DR, Bove KE: Imaging of nephroblastomatosis: An overview. *Radiology* 1992; 182:1-5.

White KS, Grossman H: Wilms and associated renal tumors of childhood. *Pediatr Radiol* 1991; 21:81-88.

# 26
# Genital Development and Disorders

---

**Key Concepts**

1. In the girl with primary amenorrhea, Turner syndrome, hydrometrocolpos, and Mayer-Rokitansky-Küster-Hauser syndrome should be considered.
2. Ovarian torsion can mimic appendicitis in a girl.
3. The vast majority of ovarian neoplasms in girls are of germ cell origin, such as the teratoma (benign or malignant) or dermoid.
4. Hydrocele is very common in boys, usually related to a patent tunica vaginalis that communicates with the peritoneal cavity. Inguinal hernia is also commonly associated (usually manually reduced) but bowel incarceration is a concern.
5. Testicular torsion is an emergency. Twisting of the testicle can lead to infarction if not surgically repaired. Ultrasound (US) or nuclear medicine can determine the absence of blood flow to the affected testicle.

## EMBRYOLOGY OF THE GONADS

Formation of the cloacal folds (midline protuberance just distal to the end of the cloaca). These folds will form either the labia in the female (due to absence of androgenic stimulation) or the scrotum in the male (swelling and fusion of the folds due to androgen stimulation).
A. Female.
  1. Normal anatomy.
     a. Neonatal.
        *1.* Enlarged uterus and ovarian follicles related to maternal hormones.
        *2.* Ovarian cysts can become quite large and are common cause of palpable cystic mass in female neonate (again, related to maternal hormonal surge).
     b. Prepubescent.
        *1.* Small tubelike uterus; often difficult to even locate ovaries (sometimes small follicles can be seen).
        *2.* As menarche approaches, uterine fundus preferentially enlarges; ovaries become more apparent with appearance of follicles.
     c. Pubertal.
        *1.* Uterus enlargement, especially fundus.
        *2.* Ovaries also enlarged with obvious follicular development.
        *3.* Can see ovarian cysts and/or free fluid.
  2. Congenital.
     a. Primary amenorrhea.
        *1.* Mayer-Rokitansky-Küster-Hauser syndrome.
           *a.* Absent or rudimentary uterus (often bicornuate) with vaginal agenesis.
           *b.* After Turner syndrome, most common syndrome to cause primary amenorrhea.
           *c.* Strong association with upper urinary abnormalities (up to 40%, including renal agenesis, ectopia, or obstruction of ureteropelvic junction [UPJ]).
        *2.* Hydrometrocolpos.
           *a.* Etiology.
              *1)* Vaginal atresia.
              *2)* Transverse vaginal septum.
              *3)* Imperforate hymen.
           *b.* Clincial presentation.
              *1)* Can be found in neonate as pelvic mass (uterine or vaginal secretions related to maternal hormones).
              *2)* Pelvic mass seen on neonatal abdominal radiograph (often mistaken for full bladder).

### Genital Development and Disorders   **237**

       *3)* Amenorrheic girl.

**Imaging**  Cystic midline mass (occasionally with debris), is readily noted on US and magnetic resonance imaging (MRI); must differentiate from full bladder.

    b. Uterine malformations.
       *1.* Etiology is due to incomplete fusion of distal segments of müllerian duct.
       *2.* Various anatomic forms (Fig. 26-1).
       *3.* Obstruction or pregnancy can occur in one limb of uterine malformation.
3. Acquired.
    a. Ovarian torsion.
       *1.* Most common in prepubertal girl; can, however, occur at any age, including newborn.
       *2.* Twisting of ovarian pedicle with vascular and lymphatic compromise.
       *3.* Often associated with tumors or cysts.
       *4.* Differential diagnosis.
         *a.* Appendicitis.
         *b.* Hemorrhagic ovarian cyst.
         *c.* Ectopic pregnancy.
         *d.* Pelvic inflammatory disease (PID).

**Imaging**  Variable appearance; can see enlarged, swollen, inhomogeneous ovary on US, often with eccentric follicles. Doppler can be helpful to document reduced or absent flow.

    b. Precocious puberty.
       *1.* Clinical presentation.
         *a.* Early appearance of secondary sex characteristics, such as breast development and pubic hair.
         *b.* Can have onset of inappropriate menarche.
       *2.* Do not mistake for thelarche.
         *a.* Prominent breast tissue in small child.
         *b.* Usually seen around age 2 and resolves.
       *3.* Etiology is due to hormonal surge.
         *a.* Central source.
           *1)* Pituitary.
           *2)* Most common reason.
           *3)* Treatment is hormonal suppression until child reaches age of onset of puberty.
         *b.* Related to adrenal (adenoma, carcinoma).

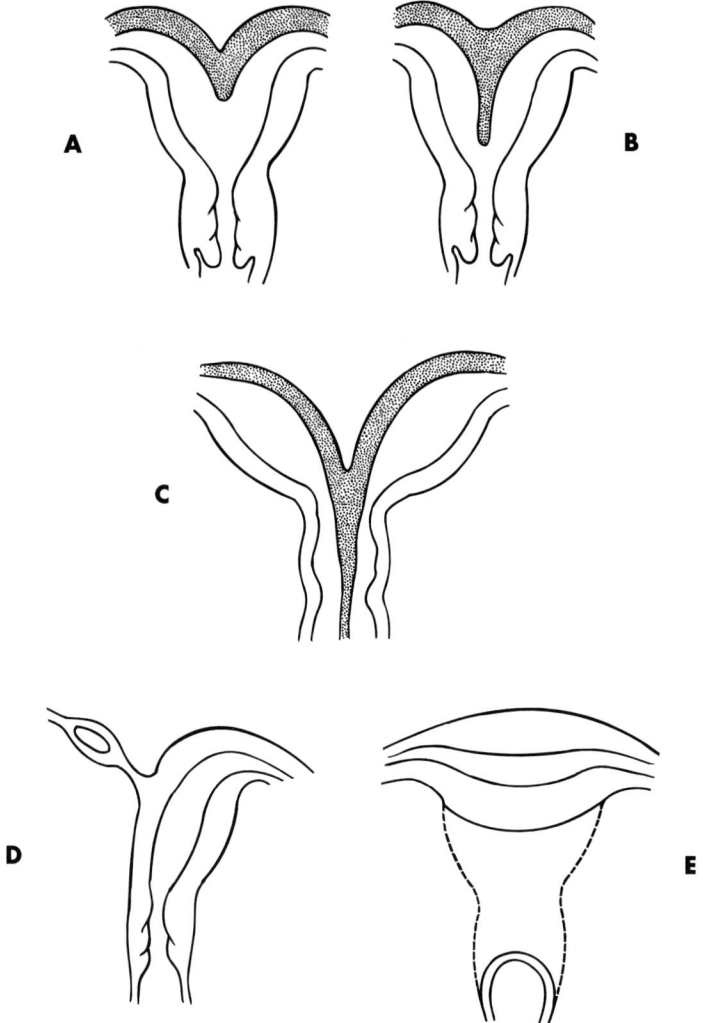

**Fig. 26-1** Types of uterine malformations. **A,** Septated uterus. **B,** Bicornuate uterus. **C,** Uterine didelphia. **D,** Unicornuate. **E,** Atresia.

    *c.* Ovarian source (granulosa cell tumor).

**Imaging** US of pelvis can document pubertal appearance of uterus and ovary. Look for ovarian mass (granulosa cell tumor) as source of hormonal surge. Do not forget to check adrenals as another source of abnormal hormonal production. MRI can be done to search for presence of pituitary tumor.

- c. Always keep in mind "adult" entities such as PID, tuboovarian abscess, intrauterine or ectopic pregnancy, and hemorrhagic cysts, which can all be seen in adolescent.
4. Neoplasms.
   a. Ovarian.
      1. Classified according to cell type.
         a. Mesenchymal (stromal).
            1) Granulosa cell.
               a) Predominantly cystic mass.
               b) Estrogen-producing tumor.
               c) Can result in precocious puberty.
            2) Sertoli-Leydig cell.
               a) Testosterone-producing tumor.
               b) Virilization of prepubescent girls.
            3) Fibroma (seen in older women; rare in children).
         b. Epithelial (rare in children).
            1) Cystadenoma.
            2) Cystadenocarcinoma.
         c. Germ cell.
            1) Majority of pediatric ovarian neoplasms (60% to 90%).
            2) Teratoma (benign or malignant); dermoids.
               a) Most common germ cell tumor overall (almost 50% of all pediatric germ cell tumors).
                  (1) Common location is sacrococcyx or pelvis.
                  (2) Look for cysts, calcifications, fat, or teeth.
            3) Embryonal cell.
            4) Dysgerminoma.
               a) Second most common germ cell tumor after teratoma.
               b) Can be found in unusual locations (mediastinum or pineal region) because of aberrant stem cell migration from gonadal ridge during embryogenesis.
            5) Yolk sac tumor (endodermal sinus).
            6) Choriocarcinoma.
               a) Secretes human chorionic gonadotropin.
               b) Highly malignant.
      2. Mixed germ cell tumor (variety of cell types previously listed); most common malignant ovarian neoplasm in older girls and adolescents.
      3. Increased alpha-fetoprotein may be present.

         a. Endodermal sinus tumor.
         b. Embryonal.
      b. Vaginal.
         1. Endodermal sinus (yolk sac).
            a. Seen in infants.
            b. Can present with painless, vaginal bleeding.
         2. Rhabdomyosarcoma.
            a. Usually in small children.
            b. Often presents with "bunch of grapes" appearance (sarcoma botryoides).
            c. Mass can sometimes be seen protruding from vaginal orifice.
         3. Clear cell adenocarcinoma.
            a. Association with diethylstilbestrol ingestion by mother during early pregnancy.
            b. Rare; seen in young adults.

> **Imaging** Mass lesion can be seen on US or CT, often filling and expanding vaginal lumen. Imaging for distant metastases is important; all of previously mentioned tumors are aggressive (particularly endodermal sinus and rhabdomyosarcoma).

B. Male.
   1. Congenital.
      a. Cryptorchidism.
         1. Incomplete descent of testicle.
         2. In term infants (3% or 4%); less than 1% by 1 year of age.
         3. On right (70%); bilateral, (30%).

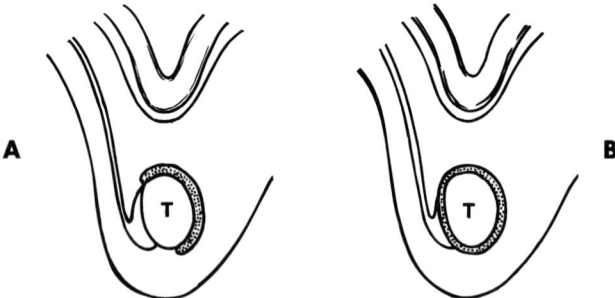

**Fig. 26-2** Testicular torsion: testicle (T). **A,** Normal testicle within scrotum, with normal tunica vaginalis (stippled). **B,** Bell-clapper anomaly of testicle with circumferential tunica vaginalis (stippled); high risk for testicular torsion.

4. Increased incidence of carcinoma with intraabdominal testes. (Therefore, surgical intervention is required to either remove testicle or place it in proper position within scrotum).
5. Associated with renal abnormalities, including prune-belly syndrome (Eagle-Barrett syndrome).

**Imaging** US of scrotum reveals absent testicles. Often, testicle can be located in inguinal canal. Intraabdominal testicle can be difficult to locate; CT or MRI is much better than US for this latter task.

b. Hydrocele (Fig. 26-2).
  1. Very common; usually related to patent tunica vaginalis that communicates with peritoneal cavity.
  2. Inguinal hernia is common association (found on left side more commonly than on right); usually can be manually reduced, but bowel incarceration is concern.

**Imaging** US is modality of choice, easily imaging anechoic fluid of hydrocele and echogenic testes. Look for bowel loops floating within scrotum (inguinal hernia).

c. Testicular torsion.
  1. Twisting of testicle that can lead to infarction if untreated.
  2. Can occur at any age; occurs most commonly between 10 and 16 years of age; found in right testicle more often than in left.
  3. Emergent condition; need to "de-torse" testicle within 12 to 24 hours to prevent infarction.
  4. Etiology.
      a. Congenital torsion.
          1) Testicle infarcts in utero.
          2) "Bell-clapper" deformity is not present, therefore, no contralateral risk for torsion.
      b. Childhood.
          1) No testicular attachment to scrotum; bell-clapper deformity (Fig. 26-3).
          2) Results in freely twisting testicle that can undergo torsion, causing vascular compromise.
          3) Need to intervene on contralateral side because of high risk of contralateral torsion (orchiopexy or "tack-down" procedure to overcome bell-clapper deformity).
  5. Differential diagnosis includes epididymitis, which would demonstrate increased flow on both nuclear medicine study and US.

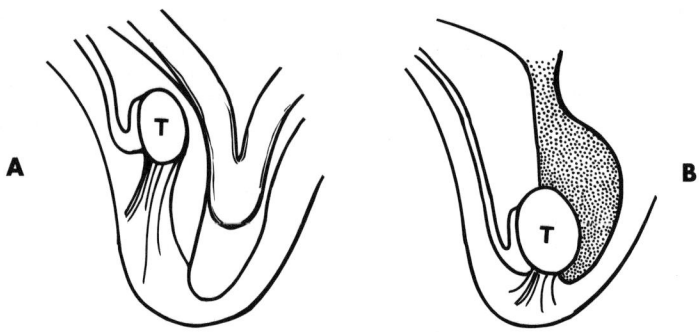

**Fig. 26-3** Inguinal hernia and hydrocele. **A,** Bowel loops can slip into patent processus vaginalis, causing inguinal hernia, which can become incarcerated. **B,** Fluid can also fill patent processus vaginalis *(stippled);* can lead to hydrocele.

> **Imaging** US (color, duplex, or power Doppler) of swollen testicle demonstrates decreased blood flow (be careful, as it can be difficult to document flow in testicle because of small vessels, not necessarily because of torsion. Need to establish normal contralateral blood flow). Nuclear medicine may document absent flow on Tc-99m study (central photopenic area within scrotum). Also difficult study to interpret owing to small size of pediatric testicle.

2. Neoplasms.
    a. Primary testicular neoplasm is uncommon in boys; usually seen in young adults (see previous list of germ cell types).
    b. Far more common is acute leukemic testicular involvement.
        1. Enlarged testicles, often bilateral.
        2. Can be first sign of relapse, since scrotum (with pampiniform plexus) is "sanctuary site" that chemotherapeutic drugs can not penetrate.
    c. Rhabdomyosarcoma.
        1. Most common genital tumor of pediatric pelvis, often perineal, bladder base, prostate, vagina, or retroperitoneum (can also be seen as head and neck tumor, particularly orbital).
        2. Very rapidly growing, aggressive ("small blue cell tumor").
        3. Usually seen in children less than 3 years of age.
C. Abnormal sex differentiation.
    1. Normal external genitalia.
        a. Turner syndrome.
            1. Most common.
            2. 45,XO karyotype.

3. Streak gonads, webbed neck, shieldlike chest with widely spaced nipples.
4. Renal abnomalities.
   a. Horseshoe kidney.
   b. UPJ obstruction.
   c. Duplication.
5. Cardiac abnormalities.
   a. Coarctation of aorta.
   b. Bicuspid aortic valve.
  b. Klinefelter syndrome.
   1. 1:1000 males.
   2. 47,XXY.
   3. Normally formed but small genitalia; sterile.
   4. Gynecomastia with increased risk of breast carcinoma.
  c. Testicular feminization.
   1. Androgen receptor abnormality.
   2. Leading to feminization, resulting male karyotype with female phenotype.
 2. Ambiguous external genitalia.
  a. Wide range from pseudohermaphrodites to true hermaphrodites (both testicular and ovarian tissue).
  b. Congenital adrenal hyperplasia.
   1. Inherited enzymatic defect.
   2. Leads to increased androgen production and virilization.

---

**Imaging** If ambiguous external genitalia are present, neonatal US of pelvis could determine correct sex, because enlarged uterus is so readily visible. Also, US may visualize diffusely enlarged adrenal glands.

---

## SUGGESTED READINGS

Brammer HM, Buck JL, Hayes WS, Sheth S, Tavassoli FA: Malignant germ cell tumors of the ovary: Radiologic-pathologic correlation. *Radiographics* 1990; 10:715-724.

Burks DD, Markey BJ, Burkhard TK, Balsara ZN, Haluszka MM: Suspected testicular torsion and ischemia: Evaluation with color Doppler sonography. *Radiology* 1990; 175:815-821.

Carrington BM, Hricak H, Nuruddin MD, Secaf E, Laros RK, Hill EC: Müllerian duct anomalies: MR imaging evaluation. *Radiology* 1990; 176:715-720.

Gilsanz V, Cleveland RH: Duplication of the müllerian ducts and genitourinary malformations. *Pediatr Radiol* 1982; 144:793-796.

Helvi M, Silver TM: Ovarian torsion: Sonographic evaluation *J Clin Ultrasound* 1989; 17:327-332.

Kier R, McCarthy S, Rosenfield AT, Rosenfield NS, Rapoport S, Weiss RM: Nonpalpable testes in young boys: Evaluation by MR imaging. *Radiology* 1988; 169:429-433.

Kornreich L, Horev G, Blaser S, Daneman D, Kauli R, Grunebaum M: Central precocious puberty: Evaluation by neuroimaging. *Pediatr Radiol* 1994; 25:7-11.

Malini S, Valdes C, Malinak LR: Sonographic diagnosis and classification of anomalies of the female genital tract. *J Ultrasound Med* 1984; 3:397-404.

Middleton WD, Siegel BA, Melson GL, Yates CK, Andriole GL: Acute scrotal disorders: Prospective comparison of color Doppler US and testicular scintigraphy. *Radiology* 1990; 177:177-181.

Sheth S, Fishman EK, Buck JL, Hamper VM, Sanders RL: The variable sonographic appearance of ovarian teratomas: Correltation with CT. *AJR* 1988; 151:331-334.

Siegel MJ: Pediatric gynecologic sonography. *Radiology* 1991; 179:593-600.

Sivit CJ, Hung W, Taylor GA, Catena LM, Brown-Jones C, Kushner DC: Sonography in neonatal congenital adrenal hyperplasia. *AJR* 1991;156:141-143.

Thind CR, Carty HML, Philling DW: Role of ultrasound in the management of ovarian masses in children. *Clin Radiol* 1989; 40:180-182.

Wells RG, Sty JR: Imaging of sacrococcygeal germ cell tumors. *Radiographics* 1990; 10:701-713.

Wheeler MD, Styne DM: Diagnosis and management of precocious puberty. *Pediatr Clin North Am* 1990; 37:1255-1271.

# SECTION V
Trauma

# 27
# Musculoskeletal Trauma

### Key Concepts

1. The type of fractures seen in children are different from the type seen in adults, because of the presence of the growth plate in the child and the inherent "plasticity" of pediatric bone.
2. Distinct types of fractures that occur in children include: bowing ("plastic"), "greenstick," torus, and Salter-Harris–type physeal injuries.
3. "Toddler's fracture" (nondisplaced tibial fracture) is the most common etiology for the child who refuses to walk or has a limp. However, such an isolated clinical history can also occur with more serious entities (such as septic hip, osteomyelitis, metastatic disease, or Langerhans cell histiocytosis). As a result, the child with history of "refusing to walk" should be imaged from the hip to the foot.
4. Fractures of the pediatric elbow can be notoriously difficult to evaluate; a common injury site for the elbow is the supracondylar region in the skeletally immature child.
5. Elevation or obliteration of fat pads or planes can be a sensitive sign for injury, especially occult or subtle fracture. Look for elevation of the posterior fat pad (elbow), pronator quadratus (forearm), and patellar fat pads (knee).

A. Incomplete fractures.
   1. Fracture that does not completely cross bone shaft.
   2. Can be very subtle; look for hints of injury in soft tissues.
      a. Soft-tissue swelling.
      b. Loss of fat planes.
      c. Deformity.
      d. Remember, you can always ask patient where it hurts.
   3. If clinical suspicion remains high in light of negative plain films and bone scan, even magnetic resonance imaging (MRI) (especially for knee or elbow injuries) can be done as more sensitive examination for pathology.
   4. Types (Fig. 27-1).
      a. Bowing.
         *1.* Also called "plastic" fracture.
         *2.* Bending of bone without visible fracture line; comparison views are often helpful.
         *3.* Commonly occurs in forearm, usually with fracture of one bone (radius) and bowing of other (ulna).
         *4.* This type of fracture is often seen in bone dysplasias (osteogenesis imperfecta).

**Imaging** Can be subtle radiographic finding with visible bowing of long bone. Nuclear medicine bone scan results are positive; delayed radiographs may demonstrate periosteal reaction, indicative of healing.

      b. Greenstick.
         *1.* Fracture penetrates one cortex only (name comes from moist spring tree branches that readily bend but do not easily break).
         *2.* Uncommon fracture.

**Imaging** On plain radiograph, fracture line is seen penetrating one cortex only (bowing of bone is often present).

      c. Stress.
         *1.* In bone, reactive change to repeated stresses.
         *2.* Microfractures are present with no visible fracture line.
         *3.* Stressed normal bone leads to "fatigue fracture."
         *4.* Stressed abnormal bone leads to "insufficiency fracture."
            *a.* Osteomalacia.
            *b.* Osteoporosis.
            *c.* Osteogenesis imperfecta.
         *5.* Common sites.
            *a.* Tibia.
            *b.* Base of metatarsals.

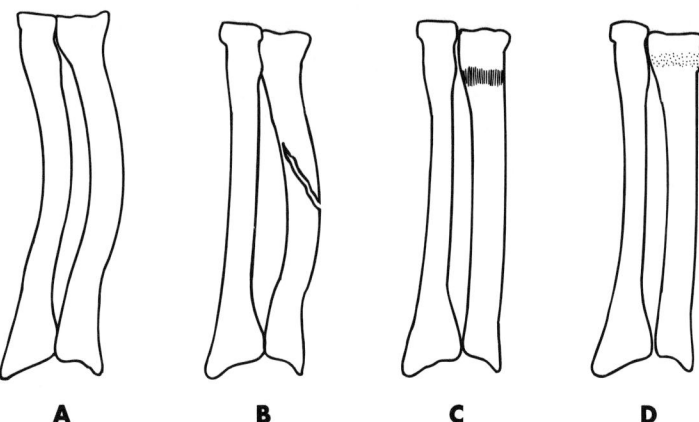

**Fig. 27-1** Types of fractures. **A,** Plastic or bowing fracture. **B,** Greenstick fracture. (Note fracture line only crosses one shaft). **C,** Stress fracture (shaded area denotes sclerosis or callus of healing). **D,** Torus or buckle fracture (stippled area depicts "trabelcular wrinkle" in area of impaction injury).

   *c.* Calcaneus.
   *d.* Femoral neck.

**Imaging** Usually subtle sclerosis or periosteal reaction can be seen on plain radiograph. Bone scan is positive ("hot spot" at site of stress fracture).

  *d.* Torus (buckle fracture).
   *1.* Cortical fracture with buckling deformity of cortex (torus in Latin means "protuberance" or "swelling").
   *2.* Common sites.
    *a.* Distal forearm.
    *b.* Proximal and distal tibia.

**Imaging** On plain radiograph, torus fractures may be subtle, because buckling cortex may be seen only in one plane (often the lateral). Look for "step-off" and sudden curve to bony cortex. Also, look for trabecular "wrinkle" (irregular trabecular pattern especially seen on anteroposterior [AP] view).

  *e.* Toddler's fracture.
   *1.* Nondisplaced fracture of tibia.
   *2.* Presents with child (between 9 months and 3 years of age) refusing to walk, usually with no definite history of trauma.

3. Because etiology of child refusing to walk includes septic hip, osteomyelitis, metastatic disease, Langerhans cell histiocytosis, and stress injuries of calcaneus and cuboid, this child should be imaged from hip to foot, rather than just obtaining tibia and fibular films (just looking for more common Toddler's fracture).

> **Imaging** Radiographs demonstrate spiral or oblique fracture of inferomedial tibia, often seen on one projection only. Fracture can be occult, manifesting as periosteal reaction on delayed films.

5. Fracture "foolers."
    a. Accessory ossification centers.
        1. Especially noted around ankle.
            a. Os subtibiale.
            b. Os subfibulare.
            c. Os trigonum tarsi.
        2. Can easily be mistaken for fracture and vice versa.
    b. Sesamoids.
        1. Function to relieve tension in tendons, especially noted around first and second digits of hands and feet.
        2. Largest is patella; also includes fabella (lateral head of gastrocnemius).
        3. Can be bipartite or tripartite and can mimic fracture.
B. Growth plate or epiphyseal injuries (see box on p. 250).
    1. Up to 15% of all pediatric fractures; often related to athletics.
    2. Growth plate is weakest part of bone, and therefore easily injured, particularly with shearing forces.
    3. Most common sites.
        a. Wrist.
        b. Ankle.
    4. More common in boys than in girls (not because boys are more active, but rather because male growth plate persists for longer period than does female growth plate).
    5. Clinical presentation.
        a. Local pain and swelling.
        b. Often point tender at site of growth plate.
    6. Prognosis of growth plate injuries.
        a. Types I, II, and III have excellent prognosis and usually heal with no sequelae.
        b. Types IV, V, and VI can disrupt growth plate with slowed, asymmetric, or interrupted growth, leading to limb shortening or angulation.

## Classification of Growth Plate or Epiphyseal Trauma

Type I (Fig. 27-2, *A*).
- Fracture involves growth plate only; usually shearing or avulsive injury.
- Local soft-tissue swelling.
- Classic locations include distal radius and ulna.
- Other locations.
  - Femoral head: slipped capital femoral epiphysis (SCFE).
  - Slipped medial epiphysis of elbow ("Little Leaguer" injury).
- In infancy, suspect child abuse.

> **Imaging** Plain radiographs demonstrate slight widening of growth plate (can be subtle finding); comparison views may be helpful. Growth plate may also be displaced (as is seen in SCFE and "Little Leaguer" elbow injury.

Type II (Fig. 27-2, *B*).
- Fracture involves growth plate and corner of metaphysis.
- Most common growth plate injury (50% to 75%).
- Common sites.
  - Distal radius.
  - Tibia.

> **Imaging** Radiographs reveal widening of growth plate with metaphyseal fragment (often triangular); often epiphyseal displacement.

Type III (Fig. 27-2, *C*).
- Fracture involving growth plate and epiphysis.
- Common site is distal tibia (also known as juvenile Tillaux fracture); growth plate separates laterally, since medial portion fuses first.

> **Imaging** Radiographs show lucency extending from epiphysis through growth plate.

Type IV (Fig. 27-2, *D*).
- Fracture involving epiphysis, growth plate, and metaphysis.
- Ten percent of growth plate injuries.
- Common sites.
  - Distal humerus.
  - Tibia.
- May require open reduction to restore articular surface.
- Can be difficult to diagnose; fracture lines evident only on certain projections.

> **Imaging** Radiographs reveal lucency extending from metaphysis, through growth plate, into epiphysis.

## Classification of Growth Plate or Epiphyseal Trauma—cont'd

Type V (Fig. 27-2, *E*).
- Crush injury; compressive force that injures growth plate, adjacent epiphysis, and metaphyseal vascular supply.
- Less than 1% of growth plate injuries.
- Common sites.
  - Distal femur.
  - Proximal tibia.

Type VI.
- Trauma to perichondrium, with reactive bone formation tethering growth plate.
- Very rare.

Type VII.
- Injury to epiphysis alone.
- Cartilaginous fracture.
- Osteochondritis dissecans.
  - Osteochondral fracture; commonly seen along lateral aspect of medial condyle of femur, talar dome, or elbow.
  - Articular cartilage fragment can become loose body.
  - Found more commonly in males than in females (3:1); bilateral (25%).

**Imaging** Radiographs may reveal often subtle defect along epiphyseal surface, especially medial condyle of femur. MRI is more sensitive and may better delineate injury.

**Imaging** Growth plate dysfunction can manifest as:
- Segmental loss of continuous lucent growth plate.
- Premature growth plate fusion, often asymmetric (Madelung deformity).
- Angulation of growth plate or articular surface.
- Localized sclerosis of adjacent metaphysis or epiphysis.
- Avascular necrosis of epiphysis.
- Limb shortening.

C. Elbow trauma.
  1. Pediatric elbow can be notoriously difficult to evaluate.
  2. Common injury sites for elbow (often determined by age).
     a. Supracondylar in skeletally immature.
     b. Radial head in young adults.
     c. Olecranon (more common in elderly patients).
     d. Traumatic dislocation is almost always posterior in direction.

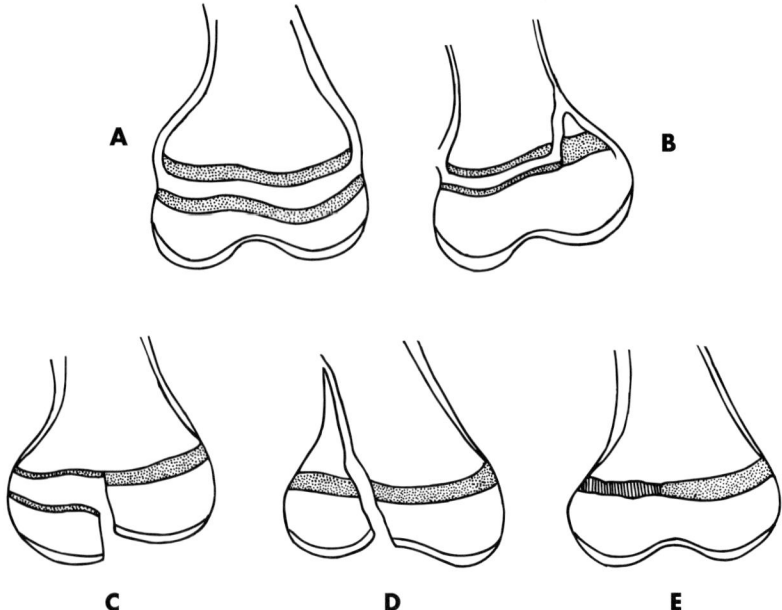

**Fig. 27-2** Salter-Harris classification (stippled area is growth plate). **A,** Salter I. **B,** Salter II. **C,** Salter III. **D,** Salter IV. **E,** Salter V (shaded area is region of crush injury).

> **Imaging** Posterior fat pad.
> - On lateral radiograph of elbow, elevation of fat pad (lucency posterior to distal humerus) is highly suspicious for fracture.
> - In light of this finding (even if exact fracture line cannot be definitively demonstrated) child's arm is often immobilized; repeat films can be obtained in 7 to 10 days.
> 
> Humeral or capitellar lines (Fig. 27-3, A).
> - On lateral view, line drawn along anterior cortex of humerus should intersect middle third of capitellum.
> - Line drawn through middle of proximal radial shaft should go through middle third of capitellum.
> - If above lines are not intact, consider supracondylar fracture with dislocation.
> 
> Appearance of elbow epiphyses ("CRITOE Mneumonic").
> - Helpful when trying to evaluate for fracture fragment versus normal epiphysis.
> - CRITOE represents order of appearance of elbow epiphyseal centers (Fig. 27-3, B).

- *C* (capitellum).
- *R* (radial head).
- *I* (internal or medial epiphysis).
- *T* (trochlea).
- *O* (olecranon).
- *E* (external or lateral epiphysis).
- Example of how to use CRITOE.
  - If fragment in usual position of lateral condyle is seen but olecranon, trochlea, and medial epiphysis have not yet appeared, then aforementioned fragment can not be epiphysis and is, in fact, fracture.

3. "Nursemaid's elbow" (Fig. 27-4).
   a. Very common in infants and small children.
   b. Mechanism of injury.
      1. Pulling of child's arm.
      2. Results in radial head slippage from annular ligament that encircles ulna or radial head.
   c. Typical history is child refusing to move afflicted arm with no history of trauma or swelling.
   d. Treatment.
      1. Reducing radial head by supination of forearm with flexion of elbow.
      2. Often radiologic technologists "accidentally" reduce this type of injury when positioning child for lateral film.

**Imaging** Radiographs are obtained to rule out other injury (such as fracture or dislocation), since "nursemaid's elbow" is radiographically occult.

4. "Little Leaguer's elbow" (Fig. 27-3, *C*).
   a. Avulsion of medial epicondyle (up to 15% of all elbow injuries).
   b. Traumatic lesion.
      1. Associated with pitching too hard, too early in life.
      2. Snapping wrist motion of throwing a curveball is main culprit, as flexor carpi ulnaris tendon pulls off medial epicondyle.
   c. Salter-Harris, type I injury; can require pinning and relocation of fragment into position to ensure proper growth.
   d. Occasionally, avulsed epicondylar fragment can become loose body, becoming entrapped within joint space itself.

**Imaging** Plain radiograph of elbow can demonstrate avulsion of medial epicondyle with widening of distance between epiphysis and medial humeral condyle.

D. Knee trauma.

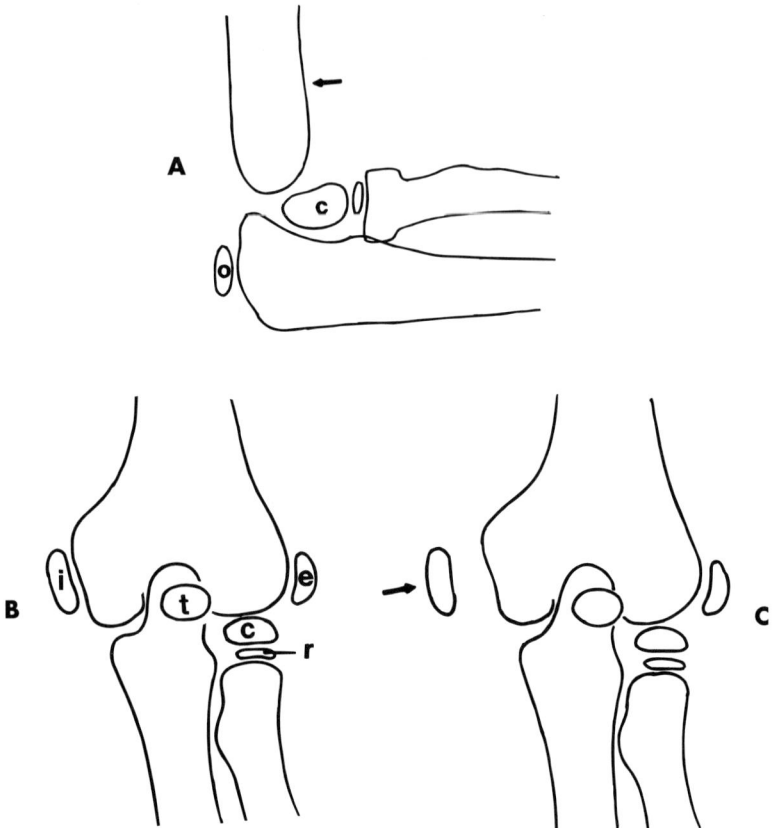

**Fig. 27-3** Elbow. **A,** Lateral view of elbow: In normal elbow alignment, anterior humeral line *(arrow)* and line drawn through midradius should bisect middle third of capitellum *(c)*. **B,** CRITOE: Mneumonic for order of appearance of epiphyseal centers of elbow. Capitellum *(c)*, radial head *(r)*, "internal" or medial epicondyle *(i)*, trochlea *(t)*, olecranon *(o* seen in **A**), "external" or lateral condyle *(e)*. **C,** Little leaguer's elbow: Displacement of medial epicondyle *(arrow)*. Compare to normal position of medial epicondyle, as seen in **B.**

    1. Internal derangement of knee (found especially in young athletes).
        a. Meniscal injuries.
        b. Ligamentous.
            *1.* Anterior cruciate ligament.
            2. Posterior cruciate ligement.
        c. Radiographically occult, MRI much more sensitive for knee injury.

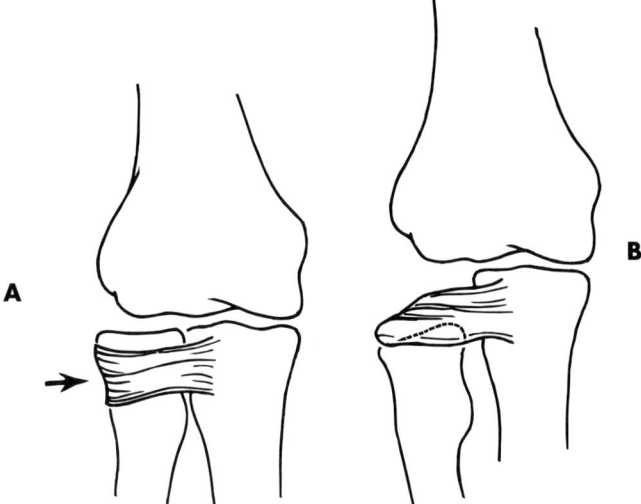

**Fig. 27-4** Nursemaid's elbow. **A,** Normal alignment of ulna and radius within annular ligament *(arrow)*. **B,** Nursemaid's elbow: Slippage of radius (radiographically occult injury).

2. Osgood-Schlatter disease.
   a. Tibial tuberosity avulsion.
      1. Tearing of patellar tendon insertion.
      2. No inflammatory response.
   b. Found more commonly in boys than in girls, peak age range is 10 to 12 years.
   c. Clinical diagnosis.

> **Imaging** Knee radiograph can suggest diagnosis: look for soft-tissue swelling, loss of infrapatellar fat pad, excessive tibial fragmentation, and thickening of patellar tendon.

3. Chondromalacia.
   a. Common abnormality of patella (can be seen in up to 30% to 50% of adults).
   b. Cartilaginous softening leads to central patellar posterior articular surface irregularity, cratering, and sclerosis.
   c. Etiology unknown; perhaps related to repeated trauma.

> **Imaging** Lateral radiograph of knee reveals sclerosis and irregularity of posterior surface of patella. Joint space loss is not usually present.

E. Muscular or soft tissue trauma.
  1. Hematoma.
     a. Soft-tissue swelling.
     b. Elevation or obliteration of fat pads or planes.
        *1.* Sensitive sign for injury, especially fracture.
        *2.* Common regions.
           *a.* Posterior fat pad (elbow).
           *b.* Pronator quadratus fat pad.
              *1)* Normally seen along volar aspect of distal forearm.
              *2)* Normally has concave appearance, matching curve of distal radius.
              *3)* With fracture and hematoma, this fat pad elevates and becomes convex to bone underneath.
           *c.* Patellar fat pads.
              *1)* Suprapatellar.
              *2)* Infrapatellar.
              *3)* Obliteration or elevation of these fat pads suggests joint effusion and knee injury.
  2. Myositis ossificans.
     a. Myositis ossificans traumatica.
        *1.* Ossification of soft tissues often seen near hips, buttocks, and elbows.
        *2.* Heterotopic bone forms in posttraumatic areas; exact pathogenesis is uncertain.
           *a.* No inflammatory component.
           *b.* Osteoblasts in soft tissue are stimulated (perhaps by traumatic incident) to form osteoid or bone.
        *3.* Should not be biopsied, since it can resemble sarcoma; also "trauma" of biopsy can be detrimental (can increase amount of ossification).
        *4.* No treatment, since it will slowly recede on its own; may take 6 to 12 months.

**Imaging** Radiographs may show soft-tissue swelling with heterotopic bone formation (often with cortical shell). No adjacent bony lesion.

     b. Myositis ossificans progressiva.
        *1.* Also known as fibrodysplasia ossificans progressiva.
        *2.* Rare disorder (possibly autoimmune).
        *3.* Progressive replacement of fascia, muscle, tendons, and ligaments by bone tissue.
        *4.* Progressive ossification results in joint ankylosis and severe limitation of motion.

5. Any trauma (such as attempt at surgical resection or release) only accentuates and worsens condition.
6. Restrictive lung disease ensues because of rib cage involvement; is often cause of early death.

## SUGGESTED READINGS

Aronson J, Garvin K, Seibert JJ, Glasier C, Tursky EA: Efficiency of the bone scan for occult limping toddlers. *J Pediatr Orthop* 1992; 12:38-44.

Berger PE, Ofstein RA, Jackson DW, Morrison DS, Silvino N, Amador R: MRI demonstration of radiographically occult fractures: What have we been missing? *Radiographics* 1989; 9:407-436.

Blumberg K, Patterson RJ: Toddler's cuboid fracture. *Radiology* 1991; 179:93-94.

Daffner RH, Pavlov H: Stress fractures: Current concepts. *AJR* 1992; 159:245-252.

Elgazzar AH, Kriss VM, Gelfand MJ: Advanced fibrodysplasia ossificans progressiva. *Clin Nucl Med* 1995; 20(6):519-521.

Harris JH: The importance of soft tissues in certain skeletal traumatic lesions. *Radiol Clin North Am* 1981; 19:601-624.

Horev G, Korenreich L, Ziv N, Grunebaum M: The enigma of stress fractures in the pediatric age group: Clarification or confusion through new imaging modalities. *Pediatr Radiol* 1990; 20:469-471.

Jaramillo D, Hoffer FA, Shapiro F, Rand F: MR imaging of fractures of the growth plate. *AJR* 1990; 155:1261-1265.

Mabry JD, Fitch RD: Plastic deformation in pediatric fractures: Mechanism and treatment. *J Pediatr Orthop* 1989; 9:310-314.

Michaels MG: A case of bilateral nursemaid's elbow. *Pediatr Emerg Care* 1989; 5:226-227.

Mink JH, Deutsch AL: Occult osseous and cartilaginous injuries about the knee: MR assessment, detection, and classification. *Radiology* 1989; 170:823-829.

Resnick CS: Diagnostic imaging of pediatric skeletal trauma. *Radiol Clin North Am* 1989; 27:1013-1022.

Rogers LF: Fractures and dislocations of the elbow. *Semin Roentgenol* 1978; 13:97-107.

Salter RB, Harris WR: Injuries involving the epiphyseal plate. *J Bone Joint Surg Am* 1963; 45:587-622.

Silverman FN: Problems in pediatric fractures. *Semin Roentgenol* 1978; 13:167-176.

# 28
# Nonaccidental Trauma (Child Abuse)

### Key Concepts

1. The diagnosis of child abuse is often made clinically; high suspicion for nonaccidental trauma occurs when the degree of injury does not match the history.
2. The most common radiologic manifestations of child abuse (discovered via skeletal survey or bone scan) are sketetal injuries.
3. Fractures of varying ages are highly suspicious for abuse, especially posterior rib fractures, corner metaphyseal fractures ("bucket-handle"), and long-bone fractures in nonambulatory children.
4. "Shaken-baby" central nervous system (CNS) injury is due to rapid acceleration and deceleration of an infant's cranium, which can cause retinal hemorrhages, parenchymal "shear" injury, and the hallmark subdural hemorrhage.
5. The most common etiology of duodenal hematoma is trauma, often nonaccidental in nature, as blunt blow of a fist or foot can compress duodenum against spine causing injury.

A. Statistics.
   1. Child abuse and neglect (also known as nonaccidental trauma or "battered babies") involves estimated 1.5 million victims per year; 150,000 of whom have severe or life-threatening injuries.
   2. Several thousand yearly fatalities occur (even higher percentage of permanent CNS damage; about 10% of cerebral palsy results from abuse).
   3. Typical age of victim is less than 2 years of age (25%); majority of victims are less than 6 years of age (80%).
   4. As much as 10% of "trauma" seen in emergency room setting in children less than 5 years of age is nonaccidental in nature.
   5. Sadly, mortality rate from child abuse in infants aged 1 to 6 months is second only to sudden infant death syndrome.
B. Skeletal manifestations.
   1. Most commonly discovered radiologic manifestation of child abuse.
   2. Skeletal findings are present in only about one third of child abuse cases.
   3. Look for multiple skeletal findings of varying ages, using skeletal survey or even bone scan.
   4. In children older than 5 years of age, skeletal survey has limited value, unless history or physical examination warrants specific imaging.
   5. Skeletal survey.
      a. Simple "babygram" is not adequate.
      b. At minimum following films are required.
         *1.* Anteroposterior (AP) chest, abdomen, and pelvis.
         *2.* AP humeri, forearms, and hands.
         *3.* AP femurs, tibias, and feet.
         *4.* AP and lateral skull.
         *5.* Also lateral chest and lateral spine in infants less than 1 year of age.
      c. All potentially positive sites need to be viewed in two projections.
   6. Bone scan.
      a. Use in child abuse screening is still controversial.
      b. Sensitive (especially for rib fractures); however, not specific (especially problematic in evaluation of metaphysis of long bones because of "hot" adjacent growth plate).
      c. Often used when plain radiographs (skeletal survey) are negative, but clinical suspicion remains high.

---

**Imaging** Long-bone fractures.
- Particularly spiral fractures.

*Continued*

*Continued from previous page*

- Highly suspicious in infant or nonambulatory child, especially femur fractures.
- Even in ambulating toddlers, 60% of femur fractures are nonaccidental.

Subperiosteal hemorrhage.
- In infancy, vascular periosteum is only loosely attached; therefore, separates and bleeds easily with twisting stresses.
- Hematoma accumulates under periosteum, ballooning out centrally, but remains contained by tight metaphyseal attachments.

Corner fracture ("bucket-handle" fracture).
- Transverse injury to metaphysis immediately adjacent to growth plate.
- Results in ringlike fracture (possibly due to avulsive forces).

Posterior rib fractures.
- Result from thoracic compression.
- Pediatric rib cage is normally resilient; therefore, true accidental fracture of ribs is rare in normal (nonpremature) infants and small children.
- Fractures are seen at costovertebral junction and also along lateral margins of ribs.
- Look for callus formation ("round ball" at costovertebral junction).
- High risk of associated CNS "shaken-baby" injury.

Periosteal reaction.
- Sign of healing bone.
  - Nonspecific.
  - Can also be due to trauma, infection, or tumor.
- Initially appears within 10 days of original injury.
- Can be used to date injury.
- Physiologic periosteal reaction.
  - Occurs in infants, peak age is about 6 months.
  - Hallmark.
    - Bilateral, thin, symmetric, periosteal reaction.
    - Only along one side of bone (usually medial cortex).
  - Usually seen involving long bones.
  - Can be mistaken for periosteal reaction from nonaccidental trauma.

Skull fractures.

- Can be relatively common in true accidental trauma (often seen as linear, parietal fracture).
- Occipital fractures are more suspicious.
  - Particularly multiple and complex ("eggshell") fractures.
  - Depressed component may be present.
- Widened sutures (associated with intracranial injury and hemorrhage that result in increased intracranial pressure).

7. Radiographic findings can be classified according to levels of suspicion of abuse.
   a. High specificity.
      1. Metaphyseal ("corner") fractures.
      2. Posterior rib fractures.
      3. Scapular fractures.
      4. Spinous process fractures.
      5. Sternal fractures.
      6. Humeral epiphyseal displacement.
   b. Moderate specificity.
      1. Multiple fractures (especially bilateral).
      2. Epiphyseal separations.
      3. Digital fractures.
      4. Complex skull fractures.
      5. Fractures of different ages.
   c. Low specificity.
      1. Clavicular.
      2. Long-bone fractures in ambulating children.
      3. Linear skull fractures.
8. Differential diagnosis of multiple fractures or periosteal reaction (child abuse foolers).
   a. Osteogenesis imperfecta.
   b. Osteopetrosis.
   c. Copper deficiency, Menkes' ("kinky hair") syndrome.
   d. Rickets.
   e. Scurvy.
   f. Caffey syndrome (infantile cortical hyperostosis).

C. CNS manifestation.
   1. Make up about 20% of child abuse cases; is leading cause of death.
   2. First described by John Caffey in 1946 as long-bone fractures with subdural hematomas; he called this syndrome "battered-baby syndrome."*

---

*From Caffey J: Multiple fractures in the long bones of infants suffering from chronic subdural hematoma. *AJR* 1946; 56:163-167.

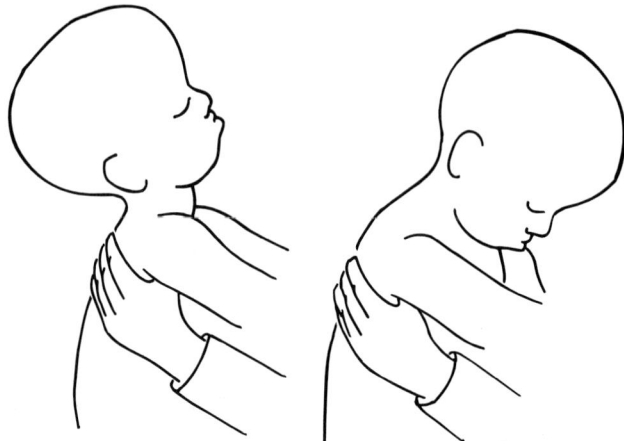

**Fig. 28-1** Mechanism of shaken-baby injury.

3. Often presents with vomiting or obtunded infant.
4. Mechanism.
   a. Direct blow.
      *1.* Skull fractures.
         *a.* Eggshell fractures.
         *b.* Can have simple linear fractures, especially occipital.
         *c.* Extracranial hemorrhage.
         *d.* Cerebral contusion.
   b. "Shaken baby" (Fig. 28-1).
      *1.* Rapid cranial acceleration and deceleration coupled with inability of child's weak neck muscles to support head and bear force (seen especially in children less than 1 year of age).
      *2.* Prominent subarachnoid space in infants.
         *a.* Protection from direct trauma.
         *b.* Yet allows more cerebral movement; therefore, increases injury with shaking.
      *3.* Ocular findings.
         *a.* Retinal hemorrhages.
         *b.* Practically pathognomonic of "shaken-baby" injury.

**Imaging** Subdural hemorrhage (most common manifestation).
- Acute; increased lentiform density.
- Chronic.
  - Low density; extraaxial collection.
  - Associated with general atrophy.

- If repeated abuse has occurred, synchronous, chronic, and acute findings may be present.
- Computed tomography (CT) is initial examination of choice, although magnetic resonance imaging is more sensitive to small hemorrhages of differing ages.

Parenchymal hemorrhagic lesions.
- Contusion (either direct blow or shaken-baby injury).
- Shearing injury.
  - Gray-white matter injury.
  - Implies severe cerebral injury with poor prognosis.
    - Seizures.
    - Mental retardation.
    - Developmental delay.

Cerebral edema or infarction.
- Hypoxia
  - Smothering.
  - Strangulation.
  - Carotid injury (dissection).
- Diffuse hypoxic injury can be seen with sparing of brainstem and basal ganglia ("reversal sign" on CT).
- Focal hypoxia (strangulation).
  - Preservation of posterior circulation.
  - Because vertebral arteries are protected in bony transverse foramina.

D. Abdominal manifestations.
  1. Duodenal hematoma.
     a. Blunt trauma to abdomen.
        *1.* Punched (fist).
        *2.* Kicked (foot).
     b. Hemorrhage into bowel wall with resulting thickened bowel folds.
     c. Can present with vomiting from obstruction.

**Imaging** Abdominal radiographs may demonstrate mass effect or paucity of central gas. Upper gastrointestinal contrast study reveals characteristic "coiled-spring" appearance or bowel fold thickening ("stacked-coin" appearance), presenting in horizontal portion of duodenum, as it passes over the spine. Partial obstruction from duodenal hematoma is often present.

  2. Visceral organ injury.
     a. Blunt blow to abdomen can result in visceral organ injury.
     b. Organs involved.

       1. Pancreas.
       2. Liver.
       3. Spleen.
       4. Renal.
    c. Type of injury.
       1. Contusion and/or laceration.
       2. Fracture.
       3. Pseudocyst formation.
    d. Best evaluated on CT.

> **Imaging** On CT, look for hypodense regions within visceral organ in question; can often see linear lacerations. Helpful secondary signs include pleural effusions, abdominal ascites, and adjacent bowel injury. Specific pancreatic injury can present with pancreatitis (late complication is pseudocyst formation).

## SUGGESTED READINGS

Albin DS, Greenspan A, Reinhart M, Grix A: Differentiation of child abuse from osteogenesis imperfecta. *AJR* 1990; 154:1035-1046.

Albin DS, Sane SM: Non-accidental injury: Confusion with temporary brittle bone disease and mild osteogenesis imperfecta. *Pediatr Radiol* 1997; 27:111-113.

Ball WS: Non-accidental craniocerebral trauma (child abuse): MR imaging. *Radiology* 1989; 173:609-610.

Bernardi B, Zimmerman RA, Bilaniuk LT: Neuroradiographic evaluation of pediatric craniocerebral trauma. *Top Magn Reson Imaging* 1993; 5:161-173.

Caffey J: Multiple fractures in the long bones of infants suffering from chronic subdural hematoma. *AJR* 1946; 56:163-167.

Chapman S, Hall CM: Non-accidental injury or brittle bones. *Pediatr Radiol* 1997; 27:106-110.

Conway JJ, Collins M, Collins M, Tanz RR, Radkowski MA, Andandappa E, Hernandez R, Freeman EL: The role of bone scintigraphy in detecting child abuse. *Semin Nucl Med* 1993; 23:321-333.

Dalton HJ, Slovis TL, Helfer RE, Comstock J, Scheurer S, Riolo S: Undiagnosed abuse in children younger than 3 years with femoral fracture. *AJDC* 1990; 144:875-878.

Haller JO, Kleinman PL, Merten DF, Cohen HL, Cohen MD, Hayden PW, Keller M, Towbin R, Sane SM: Diagnostic imaging of child abuse. *Pediatrics* 1991; 87:262-264.

Kleinman P: Diagnostic imaging in infant abuse. *AJR* 1990; 155:703-712.

Kleinman PK, Brill PW, Winchester P: Resolving duodenal-jejunal hematoma in abused children. *Radiology* 1986; 160:747-750.

Kleinman PK, Marks SC: Inflicted skeletal injury: Post mortem radiologic/histopathologic study in 31 infants. *AJR* 1995; 165:647-650.

Krugman RD, Bays JA, Chadwick DL, Kanda MB, Levitt CJ, McHugh MT: Shaken baby syndrome: Inflicted cerebral trauma. *Pediatrics* 1993; 92:872-875.

Merten DF, Carpenter BLM: Radiologic imaging of inflicted injury in the child abuse syndrome. *Pediatr Clin North Am* 1990; 37:815-837.

Merten DF, Radkowski MA, Leonidas JC: The abused child: A radiological reappraisal. *Radiology* 1983; 146:377-381.

Pergolizzi R, Oestreich AE: Child abuse fracture through physiologic periosteal reaction. *Pediatr Radiol* 1995, 25:566-567.

Sato Y, Yuh WTC, Smith WL, Alexander RC, Kao SCS, Ellerbroek CJ: Head injury in child abuse: Evaluation with MR imaging. *Radiology* 1989; 173:653-657.

Sivit CJ, Taylor GA, Eichelberger MR: Visceral injury in battered children: A changing perspective. *Radiology* 1989; 173:659-661.

Thomas SA, Rosenfield NS, Leventhal JM, Markowitz RI: Long bone fractures in young children: Distinguishing accidental injuries from child abuse. *Pediatrics* 1991; 88:471-476.

# 29
# Abdominal Trauma

---

### Key Concepts

1. Plain radiographs are often not very helpful in the evaluation of pediatric abdominal trauma, particularly when looking for visceral organ injury. However, radiographs (especially decubitus views), can reveal free air or an ileus-like bowel pattern, which may indicate injury to either the bowel or adjacent viscera.
2. Currently, computed tomography (CT) is the most sensitive examination for abdominal trauma because of its ability to demonstrate visceral organ trauma, free fluid, and even bowel injury. Ultrasound (US) is often limited in the initial evaluation of the abdomen because of overlying bowel gas; but it can ascertain free fluid and visceral organ injury.
3. Splenic injury is one of the more common of the visceral organ injuries with resulting contusion, laceration, or rupture occurring, depending on the severity of the trauma.
4. Trauma is the most common cause of pancreatitis and duodenal hematoma in childhood, especially blunt abdominal trauma (including nonaccidental trauma).
5. Abdominal ecchymoses corresponding to the lap belt are suspicious for "seat-belt" injury: avulsion injury of the bowel (especially at the ligament of Treitz).

A. Hepatic.
   1. Trauma commonly involves more-exposed right lobe of liver.
   2. Elevated liver enzymes.
      a. Contusion and/or hematoma.
         *1.* Parenchymal.
         *2.* Subcapsular.
      b. Laceration and/or fracture.
         *1.* More linear injury, extending to hepatic surface.
         *2.* Free fluid can indicate rupture or injury to capsule.
      c. Periportal fluid.
         *1.* Linear hypodense areas that track along route of portal vessels.
         *2.* Can be indicative of more subtle hepatic injury.
   3. Treatment is often conservative management, unless there is significant vascular injury with continued blood loss.

   **Imaging** CT can image variety of hepatic injuries from irregular, often subtle hypodensity of small contusion or periportal fluid, to subcapsular hematoma, laceration, and free fluid. Look for adjacent right-sided injuries (ribs, kidney, or adrenal).

B. Splenic.
   1. One of more commonly injured of visceral organs.
   2. Similar to hepatic injuries listed above; contusion, laceration, or rupture are possible.
   3. Treatment is usually conservative, unless ongoing blood loss requires intervention.
   4. Complications.
      a. Delayed rupture from subcapsular hematoma.
      b. Cyst formation.
      c. Splenosis.

   **Imaging** CT can demonstrate low-density areas of contusion or more linear laceration. Rupture of spleen with free fluid can also be seen. Be careful, however, since following contrast bolus (especially on fast, spiral CT scans), splenic enhancement can be irregular and may mimic splenic injury.

C. Pancreas.
   1. Trauma is most common cause of pancreatitis in childhood, especially blunt abdominal trauma.
      a. Motor vehicle accident.
      b. Bicycle handle bars.
      c. Human fist or foot (child abuse).

2. Pancreas can be contused, lacerated, or fractured, depending on type and force of injury.
3. Often associated with duodenal injury.
4. Elevated amylase and lipase is often present.
5. Complications.
    a. Pseudocyst formation.
    b. Usually within few weeks of injury.

> **Imaging** On abdominal radiograph, sentinel loops of dilated bowel may be seen in upper midabdomen or left upper quadrant. US may show enlarged, hypoechoic pancreas. CT best demonstrates pancreatic injury and possible resulting pancreatitis. Look for hypodense areas and/or peripancreatic fluid collections.

D. Bowel.
  1. Seat-belt injury.
     a. Abdominal ecchymoses corresponding to lap belt.
     b. Worrisome for avulsion injury of bowel, especially at ligament of Treitz.
     c. Also remember to look for vertebral fractures; chance fracture at L2.
  2. Duodenal injury.
     a. Often seen in conjunction with pancreatic injury.
     b. Hematoma (see Chapter 28).
     c. Rupture (retroperitoneal free air can be difficult to discern on radiographs).
  3. Mesenteric injury.
     a. Often focal hematoma.
     b. Can cause compression or obstruction of adjacent bowel.
  4. "Shock bowel."
     a. Vascular insufficiency to bowel, usually related to systemic hypotensive episode.
     b. Dilated, ileus-like bowel pattern with diffusely enhancing bowel walls.

> **Imaging** Abdominal radiographs may demonstrate ileus-like pattern; free air may be difficult to discern. CT can show thick folds of bowel hematoma; again free air may be subtle. Free fluid without demonstrable source (namely visceral organ injury) is also suspicious for occult bowel injury.

E. Urinary tract.
  1. Renal (Fig. 29-1).

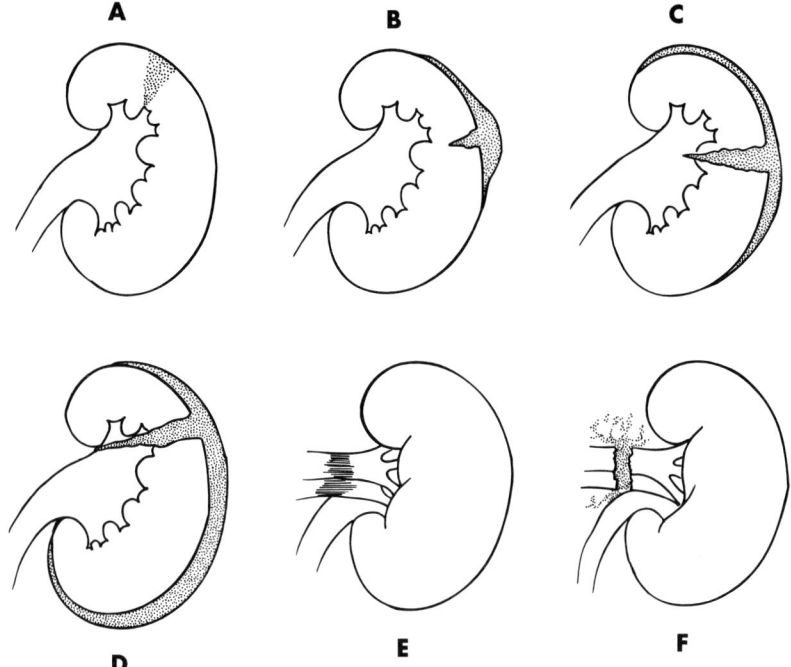

**Fig. 29-1** Renal trauma. **A,** Renal contusion *(stippled area).* **B,** Laceration and subcapsular hematoma. **C,** Laceration and subcapsular hematoma extending to collecting system. **D,** Laceration and subcapsular hematoma extending through collecting system. **E,** Vessel thrombosis *(shaded region).* **F,** Vessel rupture and avulsion with hemorrhaging into abdomen.

    a. Minor.
        *1.* Contusion.
        *2.* Laceration without extension to capsule or collecting system.
    b. Major.
        *1.* Laceration with extension to capsule.
            *a.* Capsular hematoma.
            *b.* Page kidney.
                *1)* Hypertension.
                *2)* Related to compressive effect of hematoma.
                *3)* Increased renin production.
            *c.* Laceration with extension to collecting system.
            *d.* Ruptured kidney.
            *e.* Vascular pedicle injury.
                *1)* Thrombosis.

2) Avulsion.
   f. Disruption of ureteropelvic junction (UPJ) or ureteral disruption.
      1) Extravasation of urine and contrast.
      2) Can lead to formation of urinoma.
   c. Treatment is conservative, if hemodynamically stable.

> **Imaging** CT best evaluates potential renal injury. With minor injury, look for hypodense areas of kidney (contusion). Capsular and perirenal fluid collections signal laceration that extends to or through renal capsule and may involve disruption of collecting system. Lack of contrast enhancement within kidney, coupled with perirenal fluid, is suggestive of vascular pedicle avulsion.

2. Bladder, ureters, and urethra.
   a. Ureters.
      1. Uncommon injury.
      2. Most commonly disrupted near UPJ.
   b. Bladder.
      1. Intraperitoneal.
         a. Usually full-bladder rupture with free spillage into peritoneal cavity.
         b. Surgical emergency.
      2. Extraperitoneal.
         a. More common injury.
         b. Usually associated with pelvic fractures; look for bladder displacement by pelvic hematoma.
         c. Conservative management with prolonged catheterization.

> **Imaging** Contrast cystogram can demonstrate leak of contrast following bladder injury. Remember to adequately fill out bladder on cystogram examination; sometimes rupture is only evident at large volumes. Intravenous pyelography examination best evaluates integity of ureters.

   c. Urethra.
      1. Usually related to "straddle-type" injuries, often occurring with pelvic fractures.
      2. Common locations for injury.
         a. Posterior urethra (at bladder neck).
         b. Bulbous portion of urethra.
      3. Distal urethral injuries can occur.
         a. Following instrumentation.
         b. Following catheter placement.

4. Long-term complication of urethral injury includes subsequent stricture formation.

| |
|---|
| **Imaging** Retrograde urethrogram (catheter in distal portion of urethra with injection of contrast to opacify urethral course) can demonstrate extravasation of contrast, when urethra has been disrupted. |

## SUGGESTED READINGS

Abdalati H, Bulas DI, Sivit CJ, Majd M, Rushton HG, Eichelberger MR: Blunt renal trauma in children: Healing of renal injuries and recommendations for imaging followup. *Pediatr Radiol* 1994; 24:573-576.

Brick SH, Taylor GA, Potter BM, Eichelberger MR: Hepatic and splenic injury in children: Role of CT in the decision for laparotomy. *Radiology* 1987; 165:643-646.

Brody AS, Seidel FG, Kuhn JP: CT evaluation of blunt abdominal trauma in children: Comparison of ultrafast and conventional CT. *AJR* 1989; 153:803-806.

Bulas DI, Taylor GA, Eichelberger MR: The value of CT in detecting bowel perforation in children following blunt abdominal trauma. *AJR* 1989; 153:561-564.

Kauzlaric D, Barmeir E: Sonography of trauamtic rupture of the bladder: "Bladder within a bladder" appearance of extra-peritoneal extravasation. *J Ultrasound Med* 1986; 5:97-98.

Luks FI, Lemire A, St. Vil D, Di Lorenzo M, Filiatrault D, Ouimet A: Blunt abdominal trauma in children: The practical value of ultrasonography. *J Trauma* 1993; 34:607-609.

Malangoni MA, Cue JL, Fallat ME, Willing SJ, Richardson JD: Evaluation of splenic injury by computed tomography and its impact on treatment. *Ann Surg* 1990; 211:592-597.

Mirvis SE: Diagnostic imaging of the urinary system following blunt trauma. *Clin Imaging* 1990; 13:269-280.

Patrick LE, Ball TI, Atkinson GO, Winn KJ: Pediatric blunt abdominal trauma: Periportal tracking at CT. *Radiology* 1992; 183:689-691.

Pollack HM, Wein AJ: Imaging of renal trauma. *Radiology* 1989; 172:297-308.

Ruess L, Sivit CJ, Eichelberger MR, Taylor GA, Bond SJ: Blunt hepatic and splenic trauma in children: Correlation of a CT injury severity scale with clinical outcome. *Pediatr Radiol* 1995; 25:321-325.

Sivit CJ, Eichelberger MR, Taylor GA: Blunt pancreatic trauma in children: CT diagnosis. *AJR* 1994; 158:1097-1100.

Sivit CJ, Eichelberger MR, Taylor GA: CT in children with rupture of bowel caused by blunt trauma: Diagnostic efficacy and comparison with hypoperfusion complex. *AJR* 1994; 163:1195-1198.

Sivit CJ, Taylor GA, Bulas DI: Blunt trauma in children: Significance of peritoneal fluid. *Radiology* 1991; 178:185-188.

Sivit CJ, Taylor GA, Bulas DI, Kushner DC, Potter BM, Eichelberger MR: Post-traumatic shock in children: CT findings associated with hemodynamic instability. *Radiology* 1992; 182:723-726.

Sivit CJ, Taylor GA, Newman KD, Bulas DI, Gotschall CS, Wright CJ, Eichelberger MR: Safety-belt injuries in children with lap belt ecchymosis: CT findings in 61 patients. *AJR* 1991; 157:111-114.

Stalker HP, Kaufman RA, Towbin R: Patterns of liver injury in childhood: CT analysis. *AJR* 1986; 147:1199-1205.

Taylor GA, Guion CJ, Potter BM, Eichelberger MR: CT evaluation of blunt abdominal trauma in children. *AJR* 1989; 153:555-559.

Taylor GA, O'Donnell R, Sivit CJ, Eichelberger MR: Abdominal injury score: A clinical score for the assignment of risk in children after blunt trauma. *Radiology* 1994; 190:689-694.

Yale-Loehr AJ, Kramer SS, Quinlan DM, La France ND, Mitchell SE, Gearfhart JP: CT of severe renal trauma in children: Evaluation and course of healing with conservative therapy. *AJR* 1989; 152:109-113.

# SECTION VI
Musculoskeletal System

# 30
# Musculoskeletal Infection

### Key Concepts

1. Osteomyelitis, diskitis, and septic arthritis can be devastating to the pediatric patient, because of the long-term complications to the growing skeleton.
2. Osteomyelitic bony changes on plain radiographs may take from 1 to 2 weeks before becoming evident (up to 50% of the bony cortex must be destroyed in order to be detected on routine radiographs). Nuclear medicine (Tc-99m bone scan) is much more sensitive.
3. Septic arthritis in children usually involves the hip or knee. Subsequent osteomyelitis is a concern in the patient with a septic hip joint, because the femoral metaphysis is positioned within the joint capsule.
4. Back pain in the child is a serious complaint until proven otherwise. General differential diagnosis for nontraumatic pediatric back pain:
   a. Diskitis or osteomyelits.
   b. Lymphoma or leukemia.
   c. Langerhans cell histiocytosis (formerly known as histiocytosis X).
   d. Spondylolysis, can be either congenital or traumatic.
   e. Bone lesion (such as osteoid osteoma or osteoblastoma).
   f. Metastases.
5. Periosteal reaction is a sign of healing bone and can be an early sign of osteomyelitis, previous trauma, or tumor. Mneumonic for a differential diagnosis of periosteal reaction is "SPOC."

A. Osteomyelitis.
   1. Mode of transmission in infancy and childhood.
      a. Hematogenous.
      b. Direct extension.
         *1.* Cellulitis.
         *2.* Sinuses.
      c. Direct implantation.
         *1.* Postoperative.
         *2.* Open fracture.
         *3.* Stubbed toe (impacted nail bed is source).
   2. Common sites.
      a. Femur (55%).
      b. Humerus (27%).
      c. Tibia (23%).
      d. Multisite involvement common in neonates and infants.
   3. Pathogens.
      a. *Staphlococcus aureus.*
      b. Group B *Streptoccocus* (neonates).
      c. *Salmonella* or *Streptococcus pneumoniae* (sickle cell anemia).
      d. Fungal or mycobacterial (immunocompromised).
   4. Occurs more commonly in males than in females (reason unknown; perhaps more trauma in males).
   5. Vascular anatomy is crucial component in evaluation of osteomyelitis, because hematogenous route is favored in pediatric patients.
      a. Blood supply flows to metaphysis, via nutrient arteries that enter diaphysis, and extend up to metaphysis.
      b. Metaphysis is common site of osteomyelitis because of slower blood flow in this region.
      c. From birth to approximately 18 months, venous channels can cross growth plate, connecting epiphysis to metaphysis. This connection is severed with appearance of epiphyseal ossification center.
      d. Osteomyelitis: most common location by age.
         *1.* Infant.
            *a.* Metaphyseal with epiphyseal extension.
            *b.* Up to age of appearance of ossification center.
            *c.* Isolated epiphyseal osteomyelitis can occur, but is rare.
         *2.* Child or skeletally immature adolescent (metaphyseal location).
         *3.* Skeletally mature adult (epiphyseal location).
   6. Other factors critical in spread of osteomyelitis.
      a. Loosely attached periosteum in children (pus can dissect and spread).

b. Presence of intraarticular metaphysis with access to joint space.
   1. Hip.
   2. Shoulder.
   3. Elbow.

> **Imaging** Osteomyelitic bony changes on radiographs may take from 1 to 2 weeks before becoming evident (up to 50% of bony cortex must be destroyed, in order to detect on routine radiography). Nuclear medicine (Tc-99m bone scan) is much more sensitive, since positive (increased uptake) scan be seen within 24 to 72 hours after symptoms. Remember: must do whole-body scanning (clinically silent foci may be present, especially in chronic multifocal osteomyelitis). Magnetic resonance imaging (MRI) is sensitive for early marrow edema (decreased $T_1$ signal with increased $T_2$ signal). Ultrasound (US) can detect joint effusion (especially in septic hip) and subperiosteal fluid.

7. Forms of osteomyelitis.
   a. Neonatal or infantile.
      1. Multisite involvement.
      2. Etiology.
         a. Related to implanted catheters.
         b. Group B *Streptococcus*.
      3. In this age group, infection can rupture into epiphysis via venous channels that cross growth plate. Can lead to joint space involvement or septic arthritis.
      4. Can cause bone infarction.

> **Imaging** Radiographs can show metaphyseal rarefaction and trabecular or cortical destruction; visible within 7 to 14 days.

   b. Childhood (postinfant).
      1. Metaphyseal focus.
         a. No epiphyseal spread.
         b. Venous channels spanning growth plate have been discontinued.
      2. S. aureus.
      3. Complication is early growth plate closure.

> **Imaging** Soft-tissue swelling, obliteration of fat planes, metaphyseal destruction, and periosteal reaction can be seen on plain radiographs of affected site.

c. Primary epiphyseal.
   1. In infants, epiphyseal involvement is via metaphyseal spread. In this uncommon form of osteomyelitis, there is direct hematogenous spread to epiphysis.
   2. Found almost exclusively in knee; presents with pain and limp.

**Imaging** Epiphyseal lucency can be present on plain radiographs; can be mistaken for chondroblastoma (see Chapter 31).

d. Chronic circumscribed (Brodie abscess).
   1. Lower extremity; femur or tibia (90%).
   2. Metaphyseal (60%); diaphyseal (33%).

**Imaging** Radiographs demonstrate focal lucency with adjacent sclerosis often present. Periosteal reaction (40%) can also occur.

e. Chronic, recurrent, multifocal.
   1. Common sites.
      a. Femur.
      b. Tibia.
      c. Unusual sites like clavicle and sacroiliac joints.
   2. 7 to 15 years of age.
   3. No organism has been isolated; antibiotics are ineffective. May in fact be autoimmune phenomenon, and not truly infectious etiology.
   4. Gradual resolution; treatment with steroids has been advocated.

**Imaging** Multiple sites of metaphyseal destruction are present on plain radiographs; bone scan shows multiple "hot spots."

B. Septic arthritis.
   1. Most are present in children less than 3 years of age.
   2. Usually involves hip and knee, can involve elbow.
   3. Presents with pain upon movement of joint.
      a. Child refuses to walk.
      b. Given this latter history, remember to image from hip to foot.
   4. Because metaphyseal to epiphyseal connection no longer exists, etiology is probably hematogenous seeding of synovial vasculature.
   5. Subsequent osteomyelitis is concern in patient with septic hip joint, because femoral metaphysis is positioned within joint capsule.

**Imaging** Pelvic radiograph is commonly normal, although joint effusion can sometimes be seen, manifesting as increased "teardrop distance" (distance from acetabular margin,
*Continued*

> *Continued from previous page*
> so-called teardrop, to femoral neck). Mild subluxation of hip can also be present. US is helpful in elucidation of joint fluid. In case of hip efffusion, image along anteriomedial thigh in sagittal plane and look for hypoechoic convex collection along femoral margin. However, US can not distinguish between infectious and noninfectious fluid (such as toxic synovitis).

C. Diskitis.
  1. Infection and/or inflammation involving vertebral disk.
     a. Usually hematogenous seeding.
     b. Often with adjacent vertebral endplate involvement.
  2. Adult disk is avascular; therefore, vertebral osteomyelitis is more common in adults; diskitis is more common in children.
  3. Average age of patient with diskitis is 6 to 8 years of age.
  4. Location.
     a. Most common location is lumbar spine (75%), especially L3 to L5.
     b. Rarely cervical spine.

> **Imaging** MR can demonstrate early changes of diskitis with decreased disk height and increased $T_1$ signal in adjacent vertebral marrow. Bone scan is also sensitive for adjacent vertebral involvement. Radiographs can demonstrate later findings, such as loss of disk height (due to disk destruction) versus disk herniation (through eroded vertebral endplates) with irregularity and sclerosis of adjacent vertebral endplates.

  5. Differential diagnosis for nontraumatic pediatric back pain.
     a. Diskitis or osteomyelitis.
     b. Lymphoma or leukemia.
     c. Langerhans cell histiocytosis (formerly known as histiocytosis X).
        *1.* Eosinophilic granuloma.
        *2.* Vertebra plana (collapsed vertebral body).
     d. Spondylolysis.
        *1.* Congenital.
        *2.* Traumatic.
     e. Benign bone lesions.
        *1.* Osteoid osteoma.
        *2.* Osteoblastoma.
     f. Metastases.
        *1.* Neuroblastoma metastases.
        *2.* "Drop mets" from central nervous system primary, often from posterior fossa.

> **Imaging** Back pain in child is serious complaint until proven otherwise. All children with back pain merit at least radiographs of lumbosacral spine; oblique views can be helpful, looking for spondylolysis (lucency through "Scotty dog"). If lumbar radiographs are negative and pain is unremitting, bone scan, especially single photon emission computed tomography (SPECT) and MRI are other options.

D. Periosteal reaction.
   1. Sign of healing bone; can be early sign of osteomyelitis.
   2. Differential diagnosis of periosteal reaction (SPOC).
      a. *S.*
         *1.* Syphilis.
            a. Congenital involvement.
            b. Diffuse symmetric periostitis; often with focal bony destruction.
            c. Look particularly at proximal femur, tibia, and humerus.
         *2.* Scurvey (subperiosteal hemorrhage).
         *3.* Sickle cell anemia.
            a. Dactylitis or hand-foot syndrome.
               *1)* Often earliest manifestation of disease.
               *2)* Sludging in small tubular bones of hands and feet cause pain and swelling with bony periosteal reaction from bony infarctions.
            b. Osteomyelitis.
               *1)* Most common is *S. aureus.*
               *2)* Salmonella.
         *4.* Stress fractures.
      b. *P.*
         *1.* Physiologic.
            a. Periosteal reaction that can be normal in infants from 4 to 8 months of age.
            b. Look for bilateral, symmetric involvement along one side of cortex only.
            c. Especially seen in long bones (tibia, humeri).
         *2.* Prostaglandin administration.
      c. *O.*
         *1.* Osteomyelitis.
         *2.* Other.
            a. Hypervitaminosis A.
               *1)* Periosteal reaction of ulna preferentially.
               *2)* Widened cranial sutures.
               *3)* Skin rash.

d. C.
1. Child abuse.
2. Cancer.
   a. Leukemia.
   b. Bone tumor.
      1) Osteogenic sarcoma.
         a) Elevation of periosteum (Codman triangle).
         b) Usually around knee.
      2) Ewing sarcoma.
         a) Lamellar or "onionskin" periosteal reaction.
         b) Often seen in diaphysis of bones or in flat bones, such as pelvis and clavicle.
   c. Metastases (often neuroblastoma).
3. Caffey syndrome.
   a. Also known as infantile cortical hyperostosis.
   b. Uncommon, self-limiting disease of infancy; usually seen in infants less than 6 months of age but has been seen in children up to 12 years of age.
   c. No known etiology.
   d. Interesting entity; rarely seen in last 20 years.
   e. Clinical presentation.
      1) Irritability.
      2) Febrile.
      3) Soft-tissue swelling.
   f. Location.
      1) Mandible.
      2) Clavicles.
      3) Ribs.
      4) Long-bone involvement is less likely.

> **Imaging** With Caffey syndrome, radiographs of affected region reveal bony cortical hyperostosis (often asymmetric). Radiographic findings may persist after clinical findings have subsided; they, too, eventually resolve.

**SUGGESTED READINGS**

Forster A, Pothmann R, Winter K, Baumann-Roth CA: Magnetic resonance imaging in nonspecific discitis. *Pediatr Radiol* 1987; 17:162-163.

Hamdan J, Asha M, Malloun A, Usta H, Talab Y, Ahmad M: Technetium bone scintigraphy in the diagnosis of osteomyelitis in children. *Pediatr Infect Dis J* 1987; 5:529-532.

Howard CB, Einhorn M, Dagan R, Nyska M: Ultrasound in diagnosis and management of acute hematogenous osteomyelitis in children. *J Bone Joint Surg Br* 1993; 75:79-82.

Gold RH, Hawkins RA, Katz RD: Bacterial osteomyelitis: Findings on plain radiography, CT, MR and scintigraphy. *AJR* 1991; 157:365-370.

Kaiser S, Rosenborg M: Early detection of subperiosteal abscesses by ultrasonography. *Pediatr Radiol* 1994; 24:336-339.

Lim-Dunham JE, Ben-Ami TE, Yousefzadeh DK: Septic arthritis of the elbow in children: The role of sonography. *Pediatr Radiol* 1995; 25:556-559.

Mirales M, Gonzalez G, Pulpeiro JR, Millan JM, Gordillo I, Serrano C, Olcoz F, Martinez A: Sonography of the painful hip in children: 500 consecutive cases. *AJR* 1989; 152:579-582.

Pazzaglia UE, Byers PD, Beluffi G, Chirico G, Rondini G, Cecilian L: Pathology of infantile cortical hyperostosis (Caffey's disease). *J Bone Joint Surg Am* 1985; Dec, 67(9):1417-1426.

Pinckney LE, Currarino G, Kennedy LA: The stubbed great toe: A cause of occult compound fracture and infection. *Radiology* 1981; 138:375-377.

Poznanski AK, Fernbach SK, Berry TE: Bone changes from prostaglandin therapy. *Skeletal Radiol* 1985; 14:20-25.

Riebel TW, Nasir R, Nazarenko O: Value of sonography in the detection of osteomyelitis. *Pediatr Radiol* 1996; 26:291-297.

Rosenbaum DN, Blumhagen JD: Acute epiphyseal osteomyelitis in children. *Radiology* 1985; 156:89-92.

Rosenberg ZS, Shankman S, Klein M, Lehman W: Chronic recurrent multifocal osteomyelitis. *AJR* 1988; 151:142-144.

Scauwecker DS: The scintigraphic diagnosis of osteomyelitis. *AJR* 1992; 158:9-18.

Zeiger MM, Dorr U, Schultz RD: Ultrasonography of hip joint effusions. *Skeletal Radiol* 1987; 16:607-611.

# 31
## Lesions of Bone—Benign and Malignant

### Key Concepts

1. As a general rule, pediatric bone lesions can be categorized according to the histology of the lesion. These categories include lesions of osteoblastic, cartilaginous, or fibrous origin, as well as cystic or marrow lesions.
2. Osteosarcoma, an osteoid-forming tumor, is the most common bone primary malignancy in children. Common location is around the knee (50% to 75%). Usual age range is adolescence to young adulthood.
3. Fibrous cortical defect (FCD) is a very common benign fibrous lesion in children and is a "leave alone" lesion. It is often cortically based near the metaphysis and usually located in the distal femur and proximal tibia.
4. Fibrous dysplasia is a benign fibroosseous lesion that usually occurs in the lower extremities; classic radiographic description is "ground glass" appearance of the medullary cavity of bone.
5. Unicameral bone cyst (simple bone cyst) is a medullary lesion in the metaphysis of the bone that often extends up to the epiphysis. Ninety percent occur in the proximal humerus or femur, often with resulting pathologic fracture ("fallen fragment" sign).

A. Categorization of bone lesions.
 1. As general rule, pediatric bone lesions can be categorized according to histology of lesion.
    a. Osteoblastic origin.
       *1.* Osteoma.
       *2.* Osteoid osteoma.
       *3.* Osteoblastoma.
       *4.* Osteosarcoma.
    b. Cartilaginous origin.
       *1.* Enchondroma.
       *2.* Osteochondroma (exostosis).
       *3.* Chondroblastoma.
       *4.* Chondromyxoid fibroma.
       *5.* Chondrosarcoma (not considered pediatric tumor).
    c. Fibrous-tissue origin.
       *1.* Fibrocortical defects (nonossifying fibroma).
       *2.* Ossifying fibroma.
       *3.* Fibrous dysplasia.
       *4.* Adamantinoma.
       *5.* Malignant fibrous histiocytoma.
    d. Cystic lesions.
       *1.* Unicameral bone cyst.
       *2.* Aneurysmal bone cyst.
       *3.* Intraosseous ganglion.
       *4.* Epidermoid cyst.
    e. Marrow tumors (round cell tumors).
       *1.* Ewing sarcoma.
       *2.* Langerhans cell histiocytosis (eosinophilic granuloma).
       *3.* Lymphoma (reticulum cell sarcoma).
       *4.* Leukemia.
       *5.* Infiltrative lesions, such as Gaucher disease or Neimann-Pick disease.
    f. Miscellaneous origin.
       *1.* Metastatic (neuroblastoma).
       *2.* Hemangioma or hemangioendothelioma.
       *3.* Rhabdomyosarcoma.
 2. General characteristics of bone lesions.
    a. Benign (leave alone) lesion.
       *1.* Well-circumscribed.
       *2.* Geographic.
       *3.* Sclerotic border.
       *4.* Periosteal reaction only if pathologic fracture coexists.
    b. Malignant, infiltrative, or progressive.

1. Moth-eaten.
2. Cortical destruction.
3. Periosteal reaction.
4. May have soft-tissue component.

B. Osseous lesions.
   1. Osteoma.
      a. Dense, compact bone, arising from membranous bone.
      b. Location.
         1. Skull.
         2. Nasal sinuses.
         3. Mandible.
      c. Asymptomatic.
      d. Gardner syndrome.
         1. Intestinal polyposis.
         2. Osteomas.
         3. Desmoid tumors.

   **Imaging** Sclerotic focus within bone seen on plain radiograph, often less than 2 cm in size.

   2. Osteoid osteoma.
      a. Location.
         1. Cortically based.
         2. Common sites.
            a. Tibia or femur (50%).
            b. Posterior elements of spine (10% to 20%) with most in lumbar spine.
      b. Often seen in 2nd and 3rd decades of life, in males more commonly than in females.
      c. Symptoms.
         1. Dull pain, worse at night; relieved by aspirin.
         2. Can cause painful scoliosis.
      d. Treatment.
         1. Computed tomography–guided percutaneous removal versus surgical removal of nidus.
         2. Conservative treatment with aspirin (will eventually regress but may take years).

   **Imaging** Central lucent osteoid nidus (less than 1 cm) with adjacent sclerosis can be seen on plain radiograph or computed tomography (CT); magnetic resonance imaging (MRI) does not image this cortical lesion as well as CT.

   3. Osteoblastoma.

a. Closely related to osteoid osteoma (also known as "giant osteoid osteoma").
b. Common location.
   1. Spine (30% to 40%).
   2. Especially in posterior elements or pedicles.
c. Often occurs during 2nd and 3rd decades of life; occurs in males more commonly than in females (2:1).
d. Main symptom is pain; often less intense than osteoid osteoma.
e. Treatment.
   1. Surgical curettage.
   2. Rare recurrence.

**Imaging** Radiographs show sclerotic, often expansile lesion; greater than 1.5 to 2 cm in size.

4. Osteosarcoma.
   a. Osteoid forming tumor.
   b. Location.
      1. Around knee (50% to 75%).
         a. Femur (40%).
         b. Tibia (16%).
      2. Metaphyseal.
      3. Cortical desmoid.
         a. Located in posteromedial distal femur.
         b. Mimicks osteosarcoma.
   c. Age range is 10 to 25 years; no gender difference.
   d. Symptoms are pain and swelling.
   e. Variety of types.
      1. Classic medullary osteosarcoma.
      2. Parosteal osteosarcoma.
         a. Usually occurs in older patients (20 to 40 years of age).
         b. Arises from periosteum.
         c. Better prognosis than classic osteosarcoma.
         d. Makes up 3% to 5% of all osteosarcoma types.
      3. Periosteal (juxtacortical) osteosarcoma.
         a. Arises from margin of periosteum and cortex.
         b. Usually occurs in older patients.
      4. Telangiectatic osteosarcoma.
         a. Worse prognosis than classic osteosarcoma.
         b. Very destructive lesion.
         c. May have extraosseous masses with fluid levels, resulting from blood-filled cysts.
      5. Radiation- or chemotherapy-induced osteosarcoma.

                a. Usually seen many years after chemotherapy or radiation treatment.
                b. Poor prognosis.
             6. Multifocal osteosarcoma.
                a. Multiple synchronous lesions; not metastatic.
                b. Poor prognosis.
          f. Treatment.
             1. Chemotherapy and wide-section excision, if possible.
             2. Limb salvage.
                a. Excision of tumor with preservation of limb.
                b. Use of artificial prosthesis.
             3. 5-year survival rate is up to 80% with aggressive chemotherapy.

> **Imaging** Radiographs and CT demonstrate metaphyseal medullary destructive lesion with periosteal reaction (can be exuberant, "sunburst" periostitis) and cortical disruption. MRI can show both bone marrow extension and soft-tissue extension of tumor. Pulmonary nodules are concern, since lung is common site for metastatic disease.

C. Cartilaginous lesions.
   1. Enchondroma.
      a. Benign medullary rests of cartilage.
      b. Location.
         1. Often seen in small tubular bones of hands and feet (50%).
         2. Also seen in humerus and femur.
      c. Common age range is 10 to 40 years; male versus female rate of incidence is equal (1:1).
      d. Lesion is usually painless unless pathologic fracture occurs.
      e. Ollier disease.
         1. Multiple enchondromatosis (not hereditary).
         2. Shortening and deformities of involved bones with up to 30% developing chondrosarcoma.
         3. Associated with multiple soft-tissue hemangiomas (Maffucci syndrome).

> **Imaging** Radiographs show geographic, lucent, medullary lesion with calcific flecks; may be expansile.

   2. Osteochondroma (exostosis).
      a. Cartilage-capped bony outgrowth from metaphysis.
      b. Usually located in long bones.
      c. Commonly seen in first 3 decades of life.

d. Usually asymptomatic.
   e. Multiple hereditary exostoses.
      1. Multiple exostoses that can cause limb deformities.
      2. Malignant degeneration.
   f. Treatment is surgical removal, if symptomatic.

> **Imaging** Smooth bony projection that usually points away from growth plate on radiographs; may have calcified cartilaginous cap. In rare instances, these outgrowths may become malignant.

3. Chondroblastoma.
   a. Rare, benign, cartilaginous lesion.
   b. Location.
      1. Only purely epiphyseal lesion; often seen in knee (50%).
      2. Proximal humerus.
   c. Commonly seen in 2nd and 3rd decades of life.
   d. Symptoms are pain and joint effusion (occasionally).

> **Imaging** Plain radiographs reveal lucent geographic lesion located solely within epiphysis, with occasional marginal sclerosis.

4. Chondromyxoid fibroma.
   a. Rare, benign, often expansile metaphyseal lesion composed of cartilage, myxoid, and fibrous tissues.
   b. Location.
      1. Usually found in lower extremity (75%).
      2. Especially tibia.
   c. Occurs at any age but peaks in adolescence.
   d. Symptoms are vague pain.

> **Imaging** Plain radiograph demonstrates eccentric, lucent, often loculated geographic metaphyseal lesion, with sclerotic rim (occasionally with calcifications).

5. Chondrosarcoma.
   a. Maligant but slow-growing tumor of cartilaginous cells.
   b. Location.
      1. Can arise anew in pelvis, femur.
      2. Can arise in preexisting benign lesion, such as enchondroma or exostosis.
   c. Not considered pediatric tumor, as average age of patients is 40 to 50 years.
   d. Symptoms are pain, often for long duration, prior to diagnosis.
   e. Treatment.

1. Surgical resection.
2. Radiotherapy.

**Imaging** Radiographs can demonstrate large soft-tissue mass with calcifications. Underlying bony destruction is often present.

D. Fibrous lesions.
1. Fibrous cortical defect.
   a. Also known as nonossifying fibroma (NOF).
   b. Very common benign fibrous lesion, estimated to be present in 30% to 40% of all children.
   c. Arises at epiphyseal plate and "migrates" down diaphysis, as child grows.
   d. Location.
      1. Cortically based near metaphysis (FCD is less than 2 cm in size).
      2. Eccentric, more medullary location; NOF greater than 2 cm in size.
      3. Common sites include distal femur and tibia.
   e. Seen in children and young adults with gradual involution of lesion.
   f. Symptoms.
      1. None, unless pathologic fracture is present.
      2. Usually incidental finding.
   g. No treatment needed (leave alone lesion).

**Imaging** Radiographs show geographic (cortical) lucent lesion with sclerotic rim.

2. Ossifying fibroma.
   a. Rare, cortical lesion, also known as "intracortical fibrous dysplasia."
   b. Location.
      1. Diaphysis of tibia along anterior cortex.
      2. Fibula.
   c. Seen during early childhood.
   d. Usually painless lesion, but can lead to tibial bowing or pathologic fractures.

**Imaging** "Bubbly," septated cortical lesion is seen on plain radiograph.

3. Adamantinoma.
   a. Rare fibrous tumor that can vary from benign to aggressive; resembles fibrosarcoma.

b. Location.
   1. Often seen in jaw.
   2. Tibia.
c. Common age of presentation is between 2nd and 5th decades of life.
d. Symptoms are local pain and swelling, often with traumatic history.

> **Imaging** Plain radiograph shows eccentric, lucent, geographic, "bubbly" lesion, often with sclerotic rim; may be expansile.

4. Fibrous dysplasia.
   a. Benign fibroosseous lesion.
   b. Location.
      1. Usually seen in lower extremities.
      2. Skull.
      3. Monostotic (75%); polystotic (25%).
   c. Presents at any age.
   d. Symptoms.
      1. Pain can be present with pathologic fracture.
      2. Bony deformities.
         a. Cherubism.
            1) Expansile lesions of jaw.
            2) Children under 4 years of age.
            3) Hereditary.
         b. Leontiasis ossea ("lion's face").
            1) Sclerosis of skull and facial bones.
            2) Assymetric thickening.
         c. McCune-Albright syndrome.
            1) Polyostotic fibrous dysplasia.
            2) Precocious puberty in female.
            3) "Café-au-lait" spots.

> **Imaging** Radiographs demonstrate medullary, occasionally expansile geographic lesion with ground-glass matrix and cortical thinning.

E. Cystic lesions.
   1. Unicameral bone cyst.
      a. Simple bone cyst.
      b. Location.
         1. Medullary lesion in metaphysis, extending up to epiphysis.
         2. Vast majority in proximal humerus or femur (90%); also calcaneus.

c. Common age is 2 to 20 years; found in males more commonly than in females (3:1).
   d. Usually asymptomatic, unless pathologic fracture is present; look for fallen fragment sign.
   e. Treatment.
      *1.* Intralesional steroids.
      *2.* Curettage and packing with bone chips.

> **Imaging** Radiograph reveals thinned cortex resulting from expansile, lucent, but often loculated bubbly lesion.

2. Aneurysmal bone cyst.
   a. Lytic, expansile lesion (hence name).
   b. Not true neoplasm; etiology is unknown (perhaps related to prior infection or trauma).
   c. Location.
      *1.* Metaphysis of long bones.
      *2.* Small tubular bones of hands and feet.
      *3.* Also seen in spine and flat bones of pelvis.
   d. Common age range is 6 to 25 years.
   e. Symptom is pain, often from pathologic fracture.
   f. Treatment.
      *1.* Curettage and drainage of blood.
      *2.* Packing of lesions.
      *3.* Frequent recurrence.

> **Imaging** Lytic, geographic, expansile "blow-out" lesion on plain radiograph, occasionally with cortical disruption. CT or MRI may detect fluid levels from blood-filled cavity of lesion.

3. Intraosseous ganglion.
   a. Benign, fibrous cystic lesion.
   b. Location.
      *1.* Most commonly in distal tibia (medial malleolus).
      *2.* Carpals.
   c. May present at any age.
   d. Symptoms.
      *1.* May have pain.
      *2.* Often newly discovered palpable lesion.

> **Imaging** Radiographs may show geographic, lucent lesion with thin sclerotic border; lesion is usually adjacent to joint surface.

4. Epidermoid cyst.

a. Lesion that contains squamous epithelium, keratin, and cholesterol.
b. Location.
   1. Skull (especially intrasutural).
   2. Terminal phalanges (associated with trauma history).
c. Common age range is between 2nd and 4th decades of life.

> **Imaging** Skull radiographs demonstrate geographic lucency with sclerotic border; lesion is often found near sutures. Similar finding is seen in terminal phalanges, except that lesion may be expansile.

F. Marrow lesions.
  1. Ewing sarcoma.
     a. Round cell malignant tumor.
     b. Location.
        1. Found in lower extremities, considered diaphyseal lesion (but only 25% of time); more often metaphyseal.
        2. Found in flat bones more frequently, if patient is less than 18 years of age.
           *a.* Pelvis.
           *b.* Spine.
           *c.* Scapula.
           *d.* Ribs.
     c. Age range of presentation is 10 to 20 years.
     d. Symptoms include local pain and swelling.
     e. Treatment.
        1. Radiation or chemotherapy.
        2. Resection if possible.
        3. Prognosis: 5-year survival rate of 70%.

> **Imaging** Permeative, bony, destructive lesion with onion-skin periostitis can be seen on CT and radiographs. Soft-tissue mass is often associated with this malignant bony tumor.

  2. Lymphoma or leukemia (see Chapter 35).
  3. Eosinophilic granuloma (see Chapter 35).
  4. Osteomyelitis (see Chapter 30).

**SUGGESTED READINGS**

Appell BG, Opperman HC, Brandeis WE: Skeletal lesions of Hodgkins disease: Review of the literature and case reports. *Pediatr Radiol* 1981; 11:61-65.

Azouz RM, Kozlowski K, Marton D, Sprague P, Zerhouni A, Assilah F: Osteoid osteoma and osteoblastoma of the spine in children: Report of 22 cases with brief literature review. *Pediatr Radiol* 1986; 16:25-31.

Bloehm J, Mulder JD: Chondroblastoma: A clinical and radiological study of 104 cases. *Skeletal Radiol* 1985; 14:1-9.

Frouge C, Vanel D, Coffre C, Corranet D, Contesso G, Sarrazin D: The role of magnetic resonance imaging in the evaluation of Ewing's sarcoma: A report of 27 cases. *Skeletal Radiol* 1988; 17:387-392.

Helms CA: Skeletal "don't touch" lesions. *Appl Radiol* July 1992: 16-21.

Kriss VM, Stelling CB: Osteosarcoma following chemotherapy for neuroblastoma. *Skeletal Radiol* 1995; 24(8):633-635.

Kroon HH, Schurmans J: Osteoblastoma: Clinical and radiographic findings in 98 new cases. *Radiology* 1990; 175:783-790.

Kumar R, Madewell JE, Lindell MM, Swischuk LE: Fibrous lesions of bone. *Radiographics* 1990; 10:237-256.

Moore TE, King AR, Travis RC, Allen BC: Post-traumatic cysts and cyst-like lesions of bone. *Skeletal Radiol* 1989; 18:93-97.

Myles ST MacRae ME: Benign osteoblastoma of the spine in childhood. *J Neurosurg* 1988; 68:884-888.

Ritschl P, Karnel F, Hajek P: Fibrous metaphyseal defects: Determination of their origin and natural history using a radiomorphological study. *Skeletal Radiol* 1988; 17:8-15.

Sundaram M, McGuire MH, Herbold DR: Magnetic resonance imaging of osteosarcoma. *Skeletal Radiol* 1987; 16:23-29.

Tucker MA, D'Angio GJ, Boice JD Jr, Strong LC, Li FP, Stovall M, Stone BJ, Green DM, Lombardi F, Newton W: Bone sarcomas linked to radiotherapy and chemotherapy in children. *N Engl J Med* 1987; 317:588-593.

Vanel D Tcheng S, Contesso G, Zafrani B, Kalifa C, Dubousset J, Kron P: The radiological appearance of telangiectatic osteosarcoma: A study of 14 cases. *Skeletal Radiol* 1987; 16:196-200.

Zilmer DA, Dorfman HD: Chondromyxoid fibroma of bone: Thirty-six cases with clinicopathologic correlation. *Hum Pathol* 1989; 20:952-964.

# 32
# Axial Skeleton: Spine and Skull

### Key Concepts

1. Pseudosubluxation and mild atlantoaxial separation are normal variants of the cervical spine in infants and small children.
2. Seen in infants and small children, spinal cord injury without radiographic abnormality (SCIWORA) is due to the unusually elastic pediatric bony spine. Direct cord trauma can occur followed by spontaneous reduction of the bony spine, resulting in a normal cervical radiograph in a child with neurologic deficit.
3. Types of scoliosis include congenital, neuromuscular (C-shaped), idiopathic (S-shaped) or can be due to bony lesions or tumors (such as neurofibromatosis).
4. Common causes for bony skull lesions are epidermoids, Langerhans cell histiocytosis (eosinophilic granuloma), hemangioma, or metastases (usually caused by neuroblastoma).
5. Craniosynostosis is premature fusion of the sutures of the skull. Depending on the type of suture and the extent of synostosis, characteristic bony skull configurations can result. Sagittal synostosis is the most common, producing the elongated skull known as dolichocephaly or scaphocephaly.

A. Spine.
   1. Normal variants.
      a. Pseudosubluxation.
         *1.* Hypermobility of upper cervical spine.
            *a.* Angulation and apparent forward slippage usually involving C2 on C3.
            *b.* Can involve C3 on C4 (14%).
         *2.* Usually seen in children.
            *a.* In normal children less than 8 years of age (40%).
            *b.* Although uncommon, can be present in adolescents.
         *3.* To rule out fracture, evaluate posterior laminar line. If pseudosubluxation is present, there is at most 1 mm gap (Fig. 32-1).
      b. Atlantoaxial subluxation.
         *1.* Up to 3 to 5 mm of C1 and C2 separation is accepted in young children; only 2 mm in adults.
         *2.* Mild movement of C1 or C2 on flexion or extension films can also be normal in infants and young children.
         *3.* Down syndrome.
            *a.* Greater than 5 mm of atlantoaxial separation can be seen in children with Down syndrome.
            *b.* These children are predisposed to subluxation presumably because of ligamentous laxity.
            *c.* In children with Down syndrome, 25% have hypoplastic arch of C1; when coupled with aforementioned ligamentous laxity can result in "double jeopardy" or increased risk of injury.

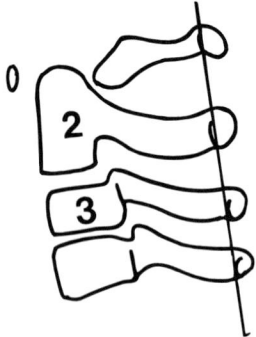

**Fig. 32-1** Posterior laminar line (pseudosubluxation): alignment of posterior lamina signals normal cervical alignment despite pseudosubluxation of C2 vertebral body in relation to C3.

    d. Imaging for "Special Olympics" participation of children with Down syndrome.
        1) Single lateral cervical spine radiograph in flexion (let child flex neck).
        2) Value of required imaging in acutally detecting patients at risk is still unproven.
  c. Vertebral configuration.
      1. Anteriorly "wedged" or compressed appearance of C3 through C7 vertebral bodies (especially C3).
      2. Normal in infants and small children.
  d. Pseudo-Jefferson fracture.
      1. "Off-set" appearance (up to 3 to 4 mm) of lateral masses of C1 on odontoid view of standard cervical spine series.
      2. Common appearance in children under age 2 (90%); can be seen in children up to age 7.
      3. True Jefferson ("burst") fractures of C1 are rare in infants and small children.
2. SCIWORA (Spinal Cord Injury without Radiographic Abnormality).
  a. Seen in infants and small children.
  b. Unusual elasticity of pediatric bony spine allows deformation of musculoskeletal structures beyond physiologic extremes; causes direct cord trauma, followed by spontaneous reduction of bony spine.
  c. Predisposing factors or risks.
      1. Unique hypermobility of infant spine.
          a. Facet joints of children are more horizontally oriented.
          b. Physiologic anterior wedging of vertebral bodies (see previous discussion).
      2. Ligamentous laxity of pediatric spine.

**Imaging** Normal cervical spine radiograph is seen, although severe clinical picture may be present. MRI is imaging modality of choice; can reveal spinal cord hematoma, edema, or transection.

3. Scoliosis.
  a. Congenital scoliosis.
      1. Developmental scoliosis induced by congenital anomalies of spine.
      2. Seen with wedge vertebrae, hemivertebrae, or butterfly vertebrae.
      3. Sharply angulated scoliosis at level of vertebral defect.
  b. Neuromuscular scoliosis (nonambulatory child).

1. C-shaped scoliosis; no compensatory curve, as is seen in idiopathic scoliosis.
2. Commonly seen in cerebral palsy.
3. Associated with coxa valga and hip dislocation.
  c. Idiopathic scoliosis.
    1. Lateral curvature of spine.
       a. S-shaped curve.
       b. Commonly presents as dextroscoliosis of thoracic spine with compensatory levoscoliosis of lumbar spine.
       c. Upright posture with normal ambulation results in lumbar compensatory component.
    2. Three types.
       a. Infantile.
          1) Associated with developmental dysplasia of hip.
          2) Associated with tethered cord.
       b. Juvenile (4 to 10 years of age).
       c. Adolescent.
          1) Most common form.
          2) Found in females more commonly than in males (up to 8:1).
    3. Treatment of idiopathic scoliosis.
       a. Nonoperative (brace) when curvatures approach 20 to 30 degrees.
       b. Surgical spinal fusion is reserved for adolescent scoliosis of 40 to 50 degrees or greater; for younger children with more rapidly progressing scoliosis, spinal fusion is considered in cases with even lesser degrees of scoliosis.

**Imaging** Scoliosis is evaluated on anteroposterior radiograph of spine in standing child; lateral is obtained for evaluation of kyphosis. Scoliosis is measured using Cobb method (Fig. 32-2).

  d. Nonidiopathic scoliosis; can be associated with pain.
    1. Intraspinal pathology.
       a. Tumors.
       b. Syrinx.
       c. Tethered cord.
    2. Neurofibromatosis; usually short, severe segments of scoliosis.
    3. Spine bony lesions.
       a. Osteoid osteoma.

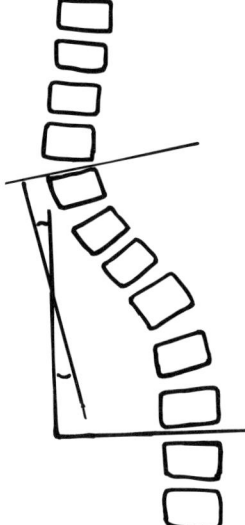

**Fig. 32-2** Scoliosis measurements (Cobb method): Line is drawn through superior and inferior endplates of vertebral bodies that encompass curve, respectively. A perpendicular line is dropped from these endplate lines and angle is measured where these lines intersect.

       b. Osteoblastoma.
       c. Vertebral body collapse.
           *1)* Osteomyelitis (tuberculosis or Pott's disease).
           *2)* Metastatic lesions.
           *3)* Langerhans cell histiocytosis.
    4. Postradiation.
    5. Associated with leg-length discrepancy.
    6. Spondylolysis or spondylolisthesis.
    7. Appendicitis; splint to right side because of pain.
    8. Scheuermann kyphosis.
       a. Greater than 40 degrees of thoracic kyphosis.
       b. Anterior vertebral wedging.
       c. Fragmented and irregular ossification of ring apophysis.
4. Schmorl node.
    a. Herniation of nucleus pulposis through vertebral body endplate.
    b. Focal defect along endplate of vertebral body, often with adjacent sclerosis.
    c. Very common; estimate over 50% present in adolescents and adults.

d. Asymptomatic.
B. Skull.
  1. Bony lesions.
     a. Epidermoids.
        *1.* Ectodermal rest within skull or inner table.
        *2.* Smooth, well-demarcated lesion with sclerotic border.
        *3.* Often intrasutural location.
     b. Langerhans cell histiocytosis (see Chapter 35).
     c. Hemangioma.
        *1.* Round lesions.
        *2.* Radial, spiculated, or striated pattern.
     d. Leptomeningeal cyst.
        *1.* Posttraumatic, also called "growing fracture."
        *2.* Skull fracture; underlying damaged dura with cerebrospinal fluid leakage can lead to formation of cyst.
        *3.* Over time (months or years), brain pulsations upon cyst can cause large defect to occur at site of fracture.
     e. Metastases.
        *1.* Usually multiple, lucent lesions of differing sizes.
        *2.* Neuroblastoma.
  2. Craniosynostosis.
     a. Premature fusion of sutures of skull.
     b. Depending on type of suture and extent of synostosis, characteristic bony-skull configurations result.
        *1.* Sagittal synostosis.
           *a.* Most common.
           *b.* Produces elongated skull known as dolichocephaly or scaphocephaly.
        *2.* Coronal synostosis.
           *a.* "Harlequin eye" can form (see following discussion).
           *b.* When bilateral, produces brachiocephalic skull (short and wide).
           *c.* Associations.
              *1)* Apert syndrome (coronal synostosis with syndactyly).
              *2)* Crouzon disease (cranial facial dysostosis).
        *3.* Metopic synostosis.
           *a.* Pointy forehead.
           *b.* Also known as trigonocephaly.
        *4.* Lambdoid synostosis.
           *a.* If bilateral, brachiocephalic skull forms.
           *b.* If unilateral, can result in plagiocephaly.
        *5.* Kleeblattschädel syndrome.
           *a.* Cloverleaf skull.

b. Universal craniosynostosis (all sutures prematurely fused).
   c. Occurs early in gestation.

> **Imaging** On skull radiographs, try to locate each suture (sagittal, coronal, lambdoid, and metopic). Ascertain if they are still patent (lucent). Sclerosis with "heaped up" margins, coupled with abnormal skull configuration, is suggestive of synostosis. Configuration of orbit is also sensitive indicator of sutural synostosis. Orbit should always be sharp and fairly round. With elongation of lateral aspect of bony orbit ("Harlequin eye"), one should consider synostosis (especially coronal). The best imaging modality for craniosynostosis is computed tomography with three-dimensional reconstruction; can directly visualize bony defects and sutural status.

## SUGGESTED READINGS

Citron N, Edgar MA, Sheehy J, Thomas DGT: Intramedullary spinal cord tumors presenting as scoliosis. *J Bone Joint Surg Am* 1984; 66B:513-517.

Deacon P, Flood BM, Dickson RA: Idiopathic scoliosis in three dimensions. *J Bone Joint Surg Am* 1985; 66B:509-513.

Gellad FE, Haney PJ, Son JC, Robinson WL, Rao KCVG, Johnston GS: Imaging modalities of craniosynostosis with surgical and pathological correlation. *Pediatr Radiol* 1985; 15:285-290.

Husson B, Pariente D, Tamman S, Zerah M: Value of MRI in the early diagnosis of growing skull fracture. *Pediatr Radiol* 1996; 26:744-747.

Kriss VM, Kriss TC: Imaging of the cervical spine in infants. *Pediatr Emerg Care* 1997; 13:44-49.

Kriss VM, Kriss TC: SCIWORA (Spinal Cord Injury WithOut Radiographic Abnormality) in infants and children. *Clin Pediatr* 1996; 35:119-124.

Madigan RR, Wallace SL: Scoliosis in the institutionalized cerebral palsy population. *Spine* 1981; 6:583-590.

Martich V, Ben-Ami T, Yousefzadeh DK, Roizen NJ: The hypoplastic posterior arch of C1 in Down syndrome—A double jeopardy. *Radiology* 1992; 183:125-128.

O'Connor JF, Cranley WR, McCarten KM, Feingold M: Commentary: Atlantoaxial instability in Down syndrome: Reassessment by the Committee on Sports Medicine and Fitness of the American Academy of Pediatrics. *Pediatr Radiol* 1996; 26:748-749.

Oda M, Rauh S, Gregory PB, Silverman FN, Bleck EE: The significance of radiographic measurement in scoliosis. *J Pediatr Orthop* 1982; 2:378-382.

Pueschel SM, Scola FH: Atlantoaxial instability in Down syndrome: Epidemiologic, radiographic and clinical studies. *Pediatrics* 1987; 80:555-560.

Ruge JR, Tomila T, Naidich TP, Hahn YS, McLone DG: Scalp and calvarial masses of infants and children. *Neurosurgery* 1988; 22:1037-1042.

Suss RA, Zimmerman RD, Leeds NE: Pseudospread of the atlas: False sign of Jefferson fracture in young children. *AJR* 1982; 140:1079-1082.

Swischuk LE: Anterior displacement of C2 in children: physiologic or pathologic? *Radiology* 1977; 122:759-763.

Swischuk LE, Swischuk PN, John SD: Wedging of C3 in infants and children: Usually a normal finding and not a fracture. *Radiology* 1993; 188:523-526.

Tandon PN, Banerji AK, Bhatia R, Goulatia RK: Craniocerebral erosion (growing fracture of the skull in children): Clincal and pathological observations. *Acta Neurochir* 1987; 88:1-9.

# 33
# Hip and Knee

---

### Key Concepts

1. Risk factors for developmental dysplasia of the hip (DDH) include:
    a. Abnormal physical examination (presence of a "hip click" or asymmetric thigh folds with abnormal position of the leg).
    b. Family history of DDH.
    c. Breech delivery (hyperflexed hip).
    d. Neuromuscular or foot abnormalities.
2. Ultrasound (US) can screen for DDH in high-risk infants. Screening examination should not be performed before 4 to 6 weeks of age, in order to reduce false-positive results related to physiologic immaturity of the hip in the neonate.
3. Hip effusion can be due to septic hip, toxic synovitis, or hematoma. US can elucidate the presence of fluid in the hip joint.
4. Avascular necrosis (AVN) of the hip is the loss of blood supply to the hip with resulting infarction of the femoral head. Idiopathic is the most common etiology in children (also known as Legg-Calvé-Perthes syndrome).
5. Juvenile rheumatoid arththritis (JRA) is a chronic polyarthritis, predominantly of larger joints, such as the knees and wrists. Radiographic findings are overgrown, hyperemic (osteopenic) epiphysis with joint space narrowing and bony erosions. Eventual bony ankylosis may occur.

A. Hip.
   1. DDH.
      a. Previously known as congenital dysplasia of hip (CDH).
      b. DDH can range from mild acetabular dysplasia, to irreducible dislocation of femoral head.
      c. Etiology: two theories.
         1. Acetabular dysplasia (too shallow; allows hip to dislocate).
         2. Joint laxity (subluxable or dislocatable hip causes acetabular dysplasia).
      d. Incidence.
         1. 1:1000 of all babies.
         2. North American Caucasian population (1% to 2%); much lower in African-American population.
         3. Found in girls much more commonly than in boys (8:1); two thirds are firstborns.
         4. Found in left hip much more commonly than in right hip (about 5:1).
      e. Clinical screening of all newborns: two maneuvers.
         1. Barlow maneuver.
            a. Progressive adduction (bring hip to midline).
            b. This maneuver flexes and stresses hip, attempting to dislocate it by posteriorly "pistoning" hip.
         2. Ortolani maneuver.
            a. Hip abduction.
            b. Attempts to relocate posteriorly dislocated hip.
            c. Hear click or feel clunk as hip relocates.
      f. Suspicious factors for DDH that merit imaging.
         1. Abnormal physical examination.
            a. Hip click (see previous discussion).
            b. Asymmetric thigh folds; abnormal position of leg.
         2. High-risk patients.
            a. Family history of DDH.
               1) Sibling with DDH; incidence is 6%.
               2) Parent with DDH; incidence in offspring is 12%.
               3) Parent with DDH and sibling with DDH; incidence in future offspring is 36%.
            b. Breech delivery (hyperflexed hip); oligohydramnios.
            c. Foot abnormalities (clubfoot, metatarsus adductus); torticollis.
            d. Neuromuscular abnormalities.
               1) Cerebral palsy.
               2) Muscular dystrophy.

**Imaging:** Radiographs.
- Lack of femoral head ossification in young infant.
  - Makes evaluation for DDH and hip subluxation difficult.
  - Normal femoral head ossification: 90% by 7 months (range: 3 to 7 months; occurs in girls sooner than in boys).
- If late or asymmetric femoral head ossification is present, DDH may be suspected.
- Rely on variety of lines and angles to approximate femoral head position (Fig. 33-1).
  - Hilgenreiner's line (line drawn through triradiate cartilage).
  - Perkin's line (line drawn perpendicular to Hilgenreiner's line that intersects outer edge of acetabulum).
  - Shenton's line (arch extending along obturator foramen to medial femoral neck). If this line is disrupted, DDH is suspected.

US.
- US can directly visualize cartilaginous femoral head and its relationship to acetabulum; acetabular shape is also evaluated.
- Dynamic study can also be done; stress Barlow maneuver is performed with direct visualization of hip stability.
- US is clearly preferable to ionizing radiation of hip radiographs.
- US can be done anytime from birth up to 8 to 10 months of age, at which time ossified femoral head interferes with examination.
- Timing of US examination.
  - Not in newborns.
    - Neonate has immature acetabulum.
    - Maternal estrogens (loosen hip and can contribute to hip joint laxity, resulting in false-positive results).
  - Fifty percent of newborn hips "tighten up" by 1 week of age; 80% tighten up by 2 months.
  - Initial newborn clinical examination for DDH will reveal 20:1000 infants are "unstable." By 3 months of age, only 1 to 2:1000 truly have DDH.

*Continued*

*Continued from previous page*
- Clinical and US examination for DDH.
  - Clinical hip screening (Barlow and Ortolani maneuvers) of all newborns at birth.
  - Sonography at 2 weeks of age for unstable hip.
  - Selective hip US screening done at 4 to 6 weeks of age.
    - Stable click.
    - High-risk factors (previously listed).
  - Advantages of US examination at 4 to 6 weeks of age.
    - Still within window of time for treatment, if positive result is obtained.
    - Decrease false-positive results related to immature acetabulum and ligamentous laxity related to maternal hormones.
    - Results in fewer repeat follow-up USs.
    - Increased detection of late presenters of DDH.
  - Dynamic US "stress" images (Harcke views) to detect hip instability (Fig. 33-2).
    - In transverse plane.
    - Do Barlow maneuver while scanning; observe femoral head movement and possible posterior displacement.

g. Treatment of DDH.
  1. Abduction devices.
     a. Pavlik harness.
     b. Casting.
     c. Surgical reduction and casting.
  2. Purpose of these abduction devices is to hold femoral head in normal position within acetabulum; acetabulum requires that femoral head be in position in order to form normally.
  3. Risk of abduction device is AVN of the hip.
  4. US of hip.
     a. Can be used to monitor progress of treatment.
     b. Can confirm correct position of femoral head during treatment.

h. Undetected (missed) DDH.
  1. Results in permanent acetabular dysplasia with delayed femoral head ossification.
  2. Long-term problems.
     a. Limp.
     b. Pain.
     c. Secondary osteoarthritis.

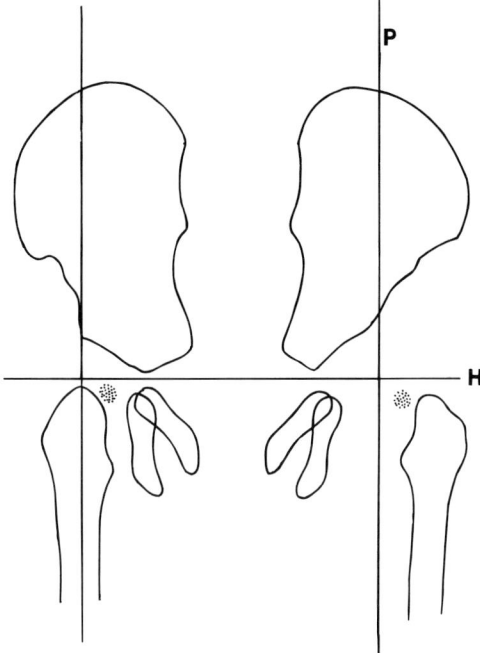

**Fig. 33-1** Radiographs of pelvis: lines and angles of DDH. Hilgenreiner's line *(H)* goes through triradiate cartilage. Perkin's line *(P)* is perpendicular to Hilgenreiner's line. The femoral head *(stippled)* should fall within lower medial quadrant. If it does not, DDH is suspected (as occurs with hip on left). Also, note steeper acetabular angle seen on left, characteristic finding with DDH.

       3. Surgical intervention.
          a. Open reduction and casting.
          b. Salter osteotomy.
             1) Ileum osteotomy to enlarge acetabulum.
             2) Procedure attempts to create a new acetabulum to "cover" subluxed hip.
  2. Hip effusion.
    a. Etiology.
       1. Septic hip.
          a. Pus in joint.
          b. Emergent condition requiring immediate hip aspiration.
       2. Toxic (transient) synovitis.
          a. Fluid in joint without evidence of bacteria, virus, or inflammatory change.
          b. Symptoms.

> **Graf US Classification of Acetabula (Detecting Shallow Acetabulum)*** (Fig. 33-3)
>
> Type I.
> - Normal acetabular morphology.
> - Alpha angle greater than 60 degrees.
>
> Type II a.
> - Child less than 3 months of age with borderline acetabular morphology and nondisplaced femoral head.
> - Alpha angle is 50 to 60 degrees, consistent with immature acetabulum.
> - Vast majority of these children progress to normal by 3 months of age (96%).
> - Repeat scanning at 3 months of age may be done to confirm this expected progression to normal.
>
> Type II b.
> - Same as II a, but child is greater than 3 months of age.
> - These children need intervention, since by 3 months, immature acetabulum should no longer be present.
>
> Type II c.
> - Acetabulum is deficient with nondisplaced femoral head (becomes II d when decentering femoral head is present).
> - Alpha angle is less than 49 degrees.
> - Intervention is required regardless of age.
>
> Type III.
> - Acetabulum is deficient.
> - Alpha angle is less than 49 degrees with subluxation of femoral head.
> - Intervention is required regardless of age.
>
> Type IV.
> - Dislocated hip.
> - Intervention warranted.

*Data from Graf R: Fundamentals of sonographic evaluation of the infant hip. *Semin Ultrasound CT MR* 1986; 4:331-338.

    *1)* Pain that subsides with rest and no other intervention.
    *2)* Limp and refusal to bear weight.
   *c.* Can be early association with Legg-Calvé-Perthes syndrome (AVN).
  3. Hematoma.
   *a.* Blood dyscrasia (hemophilia, thrombocytopenia).
   *b.* Trauma (including child abuse).
 *b.* Choice of imaging modality.
  *1.* Plain radiographs can be subtle; often not reliable modality for elucidation of effusion.
  *2.* US.

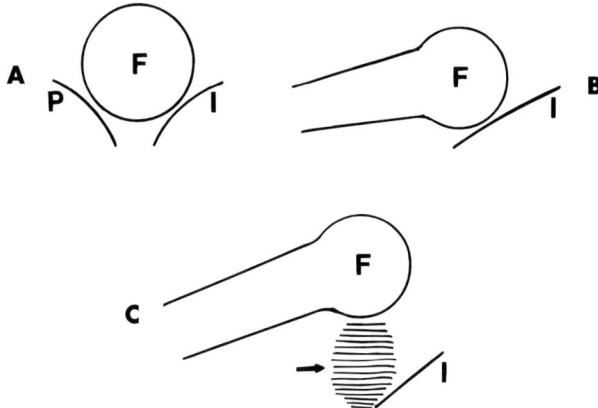

**Fig. 33-2** Dynamic US. **A,** Transverse view of hip shows normal femoral head *(F)* lying within acetabulum; ischium *(I)*, pubic bone *(P)*. Some call this "golf ball-on-a-tee" or "rose-bud" view. **B,** With hip flexed, bony femoral shaft obscures pubic bone, but femoral head *(F)* is still seen adjacent to ischium *(I)*. **C,** With subluxation of hip (after Barlow maneuver), femoral head *(F)* moves superiorly and laterally to no longer contact ischium *(I)*. Note echogenic pulvinar fat that can be apparent after hip subluxation *(arrow)*.

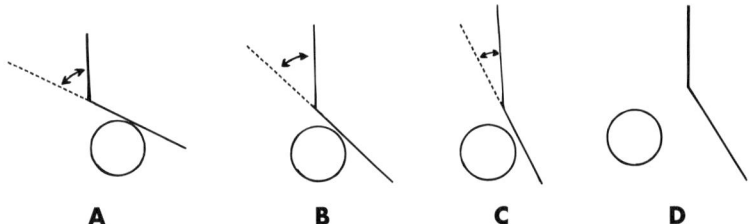

**Fig. 33-3** Graf classification (US: longitudinal view of hip). **A,** Graf I (normal). **B,** Graf II (II a or physiologic in infants less than 3 months, II b in infants greater than 3 months). **C,** Graf III (subluxed hip with steep alpha angle). **D,** Graf IV (dislocated hip). Arrows depict alpha angle.

   *a.* Sensitive for fluid collection in hip joint.
   *b.* Noninvasive, no ionizing radiation.

**Imaging** Pelvic radiographs are often normal but may show asymmetric acetabular teardrop distance indicative of fluid within joint. Adjacent bony destruction may be

*Continued*

> *Continued from previous page*
> present owing to osteomyelitis. US of hip can reveal presence of elevated joint capsule with hypoechoic fluid collection.

3. AVN.
   a. Loss of blood supply to hip with resulting infarction of femoral head.
   b. Most common etiology is idiopathic (also known as Legg-Calvé-Perthes syndrome).
   c. Risk factors for AVN.
      1. Sickle cell anemia (see Chapter 35).
      2. Trauma.
      3. Steroid use.
      4. Gaucher disease; Neimann-Pick disease.
         a. Splenomegaly.
         b. "Erlehnmeyer flask" deformity of long bones (especially femur).
      5. Blood dyscrasia (especially clotting abnormalities, such as protein C deficiency).

> **Imaging**
> - Radiograph is often first study obtained (get anteroposterior view of pelvis, and frog-leg view as well). Like osteomyelitis, early AVN is not detectable on radiograph. More advanced AVN can be seen on radiographs as femoral head sclerosis, subchondral fractures ("crescent sign"), and loss of height or collapse of femoral head.
> - Bone scan is more sensitive than radiograph but can be difficult to interpret (look for "cold spot" in normally "hot" femoral head).
> - If suspicion of AVN is high, magnetic resonance imaging (MRI) is another potential imaging modality that can render diagnosis. (Look for low-signal lesion within bright femoral head on $T_1$-weighted images.) Recent advances suggest that MRI with contrast (gadolinium) might be beneficial in early detection of AVN of hip.

4. Slipped capital femoral epiphysis (SCFE).
   a. Femoral epiphysis "falls off" of femoral shaft (posteriomedial slippage).
   b. Usually idiopathic or traumatic etiology; however, can also be seen in renal patients (rickets).
   c. Found in boys more commonly than in girls.

d. Associations.
   1. Obesity.
   2. Hypothyroidism.
   3. AVN.
   4. Rickets.
   5. Renal osteodystrophy.
e. Contralateral SCFE is present approximately 20% of time.
f. Treatment.
   1. Surgical intervention (pinning) is required, even though this is Salter I fracture (see Chapter 27).
   2. Reattaching femoral epiphysis (growth plate) to its proper position ensures continued normal growth.
g. Complications.
   1. AVN.
   2. Varus deformity with shortening of femur.
   3. Premature osteoarthritis.

> **Imaging** Hip radiographs may demonstrate widened growth plate with femoral head epiphysis no longer perched atop femoral shaft; can be subtle finding, often best seen on frog-leg view.

B. Knee: Because of rapid growth and enhanced blood supply of knee, there is increased incidence of osteomyelitis (see Chapter 30) and bone lesions, both benign (such as fibrocortical defect or nonossifying fibroma) and malignant (such as osteosarcoma) (see Chapter 31).
   1. Patella.
      a. Chondromalacia.
         1. Common abnormality of patella (some physicians estimate as high as 50% of adolescents or young adults).
         2. Cartilaginous softening leads to central patellar posterior articular surface defects.
         3. Etiology unknown; perhaps related to repeated trauma.
         4. Treatment.
            a. None; self-limiting.

> **Imaging** Knee radiographs may show central patellar posterior articular surface irregularity with cratering and sclerosis. Joint-space narrowing or osteophyte formation (degenerative-type changes) are not present.

      b. Dorsal defect of patella.
         1. Bony defect seen in upper, outer quadrant of patella.
         2. Asymptomatic; possibly type of fibrous cortical defect.
         3. No treatment or intervention is required, as defect usually fills in and remodels by adulthood.

**Imaging** Round, patellar lucency in characteristic location (superolateral) is seen on knee radiographs, often with sclerotic margin.

2. Osgood-Schlatter disease.
   a. Tibial tuberosity avulsion with tearing of patellar tendon insertion; no inflammatory response.
   b. Found in males more commonly than in females; 10 to 12 years is peak age range.
   c. Clinical diagnosis, although radiographic study can suggest diagnosis.

**Imaging** Look for soft-tissue swelling, loss of infrapatellar fat pad, excessive tibial fragmentation, and thickening of patellar tendon on knee radiographs.

3. Osteochondritis dissecans.
   a. Osteochondral fracture.
   b. Articular cartilage fragment can become loose body.
   c. Location.
      *1.* Commonly seen along lateral aspect of medial condyle of femur.
      *2.* Talar dome.
      *3.* Elbow.

**Imaging** Sharply demarcated lucency is seen along articular surface, usually in common locations (previously listed). MRI can better delineate both fracture and accompanying injuries, such as joint effusion, meniscal tear, or ligamentous tear.

4. Blount disease.
   a. Also known as tibia vara.
   b. Developmental varus deformity of tibia.
   c. Unknown etiology; could perhaps be sequlea of "developmental bowing" of child's knee that does not correct.
      *1.* Developmental bowing is normal in 2 to 3 year old; progresses normally to "knock knees" (genu valgum) in 3 to 5 year old; soon thereafter becomes normal posture.
      *2.* Abnormal stresses on tibia can result from uncorrrected bowing.

**Imaging** Knee radiograph can demonstrate marked bowing of leg, with medial joint space narrowing, medial tibial fragmentation, and "beaking" of femoral metaphysis.

5. JRA.
   a. Chronic polyarthritis, predominantly of larger joints, such as knees and wrists.
   b. Found in females more commonly than in males; onset is usually in first 5 years of life.
   c. Can have cervical spine involvement with erosion of dens and atlantoaxial subluxation.
   d. Ten percent of JRA are systemic (Still disease).
      1. Hallmark is polyarthritis.
      2. Splenomegaly.
      3. Lymphadenopathy.
      4. Fever.
      5. Pericarditis or myocarditis.

**Imaging** Radiographs reveal overgrown, hyperemic (osteopenic) epiphysis with joint-space narrowing and bony erosions. Eventual bony ankylosis may result.

6. Cortical desmoid.
   a. Avulsion of posteromedial supracondylar ridge of distal femur.
   b. Can look aggressive and mimic osteosarcoma; can even have increased uptake on bone scan.
   c. Do not biopsy, as can appear malignant; obtain follow-up films to monitor lesion, in order to confirm lack of growth and lack of progression.

**Imaging** Lateral knee radiograph shows irregularity and bony-contour loss along characteristic location (posteromedial supracondylar ridge of distal femur).

7. Growth recovery lines.
   a. Previously known as "growth arrest lines."
   b. With illness, growth slows down; can rapidly "make up for lost time," however, when illness abates. Result is sclerotic lines along growing metaphysis of long bones, especially around knee.

**Imaging** Knee radiographs of femoral and tibial metaphysis show thin, sclerotic circumferential bands (analogous to tree rings).

## SUGGESTED READINGS

Alexander JE, Seibert JJ, Aronson J, Williamson SL, Glasier CM, Rodgers AB, Corbitt SL: A protocol of plain radiographs, hip ultrasound and triple phase bone scans in the evaluation of the painful pediatric hip. *Clin Pediatr* 1988; 27:175-181.

Aronsson DD, Goldberg MJ, Kling TF, Roy DR: Developmental dysplasia of the hip. *Pediatrics* 1994; 94:201-208.

Beltran J, Herman LJ, Burk JM, Zuelzer WA, Clark RN, Lucas JG, Weiss LD, Yang A: Femoral head avascular necrosis: MR imaging with clinical-pathologic and radionuclide correlation. *Radiology* 1988; 166:215-220.

Bloomberg TJ, Nutall J, Stoker DJ: Radiology in early slipped femoral capital epiphysis. *Clin Radiol* 1978; 29:657-667.

Bluemm RG, Falke THM, Ziedses des Plantes BG, Steiner RM: Early Legg-Perthes disease demonstrated by MRI. *Skeletal Radiol* 1985; 14:95-98.

DeSmet AA, Fisher DR, Graf BK, Lange RH: Osteochondritis dissecans of the knee: Value of MR imaging in determining lesion stability and the presence of articular defects. *AJR* 1990; 155:549-553.

Eggert P, Viemann M: Physiological bow legs or infantile Blount's disease: Some new aspects on an old problem. *Pediatr Radiol* 1996; 26:349-351.

Graf R: Fundamentals of sonographic diagnosis of infant hip dysplasia. *J Pediatr Orthop* 1984; 4:735-740.

Harcke HT: Screening newborns for developental dysplasia of the hip: The role of sonography. *AJR* 1994; 162:395-397.

Harcke HT, Grissom LE: Sonographic evaluation of the infant hip. *Semin Ultrasound CT MR* 1986; 4:331-338.

Johnson JF, Brogden BG: Dorsal defect of the patella: Incidence and distribution. *AJR* 1982; 139:339-340.

King SJ, Carty HML, Brady O: Magnetic resonance imaging of knee injuries in children. *Pediatr Radiol* 1996; 26:287-290.

Krause BL, Williams JPR, Catterall: Natural history of Osgood-Schlatter disease. *J Pediatr Orthop* 1990; 10:65-68.

Mandell GA, Harcke HT: Scintigraphy of the painful hip in adolescents. *Appl Radiol* 1993; Jan:64-70.

McGoldrick F, Bourke T, Blake N, Fogarty E, Dowling F, Regan B: Accuracy of sonography in transient synovitis. *J Pediatr Orthop* 1990; 10:501-503.

Miralles M, Gonzalez G, Pulpeiro JR, Millan JM, Gordillo I, Serrano C, Olcoz F, Martinez A: Sonography of the painful hip in children: 500 consecutive cases. *AJR* 1989; 152:579-582.

Pinto MR, Peterson HA, Berquist TH: Magnetic resonance imaging in early diagnosis of Legg-Calvé-Perthes disease. *J Pediatr Orthop* 1989; 9:19-22.

Rosendahl K, Markestad T, Lie RT: Ultrasound in the early diagnosis of congenital dislocation of the hip: The significance of hip stability versus acetabular morphology. *Pediatr Radiol* 1992; 22:430-433.

Sebag G, Ducon Le Pointe H, Klein I, Maiza D, Mazda K, Bensahel H, Hassan M: Dynamic gadolinium-enhanced subtraction MR imaging—a simple technique for the early diagnosis of Legg-Calvé-Perthes disease. *Pediatr Radiol* 1997; 27:216-220.

Share JC, Teele RL: Ultrasonography of the infant hip: A practical approach. *Appl Radiol* 1992; June:27-34.

Zieger MM, Dorr U, Schulz RD: Ultrasonography of hip joint effusions. *Skeletal Radiol* 1987; 16:607-611.

# 34
# The Foot

### Key Concepts

1. There are three components in the radiographic evaluation of the pediatric foot: the hindfoot (talus and calcaneus), the midfoot (navicular, cuneiforms, and cuboid), and the forefoot.
2. Normal calcaneal-talar angle (C-T angle) is 30 to 40 degrees (as seen on the lateral projection with lines drawn through the long axis of the talus and calcaneus). On the anteroposterior (AP) projection, a talar line (through the long axis of the talus) points to the first metatarsal, while a calcaneal line (through the long axis of the calcaneus) passes through the cuboid to the fourth metatarsal.
3. Isolated metatarsus adductus is medial deviation of the forefoot with a normal hindfoot. However, metatarsus adductus can be associated with other congenital foot anomalies (such as clubfoot).
4. Equinovarus or clubfoot is a common congenital pediatric foot abnormality. Talus and calcaneus are aligned in a parallel fashion (as seen on the lateral radiograph) with varus angulation of the hindfoot and forefoot. Inversion of the foot is also present.
5. Tarsal coalition is the abnormal fusion of two or more tarsal centers. Talar and calcaneal (60%) is the most common, followed by calcaneal and navicular (30%).

A. Radiographic evaluation of the foot.
   1. Three components to evaluate.
      a. Hindfoot.
         *1.* Talus.
         2. Calcaneus.
      b. Midfoot.
         *1.* Navicular.
         2. Cuneiforms and cuboid.
      c. Forefoot.
         *1.* Metatarsals.
         2. Phalanges.
   2. Weight-bearing films, if possible.
      a. Normal AP projection (Fig. 34-1, *A*).
         *1.* Talar line (through long axis of talus) points to first metatarsal.
         2. Calcaneal line (through long axis of calcaneus) passes through cuboid to fourth metatarsal.
         3. C-T angle.
            a. 45 degrees in neonate.
               1) More vertically aligned talus is present in neonate and small child.
               2) Result: C-T angle is larger.
            b. 30 degrees by 8 years of age.

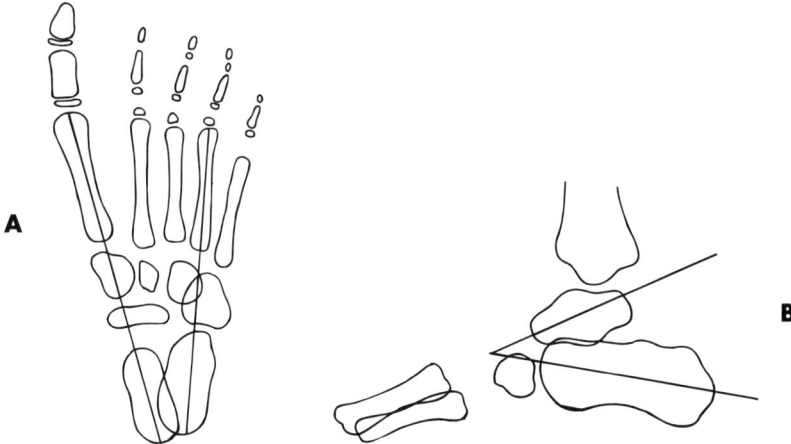

**Fig. 34-1** Normal alignment of foot. **A,** AP view with talus projecting to first metatarsal, and calcaneus projecting to fourth or fifth metatarsal. **B,** Lateral view with normal calcaneal-talar angle.

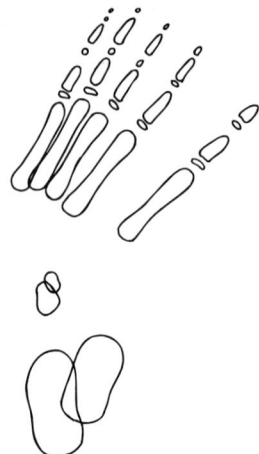

**Fig. 34-2** Metatarsus adductus, AP view. Note varus angulation of forefoot with normal hindfoot.

      b. Lateral film (Fig. 34-1, *B*).
         1. Lines drawn through long axis of talus and calcaneus.
         2. C-T angle is 30 to 40 degrees.
    3. Pathologic alignment of foot.
      a. Hindfoot: evaluate calcaneus and talus.
         1. Hindfoot varus.
           a. AP view.
              1) C-T angle is less than 30 degrees.
              2) Talus and calcaneus overlap on AP view.
           b. Lateral.
              1) Parallel talus and calcaneus.
         2. Hindfoot valgus.
           a. C-T angle is greater than 30 degrees.
      b. Forefoot: evaluate metatarsals and their relationship to talus.
         1. Varus (metatarsals point medially to long axis of talus).
         2. Valgus (metatarsals point laterally to long axis of talus).
      c. Inversion (sole of foot faces inward).
      d. Eversion (sole of foot faces outward).
B. Congenital foot abnormalities.
    1. Metatarsus adductus (varus) (Fig. 34-2).
      a. Forefoot deviates medially, but hindfoot is normal.
      b. Can often be associated with inversion of foot and clubfoot (see equinovarus).
      c. Unknown etiology.

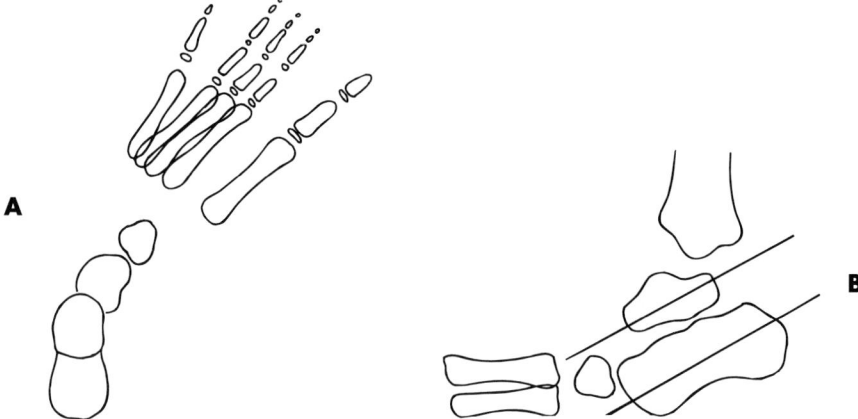

**Fig. 34-3** Equinovarus or clubfoot. **A,** AP view shows overlapping talus and calcaneus with varus angulation of forefoot. **B,** Lateral view demonstrates parallel talus and calcaneus; inversion of forefoot is also present.

2. Equinovarus (Fig. 34-3).
   a. Also known as clubfoot.
   b. 1 to 4:1000; found in males more commonly than in females.
   c. Etiology is unknown (perhaps intrauterine posturing, muscular imbalance, or central nervous system [CNS] abnormality).
   d. Treatment.
      1. Surgical correction with Achilles' tendon release.
      2. Surgical complication.
         a. Persistent equinus (or upward) position of calcaneus because Achilles' cord is too tight.
         b. "Rocker-bottom" foot (broken midfoot with abnormal relationship between hind and midfoot).

> **Imaging** Lateral foot radiograph demonstrates parallel alignment of talus and calcaneus with equinus (upward) position of calcaneus. AP view of foot shows overlap of talus and calcaneus (resulting in small C-T angle) with varus angulation of forefoot (metatarsus adductus). Inversion of foot is also present.

3. Congenital vertical talus (Fig. 34-4).
   a. Often seen with other congenital syndromes or CNS abnormalities (10% of myelomeningoceles).
   b. Essential to obtain radiograph with maximum plantar flexion of foot.

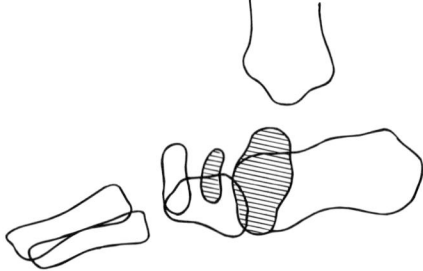

**Fig. 34-4** Congenital vertical talus. Lateral view depicts vertical alignment of talus *(shaded)* with navicular positioned along dorsal surface of talus *(shaded)*.

      c. Be aware of "oblique talus" (often mistaken for vertical talus).
         1. Vertical alignment of talus, yet normal talar and navicular articulation is maintained.
         2. Seen in cerebral palsy (CP).

> **Imaging** AP view of foot shows hindfoot valgus with forefoot valgus, while lateral view demonstrates vertical position of talus with dorsal dislocation of navicular (navicular lies along anterior portion of talus). Lateral view also shows equinus (upward) position to calcaneus with rocker-bottom deformity.

  4. Arch abnormality (Fig. 34-5).
     a. Pes planus (flat foot).
        1. Normal alignment in infants and small children.
        2. Usually asymptomatic; can be familial.
        3. Can be seen in CP; probably related to muscular inbalance and spasticity.
        4. Can be mistaken for vertical talus (see previous discussion).
     b. Pes cavus (high arch).
        1. Can be seen after clubfoot surgery.
        2. Can be sign of neurologic disorder (such as spinal cord tethering or muscle denervation).
  5. Tarsal coalition.
     a. Abnormal fusion of two or more tarsal centers.
        1. Talar and calcaneal (60%).
        2. Calcaneal and navicular (30%).
        3. Talar and navicular.
     b. Usually presents with chronic foot pain.

The Foot **319**

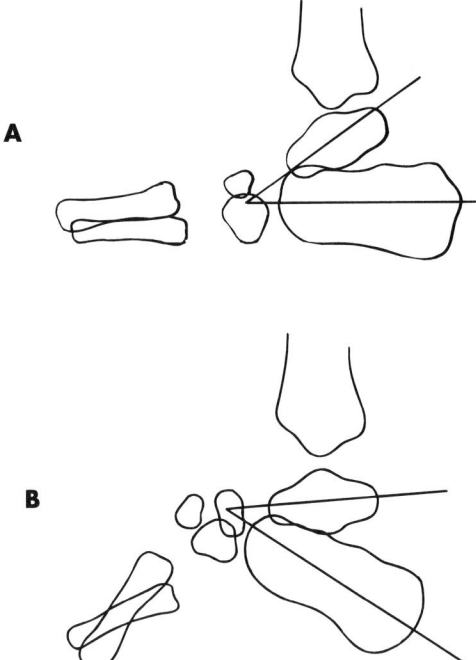

**Fig. 34-5** Arch abnormalities. **A,** Pes planus (flat foot). **B,** Pes cavus (high arch).

c. Talar osteophytes ("talar beaks") are unusual in both adults and children; should signal abnormal motion in foot, possibly related to tarsal coalition.

**Imaging** Oblique radiographs of foot may show bony connection between tarsal bones. Also, look for elongated anterior calcaneus (known as "anteater nose"). Computed tomography can confirm diagnosis by demonstrating bony bar or fibrous fusion.

## SUGGESTED READINGS

Bleck EE: Congenital clubfoot: Pathomechanics, radiographic analysis and results of surgical treatment. *Clin Orthop* 1977; 125:119-130.

Cummings RJ, Lovell WW: Current concepts review: Operative treatment of congenital idiopathic clubfoot. *J Bone Joint Surg* 1985; 670A:1108-1112.

Deutsch AL, Resnick D, Campbell G: Computed tomography and bone scintigraphy in the evaluation of tarsal coalition. *Radiology* 1982; 144:137-140.

Downey DJ, Drennan JC, Garcia JF: Magnetic resonance imaging findings in congenital talipes equinovarus. *J Pediatr Orthop* 1992; 12:224-228.

Freiberger R, Hersh A, Harrison M: Roentgen examination of the deformed foot. *Semin Roentgenol* 1970; 5:341-353.

Jacobsen ST, Crawford AH: Congenital vertical talus. *J Pediatr Orthop* 1983; 3:306-310.

Lee MS, Harcke HT, Kumar SJ, Bassett GS: Subtalar joint coalition in children: New observations. *Radiology* 1989; 172:635-639.

Oestreich AE: *How to measure angles from foot radiographs: A primer.* New York, 1990, Springer-Verlag.

Oestriech AE, Mize WA, Crawford AH, Morgan RC: The "anteater nose": A direct sign of calcaneonavicular coalition on the lateral radiograph. *J Pediatr Orthop* 1987; 7:709-711.

Resnick D: Talar ridges, osteophytes and beaks: A radiologic commentary. *Radiology* 1984; 151:329-332.

Sarno RC, Carter BL, Bankoff MS, Semine MC: Computed tomography in tarsal coalition. *J Comput Assist Tomogr* 1984; 8:1155-1160.

Simons GW: Radiography of clubfeet. *J Bone Joint Surg* 1977; 59B:485-489.

Vanderwilds R, Staheli LT, Chew DE, Malagon V: Measurements on radiographs of the foot in normal infants and children. *J Bone Joint Surg* 1988; 70A:407-415.

# 35
# Bony Abnormalities in Metabolic, Endocrine, and Hematopoietic Disorders

### Key Concepts

1. Osteopenia is a radiographic term used to describe decreased bony density caused by a disturbance in bone formation (osteoporosis), bone mineralization (osteomalacia), or bone resorption (hyperparathyroidism).
2. Osteomalacia in skeletally immature children is known as "rickets." Rickets has a variety of etiologies that are often age related; they include liver and renal malfunction, inborn enzymatic defects, and dietary causes.
3. Renal osteodystrophy (or secondary hyperparathyroidism) causes hypertrophy of the parathyroid (increased parathyroid hormone [PTH] as a compensatory mechanism for the hypocalcemia that results from renal dysfunction [elevated phosphate]). The chronic PTH stimulation results in end-organ resistance of the bones, causing osteosclerosis.
4. Sickle cell anemia has many bony manifestations that include dactylitis ("hand-foot" syndrome), osteomyelitis, bony infarctions, avascular necrosis (AVN), and the H-type vertebral body.
5. Langerhans cell histiocytosis (formerly known as histiocytosis X or eosinophilic granuloma) often presents with bone involvement, commonly seen in the skull, spine, mandible, ribs, and diaphyses of long bones.

A. Metabolic bone disease: osteopenia.
  1. Osteopenia.
     a. Radiographic term used to describe decreased bony density.
     b. Causes.
        *1.* Disturbance in bone formation (osteoporosis).
        *2.* Disturbance in bone mineralization (osteomalacia).
        *3.* Disturbance in bone resorption (hyperparathyroidism).
  2. Osteoporosis.
     a. Loss of bony substance with normal underlying bone.
     b. General osteoporosis.
        *1.* Senile (postmenopausal).
           *a.* Bony radiographic characteristics.
              *1)* Thin bony cortex.
              *2)* Coarse bony trabeculae.
              *3)* Loss of vertebral height, often with kyphosis.
           *b.* Increased incidence of fractures.
              *1)* Especially hip.
              *2)* Distal radius (Colles fracture).
        *2.* Excessive corticosteroids.
           *a.* Endogenous (Cushing syndrome).
              *1)* Adrenocortical hyperplasia.
              *2)* Adrenal adenoma or carcinoma.
           *b.* Exogenous.
              *1)* Antiinflammatory uses.
              *2)* Transplant patients.
              *3)* Crohn disease.
        *3.* Severe malnutrition or gastrointestinal malabsorption disorders.
           *a.* Celiac sprue.
           *b.* Crohn disease.
        *4.* Vitamin C deficiency.
           *a.* Scurvy.
           *b.* Imaging findings.
              *1)* Osteopenic medullary space.
              *2)* Dense epiphyseal ring (Wimberger sign).
              *3)* Periostitis (subperiosteal hemorrhage).
              *4)* Marginal metaphyseal fractures (Pelkan sign).
     c. Regional osteoporosis.
        *1.* Disuse.
           *a.* Following fracture.
           *b.* Long-term, chronic illness.
        *2.* Inflammatory.
           *a.* Periarticular (often associated with juvenile rheumatoid arthritis [JRA]).

         b. Reflex sympathetic dystrophy.
         c. Transient osteoporosis of hip.
            1) Often migratory pain; often in adolescents.
            2) Associated with pregnancy.
            3) Usually left hip.
   3. Osteomalacia.
      a. Osteopenia with underlying abnormal bone due to improper calcification of organic osteoid matrix.
      b. Rickets (pediatric form of osteomalacia).
         1. Etiology (related to age of onset).
            a. Less than 6 months of age.
               1) Neonatal rickets (found especially in premature infants).
               2) Hepatobiliary (biliary atresia).
               3) Vitamin D–dependent rickets (autosomal-recessive enzymatic defect).
               4) Hypophosphatasia (low-serum alkaline phosphatase).
            b. 6 to 18 months of age.
               1) Dietary (vitamin D deficiency).
               2) Breast-fed infants only.
               3) Limited sunlight exposure.
            c. Late onset, greater than 2 years of age.
               1) Renal disorders.
                  a) Renal tubular acidosis.
                  b) Vitamin D–resistant.
               2) Hypophosphatasia.
         2. Anticonvulsant therapy.
            a. Phenobarbitol (Dilantin).
            b. Result: increase in hepatic enzymes; this increase accelerates degradation of active vitamin D metabolites.

**Imaging** Radiographs can show loss of zone of provisional calcification with metaphyseal lucency, fraying, irregularity, and "cupping." Can also show bowing of weight-bearing bones. Rib ends may demonstrate bulbous appearance ("rachitic rosary"). There is also increased incidence of slipped femoral capital epiphysis (SCFE).

B. Osteosclerosis.
   1. Osteopetrosis.
      a. Osteoclast dysfunction with resulting abnormal bony modeling and symmetric, homogeneous skeletal sclerosis.
      b. Infantile (autosomal recessve).
         1. Hepatosplenomegaly, anemia, thrombocytopenia.
         2. Death in first decade of life.

    c. Adult (Albers-Schönberg disease, autosomal dominant).
        *1.* Varies in severity; can range from incidental finding to more severe form with repeated fractures, anemia, and/or osteomyelitis.
        *2.* "Bone within a bone" appearance.
  2. Renal osteodystrophy (see following discussion).
  3. Pyknodysostosis.
        a. Autosomal recessive.
        b. Open anterior fontanelle.
        c. Hypoplastic facial bones and paranasal sinuses.
        d. Shortened phalanges.
        e. Cranial sutural wormian bones.
        f. Anemia.
  4. Osteopoikilosis.
        a. Autosomal dominant.
        b. Multiple, scattered, small foci of sclerosis.
        c. Incidental finding.
  5. Osteopathia striata.
        a. Autosomal dominant.
        b. Linear striations involving metaphyses of long bones.
  6. Melorheostosis.
        a. Nonhereditary.
        b. Linear areas of hyperostosis oriented along long axis of tubular bones (melting wax appearance).
        c. Usually monostotic.
        d. May be associated with pain and joint stiffness.
  7. Diaphyseal dysplasia.
        a. Also known as Camurati-Englemann disease.
        b. Autosomal dominant.
        c. Symmetric hyperostosis of diaphysis of long bones.
        d. Leg pain, abnormal gait, muscular weakness.
C. Endocrine disorders.
  1. Parathyroid.
        a. Primary hyperparathyroidism.
            *1.* Increased PTH leads to increased bony resorption with increased serum calcium.
            *2.* Congenital.
                *a.* Rare, autosomal recessive.
                *b.* Hypotonicity, hypercalcemia, hepatosplenomegaly.
                *c.* Severe bony disease.
                    *1)* Subperiosteal resorption.
                    *2)* Trabecular reduction with subsequent pathologic fractures.
                *d.* Fatal, unless parathyroidectomy is performed.

3. Transient hyperparathyroidism in neonate.
    a. Related to maternal hypoparathyroidism.
    b. Self-limiting; resolves rapidly.
4. Rarely due to parathyroid adenoma or hyperplasia as is commonly seen in adults.
  b. Secondary hyperparathyroidism.
    1. Renal osteodystrophy.
        a. Hypertrophy of parathyroid (increased PTH) is compensatory mechanism for hypocalcemia, resulting from renal dysfunction (elevated phosphate).
        b. End-organ resistance of bones develops because of chronic PTH stimulation, which can result in osteosclerosis.
        c. Increased incidence of SCFE.

**Imaging** Radiographs can show bony subperiosteal resorption, general osteosclerosis, particularly of vertebral endplates "rugger-jersey" spine, acroosteolysis (resorption of distal tufts of phalanges), soft-tissue calcifications, or "brown tumors" (osteoclastoma, osteitis, fibrosa cystica).

  c. Hypoparathyroidism.
    1. No discernable bony radiographic findings.
    2. Can see basal ganglia calcifications on head computed tomography.
  d. Pseudohypoparathyroidism.
    1. Failure of end-organ response to PTH.
    2. Results in low-serum calcium.

**Imaging** Short tubular bones of hands and feet (short fourth metacarpal) on radiographs. Basal ganglia calcifications and abnormal dentition can also be present.

  e. Pseudopseudohypoparathyroidism.
    1. Normal serum calcium.
    2. Same radiographic findings as pseudohypoparathyroidism.
2. Thyroid.
  a. Thyroid problems can cause either accelerated or delayed skeletal maturity, which can be evaluated by bone age.
    1. Procedure for evaluation of bone age.
        a. Obtain anteroposterior (AP) film of left hand and compare it with examples in radiographic atlas, such as *Radiographic Atlas of Skeletal Development* by Greulich and Pyle (see Suggested Readings).
        b. Especially evaluate distal as opposed to proximal epiphyses (distal bones are more accurate). Look for epiphyseal length and curling up of distal epiphyses.

    c. Sesamoid of thumb appears by age 11 in girls and age 13 in boys.
  2. Once you have assessed your best estimate of bone age, find standard deviations (SDs) for chronologic age (also found in *Radiographic Atlas of Skeletal Development* by Greulich and Pyle). Bone age report should state chronologic age, estimated bone age, and 2 SDs in months. Make sure to comment on any bony abnormalities, such as short fourth metacarpal or cone epiphysis.
 b. Hyperthyroidism.
  1. Accelerated skeletal maturation in children.
  2. Thyroid acropachy in adults (rare).
 c. Hypothyroidism (cretinism).
  1. Delayed ossification and skeletal maturity.
  2. Delayed appearance of epiphyseal centers.
  3. Increased incidence of SCFE.

**Imaging** In addition to delayed appearance of epiphysis, plain radiographs can also show epiphyseal dysgenesis (fragmented, multicentric).

 3. Pituitary.
  a. Increased growth hormone.
  b. Results in accelerated bony growth prior to epiphyseal closure (gigantism).
  c. In adults, acromegaly may be present.
D. Toxicity.
 1. Hypervitaminosis.
  a. Vitamin D.
   1. Alternating dense and lucent metaphyseal bands.
   2. Calcifications.
    a. Soft tissue.
    b. Vascular.
    c. Renal.
  b. Vitamin A.
   1. Periostitis and hyperostosis (preferentially seen involving ulna).
   2. Widening of cranial sutures.
 2. Lead poisoning.
  a. Bony radiographic findings not evident until more than 6 months after ingestion of lead (usually from ingestion of lead paint chips).
  b. Heavy dose can cause lead encephalopathy.

**Imaging** Radiographs show dense "lead line" across metaphysis of long bones (especially distal femur, radius, and proximal tibia). Previously thought to be lead deposition, lead lines are actually caused by osteoclastic dysfunction from ingested lead, resulting in lack of bony resorption. On abdominal radiographs, lead chips can sometimes actually still be seen within gastrointestinal tract.

3. Prostaglandins.
    a. Used to maintain patency of ductus arteriosus in cyanotic neonate.
    b. Can cause periosteal reaction (often exuberant), especially of ribs and humeral shafts.
E. Hematopoietic disorders.
  1. Congenital anemias.
    a. Thalassemia (marrow hyperplasia).
       *1.* Genetic, hemoglobin-chain abnormality.
       *2.* Severe involvement (thalassemia major) versus mild involvement (thalassemia minor).
       *3.* Extramedullary hematopoiesis.
           *a.* Focal, extraosseous extensions of hematopoiesis.
           *b.* Can present as posterior paravertebral mediastinal masses; hepatosplenomegaly may also be present.

**Imaging** Bony radiographs can show expanded medullary space with thinned cortex and coarse trabeculae. Skull films demonstrate widened diploic space ("hair-on-end" skull).

    b. Sickle cell anemia.
       *1.* In United States, 1% of African-American population; 7% carry trait.
       *2.* Genetic defect resulting in sickle-shaped red blood cell.
       *3.* Hallmark is acute painful "sickle crisis," caused by ischemia or infarction from stasis and sludging of abnormal blood cells.
       *4.* Dactylitis (hand-foot syndrome).
           *a.* Onset is from 6 months to 2 years of age.
           *b.* Often first manifestation of disease.
           *c.* Clinical presentation.
               *1)* Fever.
               *2)* Soft-tissue swelling especially of hands and feet.
       *5.* Osteomyelitis.
           *a.* Diminished resistance to infections; splenic function is decreased because of autoinfarction.
           *b.* *Salmonella.*
       *6.* Bony infarctions.
           *a.* Multiple infarctions can lead to bone-in-a-bone appearance.
           *b.* Common locations.
               *1)* Femoral head.

2) Humeral head.
3) Long bones.
4) Spine.
c. H-type vertebral body.
1) Preferential collapse of central portion of vertebral body.
2) Due to sludging and subsequent ischemia of central portion of vertebra (vascular "watershed" area of spine).
d. AVN.
1) Found in 15% to 30% of sickle cell patients.
2) Vascular compromise of epiphysis.
3) Staging, based on plain radiographic findings.
  a) Stage I: no radiographic findings.
  b) Stage II: patchy sclerosis and lucency.
  c) Stage III: flattening of epiphysis with subchondral lucency or crescent sign (subchondral fracture).
  d) Stage IV: collapse and fragmentation.
4) Magnetic resonance imaging findings (95% sensitivity).
  a) Low signal on $T_1$.
  b) High intensity surrounding low signal on $T_2$.

**Imaging** Early radiographic signs of sickle cell anemia include periosteal reaction of tubular bones in hands and feet (dactylitis). Bone infarctions manifest as patchy areas of lucency and sclerosis within medullary space.

  c. Fanconi syndrome.
    1. Pancytopenia.
    2. Abnormal digits, particularly thumb (dysplastic, hypoplastic).
2. Hemophilia.
  a. Deficiency of plasma clotting factor, leading to abnormal blood coagulation.
  b. X-linked recessive: classic hemophilia (factor VIII deficiency).
  c. Christmas disease (factor IX deficiency).
  d. Better treatment available today (in form of readily available blood products) has lead to fewer complications from hemophilia; therefore, bony findings are less commonly seen.
  e. Complications.
    1. Hemarthrosis.
      a. Knee, elbow, ankle, shoulder, or hip.
      b. Joint effusion.
      c. Hemosiderin deposition.
      d. Hyperemia and epiphyseal overgrowth.

e. Synovial hyperplasia and hypertrophy.
   f. Erosive changes.
 2. "Pseudotumor."
    a. Interosseous hemorrhage, subperiosteal hemorrhage, and soft-tissue hemorrhage.
    b. Common locations.
       1) Femur and tibia.
       2) Pelvis.
       3) Small tubular bones of hands and feet.
       4) Calcaneus.
 3. From blood products used in treatment of acquired immunodeficiency syndrome.

**Imaging** Radiographs may show overall increased density of joints (due to hemosiderin deposition) as well as lucent, overgrown femoral epiphysis with femoral intercondylar notch widening (due to erosive changes). Similar findings are seen in JRA. Pseudotumor often manifests as lucent, often cystlike lesion within bone.

3. Leukemia.
   a. In children, 80% of cases are acute, lymphoblastic leukemia.
   b. Bony changes are common, present in 50% to 60% of pathologic specimens, although not usually detectable radiographically.
   c. Clinically, can be associated with fever, arthralgias, and swelling; can often be initially mistaken for JRA.

**Imaging** Radiographic findings vary, ranging from osteopenia, to lucent lesions, to permeative lesions. Lucent metaphyseal bands may be present at sites of rapid bony growth (distal femur, radius, proximal tibia, or humerus). Periostitis caused by proliferating leukemic cells can be seen. Vertebral loss of height and/or complete collapse can also occur.

4. Lymphoma.
   a. Usually non-Hodgkin type.
   b. Location.
      1. Usually in long bone.
      2. Burkitt type of non-Hodgkin lymphoma often seen in maxilla or mandible.

**Imaging** Moth-eaten, permeative lesion with periostitis can be seen on radiographs. Collapsed ("ivory") vertebra may also be present.

5. Langerhans cell histiocytosis.
   a. Histiocytic infiltration of tissues.
   b. Langerhans cell has characteristic cytoplasmic inclusion bodies with aggressive phagocytic activity.
   c. Although new name of "Langerhans Cell Histiocytosis" is preferred, following subtypes may still be used.
      1. Eosinophilic granuloma (EG).
         a. Most common form (70%).
         b. Single or multiple well-defined, lucent, medullary lesions.
         c. Location.
            1) Skull: most common site.
            2) Spine: collapsed vertebral body (vertebra plana).
            3) Other sites.
               a) Mandible ("floating teeth").
               b) Ribs.
               c) Diaphyses of long bones (femur, humerus).

> **Imaging** Radiographs show sharply demarcated lucent lesions in long bones and skull. Periosteal reaction may be present. Collapsed vertebral bodies (vertebra plana) is common manifestation of EG.

      2. Hand-Schüller-Christian disease.
         a. Chronic disseminated form (20% to 25%).
         b. "Classic" presentation, yet only seen in about 10% of cases.
            1) Diabetes insipidus.
            2) Exophthalmus.
            3) Bone lesions.
         c. Pulmonary changes.
            1) Nodular infiltrate, often in upper lobes.
            2) Can progress to fibrosis and end-stage lung disease.
      3. Letterer-Siwe disease.
         a. Acute fulminant form (less than 10%).
         b. Clinical presentation.
            1) Severe anemia.
            2) Hepatosplenomegaly.
            3) Lymphadenopathy.
         c. Because disease course is rapid (fatal in 1 to 2 years), bony changes are rarely seen.

## SUGGESTED READINGS

Ben Dridi MF, Oumaya A, Gastli H, Doggaze C, Bousnina S, Fattoum S, Ben Osman R, Gharbi HA: Radiographic abnormalities of the skeleton in patients with sickle cell anemia. *Pediatr Radiol* 1987; 17:296-302.

Bennett OM, Namnyak SS: Bone and joint manifestations of sickle cell anemia. *J Bone Joint Surg* 1990; 72:494-499.

Benz G, Brandeis WE, Willich E: Radiological aspects of leukemia in childhood. *Pediatr Radiol* 1976; 4:201-213.

Bohrer SP: Bone changes in the extremities in sickle cell anemia. *Semin Roentgenol* 1987; 22:176-185.

Brenkel IJ, Dias JJ, Davies TG, Iqbal SJ, Gregg PJ: Hormone status in patient with slipped capital femoral epiphysis. *J Bone Joint Surg* 1989; 71:33-38.

Burnstein MI, Kottamasu SR, Pettifor JM, Sochett E, Ellis BI, Frame B: Metabolic bone disease in pseudohypoparathyroidism. *Radiology* 1985; 155:351-356.

Chu T, D'Angio GJ, Farara BE, Ladisch S, Nesbit M, Pritchard J: Histiocytosis syndromes in children. *Lancet* 1987; 1:208-209.

David R, Oria RA, Kumar R, Singleton EB, Lindell MM, Shirkhoda A, Madewell JE: Radiologic features of eosinophilic granuloma of bone. *AJR* 1989; 153:1021-1026.

Dogan AS, Conway JJ, Miller JH, Grier D, Bhattathirty MM, Mitchell CS: Detection of bone lesions in Langerhans cell histiocytosis: Complementary roles of scintigraphy and conventional radiography. *J Pediatric Hematol Oncol* 1996; 18:51-58.

Eftekhari F, Yousefzadeh DK: Primary infantile hyperparathyroidism: Clinical, laboratory and radiographic features. *Skeletal Radiol* 1982; 8:201-208.

Greulich WW, Pyle SI: *Radiographic atlas of skeletal development of the hand and wrist.* Stanford, 1959, Stanford University Press.

Koo WW, Sherman R, Oestreich AE, Tsang RC, Steichen JJ, Young LW: Osteopenia, rickets and fractures in preterm infants. *Am J Dis Child* 1985; 139:1045-1046.

Lovinger RD: Rickets. *Pediatrics* 1980; 66:359-365.

MacDonald SR, Locht RC, Lindsay D, Levi C: Hemophilic arthropathy of the shoulder. *J Bone Joint Surg* 1990; 72B:470-471.

McAfee PC, Cady RB: Endocrinologic and metabolic factors in atypical presentations of slipped capital femoral epiphysis. *Clin Orthop* 1983; 130:188-197.

Miller JH, Hayon II: Bone scintigraphy in hypervitaminosis A. *AJR* 1985; 144:767-768.

Nieuwenhuyse JP, Clapuyt P, Malghem J, Everarts P, Melin J, Pauwels S, Brichard B, Ninane J, Vermylen C, Cornu G: Radiographic skeletal survey and radionuclide bone scan in Langerhans cell histiocytosis of bone. *Pediatr Radiol* 1996; 26:734-738.

Stull MA, Kransdorf MJ, Devaney LO: Langerhans cell histiocytosis of bone. *Radiographics* 1992; 12:801-823.

Wilson DA, Prince JR: MR imaging of hemophilic pseudotumors. *AJR* 1988; 150:349-350.

# 36
# Skeletal Dysplasias

---

### Key Concepts

1. Short stature in a child can be divided into two groups: proportionate (etiology is familial, endocrine, or metabolic abnormality) versus disproportionate (implies skeletal dysplasia).
2. Evaluation of skeletal dysplasia with dwarfism involves an evaluation of type of bone shortening:
   a. Rhizomelic (long bone shortening, such as femur and humerus).
   b. Mesomelic (middle bone shortening, such as tibia, fibula, radius, and ulna).
   c. Acromelic (distal bone shortening of the hands and feet).
   In addition, identify the specific part of the bones involved (metaphyseal versus epiphyseal); also identify any rib, thorax, or spine involvement.
3. The most common dwarf is the achondroplastic dwarf (autosomal dominant). Characteristic features include rhizomelic shortening, lumbar lordosis with unchanging interpedicular distance, frontal bossing, and "champagne glass" iliac bones.
4. Osteogenesis imperfecta is a heterogeneous disorder caused by abnormal collagen formation. Common characteristics include osteopenia, multiple fractures with deformities (from poor healing), and short stature (cumulative fractures).
5. Marfan syndrome is a connective-tissue disorder characterized by hypermobility of the joints, excessive height, arachnodactyly (long fingers), dislocation of the lens of the eye, and scoliosis. Major complication (including sudden death) is aortic dissection or rupture (cystic medial necrosis).

A. Dwarves.
  1. Rhizomelic (predominantly proximal-bone shortening).
     a. Achondroplasia.
        1. Most common type of dwarf; autosomal dominant.
        2. Characteristic features.
           a. Lumbar lordosis with narrow, interpedicular distance.
           b. Posterior vertebral scalloping and short pedicles.
           c. Frontal bossing with small foramen magnum.
           d. Champagne glass iliac wings.
           e. Short femoral necks.
     b. Hypochondroplasia.
        1. Often presents in later childhood; autosomal dominant.
        2. No clinical findings except for short stature.
        3. Radiographically resembles milder form of achondroplasia.
     c. Thanatophoric dwarf.
        1. Lethal, restrictive lung caused by short ribs and small thorax.
        2. Marked shortening of limbs, especially femurs ("French telephone receiver" appearance).
        3. Platyspondyly (flattening of vertebral bodies).
     d. Achondrogenesis.
        1. Lethal (type I).
        2. Severe lack of ossification of vertebral bodies.
        3. Short limbs and ribs.
     e. Chondrodysplasia punctata (stippled epiphyses).
        1. Splaying of metaphyses of markedly shortened limbs (can resemble achondroplasia).
        2. Hallmark is stippled calcifications of epiphyses with delayed epiphyseal ossification (can also be seen in cretinism and trisomy 18 syndrome).
        3. Coronal clefts (lucency between anterior and posterior ossification centers) of vertebral bodies.
        4. Conradi syndrome.
           a. Calcific deposits around epiphyseal centers and other cartilaginous areas (such as ear or trachea).
           b. Resolves by school age.
     f. Proximal femoral focal deficiency.
        1. Abnormal proximal femur with normal distal femur and knee joint.
        2. Spectrum ranging from complete absence of proximal articulation of femur to mild shortening with varus deformity.
  2. Mesomelic.
     a. Campomelic ("bent limb dwarfism").
        1. Lethal; autosomal recessive.

2. Symmetric, anterior bowing of lower extremities (especially tibia and fibula).
3. Pretibial "dimples."
4. Large cranium; micrognathia.
5. Absent thoracic pedicles and cervical spine hypoplasia.
  b. Dyschondrosteosis.
   1. Madelung deformity of forearm.
      a. Ulnar dorsal dislocation.
      b. Shortened radius.
   2. Pyramidal (V-shaped) deformity of first carpal row.
  c. Trichorhinophalangeal dysplasia.
   1. Alopecia.
   2. Pear-shaped nose.
   3. Short stature with joint laxity, avascular necrosis–like changes of hip.
   4. Cone-shaped epiphyses with shortened phalanges.
3. Acromelic.
  a. Jeune syndrome.
   1. Also known as asphyxiating thoracic dystrophy.
   2. Often lethal; autosomal recessive.
   3. Short ribs lead to long but narrow chest (causes restrictive lung disease).
   4. Polydactyly.
   5. Phalangeal, cone-shaped epiphyses that fuse prematurely (leads to shortening of phalanges).
  b. Ellis–van Creveld syndrome.
   1. Also known as chondroectodermal dysplasia.
   2. Restrictive lung from small thorax and short ribs.
   3. Seen in Amish population; autosomal recessive.
   4. Triad.
      a. Dwarfism, polydactyly, and ectodermal dysplasia.
      b. Hypoplastic nails, thin sparse hair, poor dentition.
   5. Associated with congenital heart disease (septal defects).
  c. Short rib–polydactyly syndromes.
   1. Rare.
   2. Short limbs with restrictive lung disease (from congenitally small thorax) and polydactyly.
   3. Types.
      a. Saldino-Noonan syndrome.
      b. Majewski syndrome.
      c. Naumoff syndrome.
  d. Pyknodysostosis.
   1. Osteosclerosis (multiple fractures).

2. Short phalanges.
3. Open anterior fontanelle; wormian bones.
B. Metaphyseal dysplasias.
1. Conditions with predominantly bony metaphyseal involvement (flared and irregular; often with growth plate widening).
2. Types.
   a. Jansen type.
   b. Schmid type.
   c. McKusick type.
   d. Schwachman syndrome (also know as Schwachman-Diamond syndrome).
      1. Metaphyseal dysplasia.
      2. Exocrine pancreatic dysfunction.
3. Spondylometaphyseal dysplasia (spine involvement in addition to metaphyseal abnormality).
   a. Kozlowski type.
   b. Flattened vertebral bodies.
   c. Irregular proximal femoral metaphyses with coxa vara.
   d. Delayed skeletal maturity.
C. Epiphyseal dysplasias.
1. Multiple epiphyseal dysplasia.
   a. Delayed development of irrregular and fragmented epiphyses.
   b. Autosomal dominant.
   c. Normal spine.
   d. Types.
      1. Fairbank (more severe form).
      2. Ribbing (milder form with primary involvement of hips).
2. Spondyloepiphyseal dysplasia.
   a. Autosomal dominant.
   b. Short-limbed dwarf (especially rhizomelic).
   c. Retinal detachment.
   d. Atlantoaxial instability (poor odontoid formation), flattened vertebral bodies.
   e. Fragmented and irregular epiphyses that are developmentally delayed.
3. Dysplasia epiphyseal hemimelica.
   a. Also known as Trevor disease.
   b. Usually seen in lower extremity (especially around ankle).
   c. Overgrowth of epiphysis (possibly hamartomatous overgrowth of cartilage), often with protruding calcified mass.
   d. Causes deformity of joint.
   e. Associated with hemihypertrophy.
4. Kniest syndrome.

a. Short-limbed dwarf with flexion contractures (especially of hip).
   b. Platyspondyly (flattened vertebral bodies) with scoliosis.
   c. Delayed appearance of epiphyses.
      1. Fragmented and irregular when epiphyses are present.
      2. Extra epiphysis at distal end of proximal phalanx.
   d. Ocular abnormalities (myopia, retinal detachment).
   e. Cleft palate.
D. Dysplasias with abnormal mineralization or bony density.
   1. Osteopenia (decreased bone density).
      a. Osteogenesis imperfecta.
         *1.* Abnormal collagen formation.
         *2.* Four types ranging from lethal, congenital form to late-appearing tarda variety.
         *3.* Characteristics.
            *a.* Osteopenia.
            *b.* Hallmark is multiple fractures.
               *1)* Deformities (from poor healing).
               *2)* Short stature (cumulative fractures).
            *c.* Blue sclera.
            *d.* Wormian bones.
         *4.* Can be mistaken for nonaccidental trauma (child abuse).
      b. Menkes' Kinky Hair syndome.
         *1.* X-linked.
         *2.* Defect in copper metabolism.
         *3.* Characteristics.
            *a.* Osteopenia.
            *b.* Metaphyseal spurs.
         *4.* Can be mistaken for child abuse.
      c. Hypophosphatasia.
         *1.* Inborn enzymatic defect.
         *2.* Rachitic-like changes.
            *a.* Metaphyseal fraying.
            *b.* Often deep clefts and poor mineralization are present.
            *c.* Bowing of long bones.
   2. Osteosclerosis (increased bone density) (see Chapter 35).
      a. Osteopetrosis.
         *1.* Prime defect is failure in osteoclasts resulting in poor bony remodeling and resorption.
         *2.* Generalized osteosclerosis.
         *3.* Fragile bones with frequent fractures.
         *4.* Pancytopenia.
            *a.* Due to poor bony medullary space.
            *b.* Hepatosplenomegaly (extramedullary hematopoiesis).

b. Pyknodysostosis.
3. Osteopoikilosis.
4. Osteopathia striata.
5. Melorheostosis.
6. Diaphyseal dysplasia (Camurati-Englemann disease).
E. Mucopolysaccharidoses.
   1. Incomplete degradation and storage of mucopolysaccharides.
   2. Types.
      a. Hurler syndrome.
      b. Hunter syndrome.
      c. Sanfilipo syndrome.
      d. Morquio syndrome.
   3. Characteristics.
      a. Osteopenia.
      b. Large thick cranium, often dolichocephalic (premature sagittal suture closure).
      c. Beaked ("bullet-shaped") vertebral bodies with thoracolumbar kyphosis.
      d. Short, wide metacarpals and tapering phalanges. Cortical thinning.
      e. Wide ribs that taper at costovertebral margin (paddle-shaped ribs like boat oars).
      f. J-shaped sella turcica.
F. Deposition dysplasia.
   1. "Erlenmeyer flask" deformity.
      a. Medullary deposition abnormality.
      b. Causes expansion of metaphyseal regions of long bones.
      c. Especially seen involving distal femur.
   2. Types.
      a. Pyle dysplasia.
         *1.* Also known as metaphyseal dysplasia.
         *2.* Autosomal recessive.
         *3.* Widened ribs and clavicles; mild hyperostosis of cranium.
      b. Craniometaphyseal dysplasia.
         *1.* Autosomal dominant.
         *2.* Same characteristics as Pyle dysplasia but with more cranial hyperostosis and less metaphyseal abnormality.
      c. Neimann-Pick disease (see Chapter 41).
      d. Gaucher disease.
         *1.* Deficency of glucocerebrosidase (leads to abnormal storage of cerebroside in reticuloendothelial system).
         *2.* Most common lysosomal storage abnormality.
         *3.* Organs of involvement.
            *a.* Liver and spleen (often massive splenomegaly).

  *b.* Bone marrow.
   *1)* Marrow deposition.
   *2)* Can lead to Erlenmeyer flask deformity of long bones, especially femur.
   *3)* Bony infarcts.
G. Fibrous or cartilaginous dysplasias (see Chapter 31).
 1. Fibrous dysplasia.
  a. Excessive proliferation of spindle cell fibrous tissues in medullary cavity of bone.
  b. Bony expansion, pathologic fractures, and deformity can occur.
  c. Types.
   *1.* Usually monostotic.
   *2.* Polyostotic variety (McCune-Albright disease).
    *a.* "Café-au-lait" spots.
    *b.* Precocious puberty.
   *3.* Cherubism (involves face, mandible).
   *4.* Leontiasis ossea ("lion's face").
 2. Enchondromatosis (Ollier disease).
  a. Multiple enchondromas.
  b. Expansile medullary bony lesions.
  c. Can cause pathologic fractures and deformities.
  d. Chance of malignant degeneration (chondrosarcoma) 5% to 20%.
  e. Maffucci syndrome.
   *1.* Multiple enchondromatosis.
   *2.* Soft-tissue hemangiomas (phleboliths on radiographs).
 3. Osteochondromatoses.
  a. Multiple hereditary exostoses that point away from joint.
  b. Chance of malignant degeneration 5% to 10%.
  c. Short, thick femoral neck.
H. Dislocating dysplasias.
 1. Larsen syndrome.
  a. Characteristic face (hypertelorism with depressed nasal bridge).
  b. Multiple ossification centers (calcaneus).
  c. Joint dislocations (especially knee).
  d. Cervical spine kyphosis.
 2. Arthrogryposis multiplex congenita.
  a. Fixed flexion deformities and joint dislocation (hip, knee, and elbow); patellar hypoplasia.
  b. Scoliosis.
  c. Club foot.
  d. Osteopenia.
 3. Diastrophic dwarfism.
  a. Twisted extremities and spine (short-limb dwarf).

    b. Multiple joint dislocations (hypermobile thumb) and contractures.
    c. Kyphoscoliosis.
    d. Deformed earlobes (cystic lesions).
I. Other.
  1. Cleidocranial dysostosis.
    a. Autosomal dominant.
    b. Absent clavicles.
    c. Widened cranial sutures with wormian bones.
    d. Poor dentition.
  2. Dyssegmental dysgenesis.
    a. Short, curved limbs with metaphyseal widening.
    b. Variable vertebral body shape and size (anisospondyly).
    c. Types.
      *1.* Silverman-Handmaker (lethal).
      *2.* Rolland-Desbuquois.
  3. Marfan syndrome.
    a. Connective-tissue disorder with hypermobility of joints.
    b. Autosomal dominant, with widely variable expression.
    c. Excessive height, arachnodactyly (long fingers).
    d. Dislocation of lens of eye; retinal detachment.
    e. Scoliosis.
    f. Hernias (hiatal and inguinal).
    g. Aortic dissection or rupture (cystic medial necrosis); aortic valvular insufficiency.

**SUGGESTED READINGS**

Azouz EM, Slomic AM, Marton D, Rigault P, Finidon G: The variable manifestations of dysplasia epiphysealis hemimelica. *Pediatr Radiol* 1985; 15:44-49.

Beighton P: *Inherited disorders of the skeleton,* ed 2. New York, 1988, Churchill-Livingston.

Beighton P, Cremin BJ: *Sclerosing bone dysplasias.* Berlin, 1980, Springer-Verlag.

Berdon WE (ed): Special issue: Bone dysplasia. *Pediatr Radiol* vol 27(5) May 1997; 357-454.

Felson B (ed): Dwarfs and other little people: A roentgen guide. *Semin Roentgenol* 1973; 8:135-263.

Kaitila II, Leisti JT, Rimoin DL: Mesomelic bone dysplasias. *Clinc Orthop* 1976; 114:94-106.

Kozlowski K: Metaphyseal and spondylometaphyseal chondrodysplasias. *Clin Orthop* 1976; 114:83-93.

Loria-Cortes R, Quesada-Calvo E, Cordero-Chaverri C: Osteopetrosis in children: A report of 26 cases. *J Pediatr* 1977; 91:43-47.

McAlister WH: An approach to skeletal dysplasias. Current Concepts: A categorical course in pediatric radiology. *SPR syllabus* (RSNA Publications) 1994:101-117.

Rouse GA, Filly RA, Toomet F, Grube GL: Short limb skeletal dysplasias of the fetal spine with sonography and radiography. *Radiology* 1990; 174:177-180.

Spranger J: The epiphyseal dysplasias. *Clin Orthop* 1976; 114:46-60.

Spranger J, Cremin B, Beighton P: Osteogenesis imperfecta congenita: Features and prognosis of a hetergenous condition. *Pediatr Radiol* 1982; 12:21-27.

Taybi H, Lachman R: *Radiology of syndromes, metabolic disorders and skeletal dysplasias,* ed 3. Chicago, 1990, Mosby–Year Book.

# SECTION VII
Neurologic System: Head and Neck

# 37
# Congenital Brain Malformations

### Key Concepts

1. Chiari type II malformation is a hindbrain dysgenesis with a small posterior fossa and caudal displacement of the fourth ventricle, the medulla, and the cerebellum. Myelomeningocele and hydrocephalus usually coexist (over 90% of cases).
2. Anomalies of the corpus callosum (CC) have a strong association with other congenital abnormalities, such as Chiari malformations, Dandy-Walker syndrome, or interhemispheric lipomas.
3. Neurofibromatosis (NF) is the most common of the phakomatoses (neurocutaneous syndromes). Hallmark findings include:
    a. "Café-au-lait" spots.
    b. Central and peripheral schwannomas.
    c. Optic nerve gliomas; intracranial astrocytomas.
    d. Scoliosis.
    e. Bilateral acoustic neuromas.
    f. Central nervous system (CNS) tumors, such as meningiomas.
4. Hydranencephaly is a destruction of cerebral hemispheres, resulting from bilateral internal carotid occlusion; cerebral tissue is replaced by cerebrospinal fluid–filled sacs. Hydranencephaly must be differentiated from severe hydrocephalus, such as can be seen with congenital aqueductal stenosis.

A. Stages of brain development.
   1. Neural tube closure.
      a. Also called dorsal induction; occurs at 3 to 4 weeks of gestation.
      b. Formation of neural tube.
         *1.* Thickening of embryonic ectoderm (dorsal to notochord) forms neural plate.
         *2.* This ectoderm of neural plate (neuroectoderm) invaginates to form neural groove with neural folds seen alongside groove.
         *3.* Fusion of midline neural folds begins in the thoracic region and progresses at both ends to form neural tube.
      c. Interaction between developing neural tube and adjacent mesoderm produces meningeal layer, vertebra, and skull.
   2. Diverticulation.
      a. Also called ventral induction; occurs at 5 to 6 weeks of gestation.
      b. Brain and face form during stage of diverticulation.
      c. Cephalic end of embryo forms into prosencephalon, mesencephalon, rhombencephalon, and facial structures.
         *1.* Prosencephalon divides into telencephalon and diencephalon.
            *a.* Telencephalon goes on to divide and form two cerebral hemispheres and two lateral ventricles; connection does remain between two hemispheres (CC).
            *b.* Diencephalon forms thalamus, hypothalamus, and pineal body.
         *2.* Mesencephalon (midbrain).
            *a.* Superior colliculi.
            *b.* Inferior colliculi.
         *3.* Rhombencephalon divides into metencephalon and myelencephalon.
            *a.* Metencephalon.
               *1)* Cerebellum.
               *2)* Pons.
            *b.* Myelencephalon (medulla).
      d. Result of successful completion of above first two stages: bihemispheric brain, lying within intact calvarium with complete face.
   3. Neuronal proliferation.
      a. Occurs during 8 to 16 weeks of gestation.
      b. Neuronal proliferation, differentiation, and histogenesis occur simultaneously during this time.
      c. Neuroblasts are generated within highly vascular germinal matrix along ependymal surface.
   4. Neuronal migration.
      a. Occurs from 12 to 32 weeks of gestation.

b. Neuroblasts in germinal matrix migrate from ventricular subependymal surface to form superficial cortex and nuclei of basal ganglia.
c. Brain also undergoes sulcation, increasing the surface area (occurs from 24 to 36 weeks of gestation).
d. Latter two stages of proliferation and migration are lengthy and vulnerable to variety of insults.
5. Myelination.
   a. Myelination is ongoing process that continues after birth.
   b. As general rule, myelination proceeds posteriorly to anteriorly, centrally to peripherally, and inferiorly to superiorly.
   c. At birth, dorsal pons, inferior and superior cerebellar peduncles, and thalamus are myelinated.
   d. By 2 months of age, precentral gyrus myelinates, as does ventral pons.
   e. By 3 to 5 months of age, deep white matter of cerebellum myelinates, with corpus callosum and internal capsule myelination completed by 4 to 11 months.
B. Disorders of neural tube closure: Dorsal induction.
   1. Anencephaly.
      a. Absent cranial vault and cerebral hemispheres.
      b. Skull base, midbrain, and brainstem are intact.
      c. Found in girls more commonly than in boys (4:1).
      d. Increased alpha-fetoprotein, polyhydramnios.

**Imaging** Often diagnosed on prenatal US with absence of intracranial structures beyond orbits.

   2. Encephalocele.
      a. Incidence is 1 to 3:10,000.
      b. Midline cranial and dural defect with herniation of meninges (meningocele) or brain and meninges (encephalocele).
      c. Common locations.
         *1.* Occipital (71%).
         *2.* Parietal (10%).
         *3.* Skull base lesions (18%).
            *a.* Frontoethmoidal (more common in Asian population).
               *1)* Nasofrontal.
               *2)* Nasoethmoidal.
               *3)* Nasoorbital.
            *b.* Sphenoorbital.
            *c.* Sphenomaxillary.
            *d.* Nasopharyngeal.

d. Often obvious defect in neonate, yet can be subtle with only slight herniation (especially nasofrontal herniation).

**Imaging** Magnetic resonance imaging (MRI) can image contents of cranial and dural defect, identifying presence of brain and/or cerebrospinal fluid (CSF) within herniated sac. High-resolution coronal computed tomography (CT) may be necessary to visualize osseous abnormalities in lesions involving skull base.

3. Chiari malformations.
   a. Chiari type I.
      1. Cerebellar-tonsil herniation below foramen magnum.
      2. Normal fourth ventricle.
      3. Small or nonexistent cisterna magna; can be associated with syringohydromyelia.
      4. Often incidental finding, although can be associated with headaches.

**Imaging** Sagittal MRI can demonstrate low-lying cerebellar tonsils (abnormal is greater than 6 mm below foramen magnum during first decade of life and 5 mm for second through third decades).

   b. Chiari type II.
      1. Incidence is 2 to 3:1000; found in females more commonly than in males (2:1).
      2. Hindbrain dysgenesis with small posterior fossa.
      3. Caudal displacement of the fourth ventricle, medulla, and cerebellum.
      4. Myelomeningocele and hydrocephalus (over 90%).
      5. Can be associated with agenesis of corpus callosum and syringohydromyelia.

**Imaging** MRI and CT findings include colpocephaly of ventricles (dilated posteriorly), squared off frontal horns, tectal beaking of midbrain, cervicomedullary kinking, enlarged massa intermedia, hypoplastic falx with interdigitations, and lacunar skull (primary dysplasia of membranous bone).

   c. Chiari type III.
      1. Characteristics of Chiari type II.
      2. Occipital encephalocele.
C. Anomalies of CC.

1. Can have complete versus partial absence.
2. Insult occurs prior to 20 weeks gestation.
   a. In partial absence, posterior CC defects are seen.
   b. Results from CC formation, which forms anteriorly to posteriorly.
3. Strong association with other anomalies.
   a. Chiari malformations.
   b. Dandy-Walker syndrome.
   c. Holoprosencephaly.
4. Interhemispheric lipoma (often lipoma of CC).
   a. Rare; incidence is less than 1:1000.
   b. Primitive fat incorporated in midline at 3 to 5 weeks of gestation.
   c. Common interhemispheric sites.
      *1.* CC.
      *2.* Cerebellar-pontine angle.
      *3.* Quadrigeminal plate.
   d. Forty percent of midline lipomas occur with agenesis of CC.

> **Imaging** Agenesis of CC manifests on US, CT, and MRI as straightened, medially concave, lateral ventricles that are caused by course of Probst bundles (axons that normally cross in CC, but instead course sagittally along medial aspects of lateral ventricles) (Fig. 37-1). Also present are abnormal frontal horns ("Texas longhorn" appearance). MRI sagittal midline view, however, is best at directly demonstrating complete or partial absence of CC. Look for incorporation of fat, which may occur in dysplastic CC.

D. Disorders of diverticulation.
   1. Holoprosencephaly.
      a. Incidence is 1:16,000.
      b. Spectrum of anomalies.
         *1.* Incomplete cleavage of forebrain.
         *2.* Fused cerebral hemispheres, thalami, and ventricles.
      c. Also present are midface anomalies.
      d. Types.
         *1.* Alobar (most severe form).
            *a.* Large monoventricle with thin rim of cerebral tissue anteriorly located.
            *b.* Fused thalami.
            *c.* Absent midline structures, such as corpus callosum and interhemispheric falx.
         *2.* Semilobar.
            *a.* Partial development of posterior falx and occipital horns.

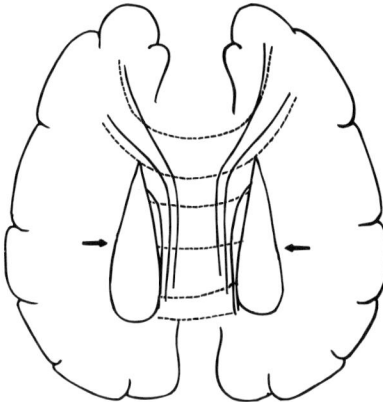

**Fig. 37-1** Probst bundles (agenesis of CC). With agenesis of CC, normal path of white-matter fibers *(dotted lines)* is disrupted and takes inferior course *(solid line)*, resulting in characteristic straightened appearance of lateral ventricles *(arrows)*.

            b. Partial separation of occipitoparietal lobes.
       3. Lobar (mildest form).
           a. Interhemispheric falx is complete but anteriorly located.
           b. Well-formed occipital, temporal, and parietal lobes; partial frontal lobe fusion.
           c. Normal thalami, ventricles.
    2. Septooptic dysplasia (De Morsier syndrome).
       a. Some consider this to be mildest form of holoprosencephaly, with forebrain anomaly limited to hypoplastic optic nerves, chiasm, or infundibulum.
       b. Patients are often blind with diabetes insipidus and hypothalamic or pituitary abnormalities.
       c. Absent septum pellucidum.
E. Disorders of neuronal proliferation, differentiation, and histogenesis.
    1. NF.
       a. Autosomal dominant; greater than 50% are spontaneous mutations.
       b. NF type I ("classic NF" or von Recklinghausen disease).
           *1.* Defect on chromosome 17; incidence is 1:2500 to 3000 births.
           *2.* "Café-au-lait" spots.
           *3.* Central and peripheral schwannomas.
           *4.* Optic nerve gliomas and intracranial astrocytomas.
           *5.* Sphenoid wing dysplasia.
           *6.* Scoliosis.
           *7.* Plexiform neurofibromas.

8. Unidentified bright objects in CNS.
   a. Common locations.
      1) Internal capsule.
      2) Basal ganglia and thalami.
      3) Brainstem.
   b. Best seen on MRI as bright lesions on $T_2$-weighted images that do not enhance.
 c. NF type II ("central CNS" NF).
    1. Defect on chromosome 22; incidence is 1:50,000.
    2. Bilateral acoustic neuromas.
    3. CNS tumors.
       a. Meningiomas.
       b. Ependymomas.
       c. Gliomas.
    4. Less-frequent cutaneous manifestations than NF type I.
2. Tuberous sclerosis (Bourneville disease).
   a. Autosomal dominant.
   b. Mental retardation, seizures, adenoma sebaceum.
   c. Hamartomas.
      1. CNS tubers.
         a. Calcified, usually subependymal nodules.
         b. Foramen of Monro giant cell astrocytoma.
         c. Cortical and subcortical foci signal abnormalities on MRI.
      2. Renal (angiomyolipoma).
      3. Cardiac (rhabdomyomas).
3. Sturge-Weber syndrome (encephalotrigeminal angiomatosis).
   a. Port-wine stain on face in trigeminal distribution.
   b. Seizures, severe mental retardation.
   c. Intracranial gyral calcifications.
      1. "Tram track" distribution.
      2. Especially occipital location.
   d. Ipsilateral enlargement and enhancement of choroid plexus.
4. Von Hippel-Lindau disease.
   a. Autosomal dominant.
   b. Hemangioblastomas.
      1. Cerebellar.
      2. Retinal.
      3. Spinal cord.
   c. Cysts.
      1. Renal.
      2. Hepatic.
      3. Pancreatic.

d. Associated with pheochromocytoma and renal cell carcinoma.
F. Disorders of sulcation and migration: Abnormal thickness, folding, and organization of cerebral hemispheres.
 1. Lissencephaly (agyria).
    a. Absent cerebral sulci and gyri due to interrupted neuronal migration from subependymal germinal matrix (12 to 16 weeks of gestation).
    b. Only four cortical layers form (normal number of layers is six).
    c. Clinical presentation.
       *1.* Seizures.
       *2.* Severe mental retardation.
       *3.* Heterotopias.
       *4.* Abnormal CC.
    d. Types.
       *1.* Type I.
          *a.* More common.
          *b.* Sporadic.
       *2.* Type II.
          *a.* Associated with genetic syndromes.
          *b.* Walker-Warburg syndrome.
    e. Be aware that premature brains (brains that have not completed sulcation) can appear "smooth" and can mimic lissencephaly.

> **Imaging** MRI, CT, and US can demonstrate hourglass- or figure 8–shaped brain with smooth surface. Only fold present is central sylvian fissure (occurs at about 20 weeks of gestation).

 2. Pachygyria.
    a. Reduced number of coarse, broad, shallow gyri.
    b. Seizures and mental retardation.
 3. Polymicrogyria.
    a. Increased number of abnormally small gyri.
    b. Etiology may be due to unequal distribution of final migrating neurons (at 20 to 24 weeks of gestation) that form most superficial cortical layers.
    c. Can have focal areas of polymicrogyria that are asymptomatic.
    d. Pathologic diagnosis; may be indistinguishable on imaging studies.
 4. Heterotopias.
    a. Arrested neuronal migration with ectopic gray-matter nodules or bandlike areas.
    b. Usually located in subependymal or subcortical regions.

c. Often asymptomatic but can be seizure focus.
d. Must distinguish from tumor, since heterotopias can mimic cerebral masses.

**Imaging** CT and MRI can show multiple small nodules, usually along ventricular (subependymal) surface. Heterotopias always match gray-matter signal on MRI and lack contrast enhancement.

5. Schizencephaly.
   a. Full-thickness clefts in cerebral hemispheres that can be bilateral; often at level of sylvian fissure.
   b. Pathogenesis uncertain; probably developmental etiology (due to aberrant migration, since clefts are lined with gray matter).
   c. Types.
      1. Type I.
         a. "Closed lips."
         b. Absent CSF cavity.
      2. Type II.
         a. "Open lips."
         b. Clefts are filled with CSF.
         c. Communication of extraaxial fluid with ventricle at site of cleft.
   d. Seizures and mental retardation.
   e. Associated with dysgenesis of CC and heterotopias.

**Imaging** MRI, CT, and US demonstrate cerebral clefts lined with gray matter, extending from cortex to ventricle. CSF within clefts may be present.

G. Disorders of cerebellum and posterior fossa.
   1. Dandy-Walker syndrome.
      a. Marked dilatation of fourth ventricle communicating with retrocerebellar posterior fossa cyst.
      b. Pathogenesis is uncertain; may be due to obstruction or atresia of outlet foramina (Magendie and Lushka foramina).
      c. No communication between fourth ventricular cyst and basal cisterns.
      d. Associated with agenesis of CC (15% to 25% of cases).
      e. Hydrocephalus need not occur but is prognostic factor if present.

**Imaging** MRI and CT demonstrate:
   • Large posterior fossa.
   • Retrocerebellar cyst communicating with fourth ventricle.

- Absent or hypoplastic cerebellar vermis.
- Hydrocephalus is often present.
- Tentorial insertion above lambdoid sutures (known as torcular-lambdoid inversion).

2. Dandy-Walker variant.
   a. More common than "true" Dandy-Walker syndrome.
   b. Smaller retrocerebellar cyst, milder vermian agenesis, normal-sized posterior fossa.
   c. Patent foramen of Magendie allows for some communication between cyst and basal cisterns.
   d. Differential diagnosis of normal-sized posterior fossa with cystic collection also includes:
      1. Retrocerebellar arachnoid cyst.
      2. Giant cisterna magna.
      3. For these two entities, look for intact cerebellum and vermis as possible distinguishing features from Dandy-Walker variant.

**Imaging** MRI and CT reveal predominantly fluid-filled, yet normal-sized posterior fossa, often with some cerebellar tissue (although tissue is hypoplastic). No hydrocephalus is present.

3. Cerebellar hypoplasia or agenesis.
   a. Failure of normal development of vermis and cerebellar hemispheres.
      1. Can be isolated (Joubert syndrome).
         a. Complete agenesis of vermis.
         b. Dysplastic cerebellum.
         c. Characteristic "triangular-shaped" fourth ventricle caused by missing vermis seen on CT and MRI.
         d. Also associated with syndactyly.
      2. Can be part of syndrome, such as Dandy-Walker syndrome or variant.
   b. Partial agenesis is more common with preservation of anterior and superior aspects of cerebellum (related to formation order, which is rostral-to-caudal).
   c. Hypoplastic cerebellar peduncles and brainstem (especially pons) is often present with ex vacuo dilatation of retrocerebellar CSF space.

H. Destructive lesions.
   1. Hydranencephaly.
      a. Destruction of cerebral hemispheres.
         1. Extreme form of porencephaly (see following discussion).

2. Caused by bilateral internal carotid occlusion.
   b. Cerebral tissue replaced by CSF-filled sacs.
   c. Thalami, brainstem, and posterior fossa preserved (posterior circulation).
   d. Must differentiate from severe hydrocephalus (such as congenital aqueductal stenosis).

> **Imaging** Fluid fills cranial vault above tentorium with no supratentorial cortical tissue present. Look on US, CT, or MRI for thin rim of cortical tissue that would help distinguish hydranencephaly from severe hydrocephalus.

2. Porencephaly.
   a. CSF cavity caused by destruction of formed brain tissue.
   b. CSF space communicates with ventricular system.
   c. Etiology is probably acquired (vascular or infectious insult in utero).

**SUGGESTED READINGS**

Altman NR, Naidich PP, Braffman BH: Posterior fossa malformations. *AJNR* 1992; 13:619-624.

Barkovich AJ, Gressens P, Evrard P: Formation, maturation and disorders of brain neocortex. *AJNR* 1992; 13:423-446.

Barkovich AJ, Fram EK, Norman D: MR of septo-optic dysplasia. *Radiology* 1989; 171:189-192.

Barkovich AJ, Kjos BO: Gray matter heterotopia: MR characteristics and correlation with developmental and neurologic manifestations. *Radiology* 1992; 182:493-499.

Barkovich AJ, Norman D: MR imaging of schizencephaly. *AJR* 1988; 150:1391-1396.

Braffman BH, Bilaniuk LT, Naidich TP, Altman NR, Post MJD, Quencer RM, Zimmerman RA, Brady BA: MR imaging of tuberous sclerosis: Pathogenesis of this phakomatoses and literature review. *Radiology* 1992; 183:227-238.

Byrd SE, Osborn RE, Bohan TP, Naidich TP: CT and MR evaluation of migrational disorders of the brain. *Pediatr Radiol* 1989; 19:151-156.

Byrd SE, Naidich TP: Common congenital brain anomalies. *Radiol Clin North Am* 1988; 26:755-772.

Kendall B, Kingsley D, Lambert SR, Taylor D, Finn P: Joubert syndrome: A clinicoradiological study. *Neuroradiology* 1990; 31:502-506.

Kollias SS, Ball WS, Prenger EC: Cystic malformations of the posterior fossa: Differential diagnosis clarified through embryologic analysis. *Radiographics* 1993; 13:1211-1231.

Mikulis DJ, Diaz O, Egglin TK, Sanchez R: Variance of the position of the cerebellar tonsils with age: Preliminary report. *Radiology* 1992; 183:725-728.

Rubenstein D, Cajade-Law AG, Youngman V, Hise JM, Baganz M: Development of the corpus callosum in semilobar and lobar holoprosencephaly. *Pediatr Radiol* 1996; 26:839-844.

Sevick RJ, Barkovich AJ, Edwards MSB, Koch T, Berg B, Lempert T: Evolution of white matter lesions in neurofibromatosis type I. *AJR* 1992; 159:171-175.

Shu HH, Mirowitz SA, Wippold FJ: Neurofibromatosis: MR imaging findings involving the head and spine. *AJR* 1993; 160:159-164.

Van Es R, North KN, McHugh K, De Silva M: MRI findings in children with neurofibromatosis type I: A prospective study. *Pediatr Radiol* 1996; 26:478-487.

Wolpert SM, Anderson M, Scott RM, Kwan ESK, Runge VM: The Chiari II malformation: MR imaging evaluation. *AJNR* 1987; 8:783-791.

# 38
# Neonatal Head

## Key Concepts

1. Because of the presence of fontanelles in infants, head ultrasound (US) in neonates can be used to evaluate for congenital brain malformations, hemorrhage, or ischemia.
2. Premature infants are at high risk for intracranial hemorrhage, which usually originates in the subependymal germinal matrix (highly vascular area of developing neuroblasts).
3. Intracranial hemorrhage is a spectrum, ranging from grade I (germinal matrix, subependymal hemorrhage, usually with no long-term neurologic sequelae) to grade IV (intraparenchymal component with 90% incidence of neurologic sequelae).
4. Periventricular leukomalacia (PVL) is necrosis of periventricular white matter, caused by hypoperfusion or ischemia, especially near the frontal horns and trigone region. Adjacent ventricular ex vacuo dilation may also be present because of the white-matter loss. Clinically, PVL can manifest as cerebral palsy (CP).
5. Macrocephaly is a common problem in the evaluation of the growing infant and child; usually a large head (out of proportion to the rest of the body) is caused by benign macrocephaly that will resolve. Hydrocephalus (either posthemorrhagic, postinfectious, or resulting from congenital aqueductal stenosis, meningomyelocele, or tumor) is another concern.

A. Neonatal head US.
   1. Possible because of presence of fontanelles (normally use anterior fontanelle as acoustic window).
   2. Anterior fontanelle can remain open for up to 2 years, but brain scanning is really only feasible up to about 1 year of age (obviously, the smaller the fontanelle, the more technically difficult the study).
   3. Standard head US examination is performed in two planes: coronal and sagittal (Fig. 38-1).
B. Prematurity.
   1. Head US screening for premature infants.
      a. Routinely performed during first week of life.
      b. Criteria for screening.
         *1.* Weight of infant is less than 1200 to 1500 g.
         *2.* Less than 32 weeks gestational age.
         *3.* Clinical signs.
            *a.* Apnea and bradycardia.
            *b.* Hypotension with decreasing hematocrit.
            *c.* Seizures.
            *d.* Increasing head circumference.
            *e.* Bulging fontanelle.
   2. Hemorrhage.
      a. Incidence of hemorrhage in premature infants.
         *1.* In infants less than 32 weeks gestation and weighing less than 1500 g, incidence can range from 30% to 50%.
         *2.* Five percent of term infants can have intracranial hemorrhage.

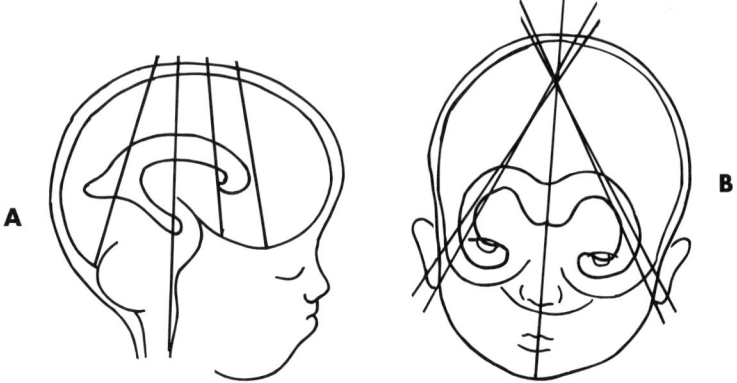

**Fig. 38-1** Transverse and coronal head US protocol. **A,** Sagittal view of brain with lines depicting US "slices" obtained through anterior fontanelle. **B,** Coronal view of brain. Again, lines depict US views obtained via anterior fontanelle.

b. Location of hemorrhage.
   1. Germinal matrix.
      a. Most common location of hemorrhage.
      b. Germinal matrix is located along wall of lateral ventricle and is most prevalent in region of caudothalamic groove.
      c. Extremely vascular germinal matrix contains developing neuroblasts that gradually migrate to form cerebral cortex. As infant approaches term, germinal matrix slowly involutes.
   2. Intraventricular.
      a. Hemorrhage originates in germinal matrix adjacent to lateral ventricle.
      b. Hemorrhage can then propagate and rupture into ventricular system.
c. Grading of intracranial hemorrhage on US (see box on facing page).
d. Incidence of different types of hemorrhage.
   1. Grade I (75%).
   2. Grades II and III (20%).
   3. Grade IV (5%).
e. Etiology.
   1. In premature infant, arterial cerebral autoregulation is poor.
   2. Result: increased cerebral blood flow or changing blood pressures (either hypertensive or hypotensive episodes) can have a dramatic effect on germinal matrix, causing hemorrhage.
   3. Coexistence of hemorrhage and ischemia in premature infant is 28% to 55%.
f. Effects of intracranial hemorrhage.
   1. Early.
      a. Ventriculitis can occur following hemorrhage and infection.
      b. Ventriculitis manifests as increased echogenicity of ventricular lining, often with ventriculomegaly.
   2. Long-term neurologic sequelae.
      a. Ventriculomegaly.
         1) Hydrocephalus that may require ventricular drain or ventricular-peritoneal shunt.
         2) Ventricular enlargement (especially following hemorrhagic or ischemic event) can also be related to cerebral atrophy and ex vacuo dilation.
         3) Can be difficult to discern obstruction versus atrophy.
            a) Clinical findings (full or bulging fontanelle or enlarging head size) are helpful criteria for determining true ventricular obstruction.

### Grading System Devised to Describe Germinal Matrix Hemorrhage (GMH) and Its Intraventricular (IVH) or Intraparenchymal Extension.*

Grade I
- Subependymal hemorrhage.
- Echogenic area in caudothalamic groove.

Grade II
- Germinal matrix hemorrhage that ruptures into ventricle.
- No ventricular dilatation is present.

Grade III
- Ventricular hemorrhage.
- Ventricular dilatation causes.
  - Poor cerebrospinal fluid resorption from pacchionian granulations (communicating hydrocephalus).
  - Direct obstruction (noncommunicating hydrocephalus) from clot or inflammatory adhesions secondary to arachnoiditis.

Grade IV
- Intraparenchymal hemorrhage.
- Often results in porencephalic cysts.
- Debate has arisen concerning status of grade IV or intraparenchymal hemorrhage.
  - Originally, intraparenchymal component was described as extending from GMH or IVH.
  - More recent theories suggest that IVH and subsequent dilatation can cause venous obstruction or congestion in periventricular white matter, resulting in venous infarction. This periventricular ischemia or infarction can have hemorrhagic component as well.

*Data compiled from Papile L, Burstein J, Burstein R, Koffler H: Incidence and evaluation of subependymal and intraventricular hemorrhage: A study of infants with birthweights less than 1500 grams. *J Pediatr* 1978; 92:529-534.

      *b)* Resistive index (RI) of middle cerebral artery may be helpful. RI = (systolic − diastolic) ÷ systolic. "Normal" is defined as $0.75 \pm 0.10$. In cases of increased intracranial pressure (obstruction), RI is abnormally high (greater than 0.85) with low diastolic flow (Fig. 38-2).
  *b.* Spastic dyplegia, CP.
  *c.* Mental retardation and developmental delay.
  *d.* Incidence of long-term neurologic sequelae.
    *1)* Grade I: 1% to 5%.
    *2)* Grade II: 5% to 10%.

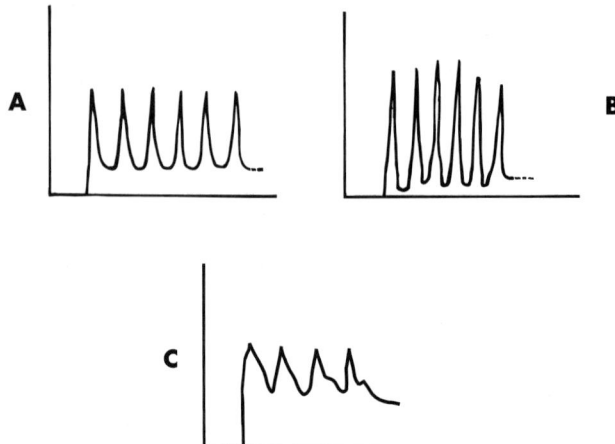

**Fig. 38-2** RI tracings: **A,** Normal (0.75 ± 0.10). **B,** Increased intracranial pressure (low diastolic flow). **C,** Ischemia (high diastolic flow).

3) Grade III: 50% to 60%.
4) Grade IV: 90%.

**Imaging** Acute hemorrhage on US appears echogenic, usually seen in region of caudothalamic groove and/or with echogenic hemorrhagic extension into ventricle or surrounding parenchyma. Look for ventricular enlargement.

g. PVL.
1. Necrosis of periventricular white matter, especially near frontal horns and trigone region (watershed areas that are most vulnerable to hypoperfusion or ischemia).
2. Findings may be subtle initially; diagnosis is often made retrospectively, once cystic areas on imaging studies (US), computed tomography (CT), or magnetic resonance imaging (MRI) appear.
3. Result of PVL is decreased volume of parietal deep white matter; this results in CP.
    a. Clinical syndrome of nonprogressive motor deficits of central origin with onset from early infancy.
    b. Spastic dyplegia.

**Imaging** US may initially be normal or may show areas of increased periventricular echogenicity. It can be difficult to distinguish initial PVL echogenicity from normal periventricular echogenic "halo." Later, cystic changes

> may be evident (3 to 4 weeks after insult). MRI can demonstrate delayed myelination, thin areas of white matter (including corpus callosum) with occasional global cerebral atrophy, and mild adjacent ventricular enlargement (ventricular ex vacuo dilatation).

C. Congenital anomalies (see Chapters 37 and 39).
 1. "TORCH."
    a. Congenital brain infections.
       1. *T*oxoplasmosis.
       2. *O*ther agents (congenital syphilis and viruses).
       3. *R*ubella.
       4. *C*ytomegalovirus (CMV).
       5. *H*erpes.
    b. Look for calcifications, especially along ventricular system.
    c. Ventriculomegaly.
    d. Echogenic, linear pattern in thalamus or basal ganglia seen on US.
       1. Mineralizing vasculopathy, especially seen in CMV.
       2. Also seen in trisomy 13 syndrome, fetal alcohol syndrome, and Down syndrome.
 2. Chiari malformation.
    a. Low-lying cerebellar tonsils.
    b. Ventriculomegaly.
 3. Agenesis of corpus callosum.
    a. "Long-horn" or "viking-helmet" appearance of frontal horns.
    b. Straightening or vertical orientation of lateral ventricles (due to vertical orientation of bundles of Probst).
 4. Dandy-Walker malformation.
    a. Cystic dilatation of posterior fossa, often with hydrocephalus.
    b. Hypoplastic vermis.
 5. Hydranencephaly.
    a. "Water bags" in head.
    b. Near-complete destruction of cerebral hemispheres.
       1. Probably caused by bilateral carotid occlusion in utero.
       2. Small portions of inferior temporal and occipital lobes can have blood supply from posterior circulation and therefore can be spared.
 6. Vein of Galen aneurysm.
    a. Arteriovenous (AV) malformation (not true aneurysm).
    b. Usually aberrant connection between anterior cerebral, choroidal arteries, or thalamoperforators and vein of Galen.
    c. Usually presents early in neonate with congestive heart failure, caused by shunting across AV malformation (poor prognosis).
    d. May attempt interventional embolization.

> **Imaging** Head US demonstrates hypoechoic, dilated vein of Galen that has very high color and duplex Doppler flow. Often surrounding encephalomalacia may be present (poorer prognosis). Malformation is signal void on MRI and intensely enhanced on CT contrast study.

D. Anoxia or ischemia.
  1. Perinatal asphyxia.
     a. Often due to hypotension (low cerebral blood flow can lead to ischemia).
     b. Hypoxia is also vasodilatory.
        *1.* After decreased blood pressure from asphyxia, vasodilatory effect can rupture delicate vessels of germinal matrix, causing them to hemorrhage.
     2. RI (as seen in US) (Fig. 38-2).
        *a.* When ischemia is present, RI of middle cerebral artery (MCA) is abnormally low (less than 0.65).
        *b.* Diastolic flow is increased in ischemia from loss of autoregulation of vessels (leads to low RI).
        *c.* Be aware of false-postive RI.
           *1)* Complete loss of diastolic flow due to patent ductus arteriosus.

> **Imaging** Head US may show increased echogenicity of parenchyma, often with slitlike ventricles that could be caused by cerebral edema from ischemia, focal hemorrhage, or both. Echogenic thalamus is particularly ominous sign of severe hypoxic or ischemic insult. However, initial qualitative head US is often negative; therefore, quantitative RI may be helpful.

E. Macrocephaly.
  1. Common problem in evaluation of growing infant and child; head is usually large (out of proportion to rest of body) but benign.
  2. Evaluation of large head.
     a. Confirm measurements and plot curve.
     b. Look for signs of increased intracranial pressure.
     c. Family history of head growth.
     d. History of headaches, nausea or vomiting, or developmental delay.
     e. Imaging of head.
        *1.* US.
           *a.* Excellent first screening test.
              *1)* Noninvasive.

*2)* No sedation needed.
  *b.* Can be used only on infants, depending on size of anterior fontanelle.
 *2.* CT.
 *3.* MRI.
 3. Causes of macrocephaly.
  a. Benign macrocrania.
   *1.* Big head in otherwise normal-growing infant or child.
   *2.* Most common reason for large head in children.
   *3.* Often family history of large heads.
   *4.* Long-term prognosis.
    *a.* Rest of body usually catches up with head.
    *b.* Results in normal development.

---

**Imaging** CT and US show normal cerebral parenchyma with top normal ventricular system, often with enlarged subarachnoid spaces (extraaxial fluid).

---

  b. Hydrocephalus.
   *1.* Congenital aqueductal stenosis.
   *2.* Posthemorrhagic (premature infants).
   *3.* Postinfectious (meningitis).
   *4.* Meningomyelocele.

---

**Imaging** Varying degree of ventriculomegaly can be seen on CT and US.

---

  c. Tumors (can often cause hydrocephalus; see Chapter 40).
   *1.* Infants (less than 1 year of age).
    *a.* Intraventricular tumors.
     *1)* Choroid plexus papilloma.
     *2)* Choroid plexus carcinoma.
    *b.* Congenital tumors.
     *1)* Teratoma.
     *2)* Primitive neuroectodermal tumors.
     *3)* Neuroblastoma.
   *2.* Children (greater than 1 year of age).
    *a.* Craniopharyngioma.
    *b.* Posterior fossa tumors.
     *1)* Cystic astrocytoma.
     *2)* Medulloblastoma.
     *3)* Ependymoma.
    *c.* Slow-growing gliomas (tectal).
    *d.* Astrocytoma.
    *e.* Dermoid or epidermoid.

d. Congenital brain malformations (see Chapter 37).
   1. Holoprosencephaly (look for facial abnormalities).
   2. Hydranencephaly.
   3. Dandy-Walker malformation (posterior fossa cyst).
   4. Arachnoid cyst.
   5. Aqueductal stenosis (hydrocephalus).
e. Congenital developmental disorders.
   1. Tay-Sachs disease.
   2. Dysmyelinating disorders (see Chapter 41).
      a. Alexander disease.
      b. Krabbe disease.
      c. Canavan disease.
   3. Skeletal dysplasias (achondroplastic dwarf).
   4. Tuberous sclerosis (foramen of Monro giant cell astrocytoma).
   5. Intrauterine growth retardation (asymmetric).
   6. Mucopolysaccharidoses.
      a. Hurler syndrome.
      b. Hunter syndrome.

**SUGGESTED READINGS**

Babcock DS: Sonography of the brain in infants: Role in evaluating neurologic abnormalities. *AJR* 1995; 165:417-423.

Bowerman RA, Donn SM, DiPietro MA, D'Amato CJ, Hicks SP: Periventricular leukomalacia in the preterm newborn infant: Sonographic and clinical features. *Radiology* 1984; 151:383.

Connolly B, Kelehan P, O'Brien N, Gorman W, Murphy JF, King M, Donoghue V: The echogenic thalamus in hypoxic ischemic encephalopathy. *Pediatr Radiol* 1994; 24:268-271.

Frank JL: Sonography of intracranial infection in infants and children. *Neuroradiology* 1986; 28:440-451.

Han BK, Babcock DS, Oestriech AE: Sonography of brain tumors in infants. *AJNR* 1984; 5:253-258.

Hay TC, Rumack CM, Horgan JG: Cranial sonography: Intracranial hemorrhage, periventricular leukomalacia and asphyxia. In Babcock DS, ed. *Neonatal and pediatric ultrasonography: Clinics in diagnostic ultrasound.* New York, 1989, Churchill Livingston.

Hernanz-Schulman M, Cohen W, Genieser NB: Sonography of cerebral infarction in infancy. *AJR* 1988; 150:897-902.

Kirks DR, Bowie JD: Cranial ultrasonography of neonatal periventricular/intraventricular hemorrhage: Who, why and when? *Pediatr Radiol* 1986; 16:114-117.

Papile L, Burstein J, Burstein R, Koffler H: Incidence and evaluation of subependymal and intraventricular hemorrhage: A study of infants with birthweights less than 1500 grams. *J Pediatr* 1978; 92:529-534.

Reeder JD, Sanders RC: Ventriculitis in the neonate: Recognition by sonography. *AJNR* 1983; 4:37-41.

Rogers B, Msall M, Owens T, Guernsey K, Brody A, Buck G, Hudak M: Cystic periventricular leukomalacia and type of cerebral palsy in preterm infants. *J Pediatr* 1994; 125:1-8.

Rosenberg HK, Kessler A: Sonography of neonatal intracranial infection. *Ultrasound Q* 1993; 11:125-133.

Rumack CM, Manco-Johnson ML, Manco-Johnson MJ, Koops BL, Hathaway WE, Apparetim S: Timing and course of neonatal intracranial hemorrhage using real-time ultrasound. *Radiology* 1985; 154:101-104.

Rypens F, Avni EF, Dussaussois L, David P, Vermeylen D, Van Bogaert, Matos C: Hyperechoic thickened ependyma: Sonographic demonstration and significance in neonates. *Pediatr Radiol* 1994; 24:550-553.

Siebert JJ, McCowan TC, Chadduck WM, Adametz JR, Glasier CM, Williamson SL, Taylor BJ, Leithiser RE, McConnell JR, Stansell CA, Rodgers AB, Corbitt SL: Duplex pulsed Doppler US versus intracranial pressure in the neonate: Clinical and experimental studies. *Radiology* 1989; 171:155-159.

Stark JE, Siebert JJ: Cerebral artery Doppler ultrasonography for the prediction of outcome after perinatal asphyxia. *J Ultrasound Med* 1994; 13:595-600.

Storr U, Rupprecht T, Bornemann A, Ries M, Beinder E, Bowing B, Harms D: Congenital intracerebral teratoma: A rare differential diagnosis in newborn hydrocephalus. *Pediatr Radiol* 1997; 27:262-264.

Volpe JJ: *Neurology of the newborn,* ed 2. Philadelphia, 1987, WB Saunders Co.

# 39
# Central Nervous System Infections

> **Key Concepts**
>
> 1. Congenital "TORCH" (*t*oxoplasmosis, *o*ther agents [congenital syphilis and viruses], *r*ubella, *c*ytomegalovirus [CMV], and *h*erpes simplex) infections can be devastating central nervous system (CNS) infections in the newborn.
> 2. Meningitis is the most common CNS infection; long-term complications include postinfectious hydrocephalus and hygroma formation.
> 3. Herpes encephalitis is commonly located in the temporal lobes and can result in a necrotic and hemorrhagic encephalitis that can cause brain destruction.
> 4. Acute disseminated encephalomyelitis (ADEM) is a postinfectious encephalitis (probably autoimmune etiology) that can lead to demyelination.

A. Congenital infections.
   1. Route of infection.
      a. Transplacental.
      b. Ascending (via cervix).
   2. Types (TORCH).
      a. Toxoplasmosis.
      b. Other agents (congenital syphilis and viruses).
      c. Rubella.
      d. CMV.
      e. Herpes.
   3. Clinical presentation depends on severity of infection.
   4. Complications.
      a. Microcephaly.
      b. Seizures; mental retardation.

   > **Imaging** Ultrasound (US), computed tomography (CT), or magnetic resonance imaging (MRI) can demonstrate ventricular enlargement (depending on amount of brain destruction), often with cortical calcifications (especially toxoplasmosis) or periventricular calcifications and migrational abnormalities (especially CMV).

B. Meningitis.
   1. Most common type of CNS infection.
      a. Viral.
      b. Bacterial.
      c. Tuberculous.
   2. Route of infection.
      a. Hematogenous.
      b. Direct, contiguous spread.
         *1.* Otitis media, mastoiditis.
         *2.* Sinusitis.
         *3.* Cortical brain abscess.
   3. Clinical presentation.
      a. Fever.
      b. Headache.
      c. Nuchal rigidity.
   4. Complications.
      a. Ventriculitis (30%).
         *1.* Inflammation of ependymal lining.
         *2.* Seen especially in neonates with meningitis or hemorrhage.
      b. Hydrocephalus.
         *1.* Disruption of cerebrospinal fluid resorption (communicating hydrocephalus).

2. Scarring or adhesions (noncommunicating hydrocephalus).
    c. Thrombosis.
        1. Venous or dural sinus thrombosis and infarction.
            a. Sagittal sinus thrombosis.
                1) More commonly seen with dehydration.
                2) Especially in infants.
            b. "Delta sign."
                1) CT finding of sagittal sinus thrombosis.
                2) "Dense" posterior falx or torcula on unenhanced CT.
                3) Low-density triangle (thrombosis) within sinus or torcula can be seen on enhanced CT.
                4) Be aware of false-positive results (neonates have physiologic "dense" posterior falx or torcula).
        2. Can lead to cerebral parenchymal spread (abscess).
    d. Hygromas (subdural effusions).
        1. Especially seen with *Haemophilus influenza* meningitis.
        2. Usually located in frontal and temporal regions.

> **Imaging** Initial CT is usually normal. Contrast scan may demonstrate meningeal enhancement. Subsequent ventriculitis can be seen on US as echogenic lining to ventricular system, often with ventricular enlargement. Hygromas are usually delayed finding.

C. Encephalitis.
  1. Viral.
     a. Herpes simplex.
        1. Types.
            a. Type I (oral herpes) is usual etiology for herpes encephalitis.
            b. Type II (genital herpes) usually causes congenital or perinatal (TORCH) infections.
        2. One third of all cases of herpes encephalitis are seen in children.
        3. Common locations.
            a. Type I.
                1) Temporal lobes.
                2) Usually unilateral.
            b. Type II (can involve any part of brain).
        4. Results in necrotic and hemorrhagic encephalitis that can cause brain destruction.
        5. Treat with acyclovir.

> **Imaging** CT may show low-density areas, preferentially in temporal lobes (type I). MRI is more sensitive to early disease with areas of high signal on $T_2$-weighted images.

    b. Subacute sclerosing panencephalitis.
        1. Due to reactivation of measles virus (can be years after primary infection).
        2. Predominantly involves white matter (demyelinating), although generalized cerebral atrophy may result.

> **Imaging** CT and MRI both demonstrate patchy, white-matter abnormalities (low density on CT and high signal on $T_2$-weighted MR images) that do not enhance.

    c. Human immunodeficiency virus.
        1. Primary finding is diffuse atrophy with occasional basal ganglia calcifications.
        2. Disseminated CMV or *Candida* meningitis or encephalitis.
        3. Progressive multifocal leukoencephalitis.
            a. Caused by reactivation of papova virus in immunocompromised patient.
            b. Results in demyelination and destruction of white matter.
        4. CNS lymphoma (rare in children).
2. Bacterial.
    a. Can be transmitted hematogenously versus directly (adjacent sinus infection).
    b. Encephalitis can progress to form abscess.
    c. Types.
        1. *Staphylococcus aureus.*
        2. *Streptococcus.*
        3. *Esherichia coli.*
        4. *H. influenza.*
            a. More commonly causes meningitis alone.
            b. Common complication is subdural hygromas.

> **Imaging** MRI or CT may reveal cerebral edema early in course of the disease. Enhancement of involved area may occur, as well as ring enhancement of any formed abscess cavity.

3. Parasitic.
    a. Cysticercosis *(Taenia solium).*
        1. Parasite is initially ingested with subsequent dissemination of eggs.

2. Seen in Latin America, India, and Africa.
3. Intracranial larvae can be parenchymal or intraventricular.
4. Often presents with seizures or hydrocephalus.
    a. Caused by intraventricular cysticercosis.
    b. Either direct obstruction or ventriculitis from infection.

> **Imaging** CT and MRI can demonstrate cystic lesion of cysticerosis (scolex is head of larvae, cystic portion is bladder), which has wall enhancement. The lesions are often seen at gray–white-matter junction or within ventricular system (usually fourth ventricle). Adjacent edema and calcifications are often present (caused by dead larvae; calcifications take years to form).

4. ADEM.
    a. Postinfectious encephalitis or myelitis (following measles, mumps, varicella, or upper respiratory infections).
    b. Probably autoimmune reaction, causing inflammatory reaction that can lead to demyelination.
    c. Often presents 1 to 2 weeks following viral illness or vaccination.
    d. Usually resolves without complications; steroids may be helpful.

> **Imaging** Bilateral, scattered, although often asymmetric, high-signal lesions in subcortical white matter, basal ganglia, and spinal cord can be seen on MRI ($T_2$-weighted images); probably caused by areas of demyelination.

**SUGGESTED READINGS**

Bale JF, Anderson RD, Grose C: MRI of the brain in childhood herpes virus. *Pediatr Infect Disease J* 1987; 6:644-647.

Byrd SE, Locke GE, Bigges S, Percy AK: Computed tomographic appearance of cerebral cysticercosis in adults and children. *Radiology* 1982; 144:819-823.

Dunn V, Bale JF, Zimmerman RA, Perdue Z, Bell WE: MRI in children with postinfectious disseminated encephalomyelitis. *Magn Reson Imaging* 1986; 4:25-32.

Haimes AB, Zimmerman RD, Morgello S, Weingarten K, Becker RD, Jennis R, Deck MDF: MRI of brain abscesses. *AJNR* 1989; 10:279-291.

Krawiecki NS, Dyken PR, El Gammel T, DuRant RH, Swift A: CT of the brain in subacute sclerosing panencephalitis. *Ann Neurol* 1984; 15:489-493.

Lukes SA, Norman D: Computed tomography in acute disseminated encephalitis. *Ann Neurol* 1983; 13:567-572.

Modi G, Campbell H, Brill P: Subacute sclerosing panencephalitis. *Neuroradiology* 1989; 31:433-434.

Preidler KW, Piepl T. Ranner G: Cerebral schistosomiasis: MR and CT appearance. *AJNR* 1996; 17:1598-1600.

Price, DB, Jacobs J, Haller JO, Inglese CM, Kramer J, Hotson GC, Loh JP, Schlusselberg D, Menez-Bautista R: Pediatric AIDS: Neuroradiologic and neurodevelopmental findings. *Pediatr Radiol* 1988; 18:445-448.

Shaw DWW, Cohen WA: Viral infections of the CNS in children: Imaging features. *AJR* 1993; 160:125-133.

Suss RA, Maravilla KR, Thompson J: MR imaging of intracranial cysticercosis. *AJNR* 1986; 7:235-242.

Taccone A, Gambaro G, Chiorzi M: Computed tomography in children with herpes simplex encephalitis. *Pediatr Radiol* 1988; 19:9-12.

Weiner LP, Fleming JV: Viral infections of the nervous system. *J Neurosurg* 1984; 61:207-224.

# 40
# Brain Neoplasms

## Key Concepts

1. In terms of incidence of pediatric malignancy, brain neoplasms are second only to leukemia and lymphoma. About 20% of all brain tumors present in children.
2. As a general rule, posterior fossa lesions are seen more commonly in children (4 to 11 years of age), with supratentorial lesions seen more commonly in toddlers and infants (less than 2 years of age). Over 11 years of age, supratentorial lesions once again predominate.
3. Presentation varies and includes increasing head circumference, headaches, nausea and/or vomiting, seizures, or focal neurologic signs.
4. Posterior fossa lesions in children include astrocytoma (juvenile pilocytic), medulloblastoma, and ependymoma.
5. Craniopharyngioma comprises 50% of pediatric suprasellar lesions. Although a benign, slow-growing, and often cystic tumor, local recurrence is common.

A. Posterior fossa.
 1. Astrocytoma.
    a. Most common overall brain tumor in children; 60% are located in posterior fossa.
    b. Glial tumor that arises from astrocytes.
    c. Often cystic with solid nodule that enhances (juvenile pilocytic).
    d. Rarely hemorrhages; 20% have calcifications.
    e. Graded 1 through 4 (based on malignant potential).
       *1.* Grade 1 is pilocytic astrocytoma.
          *a.* Excellent prognosis.
          *b.* 5-year survival rate is 90%.
       *2.* Grade 4 is highly malignant glioblastoma multiform.

> **Imaging** Computed tomography (CT) or magnetic resonance imaging (MRI) demonstrates often large, eccentric cystic lesion that may be unilocular or multilocular (fluid may appear more dense than cerebrospinal fluid [CSF] because of increased protein content). Because of size of lesion and its propensity for posterior fossa, hydrocephalus often occurs. Also, look for eccentric, solid, enhancing nodule (characteristic of juvenile pylocytic variety).

 2. Medulloblastoma.
    a. Some classify medulloblastoma as part of highly malignant spectrum of primitive neuroectodermal tumors (PNET).
    b. Arises from germ cells of medullary epithelium of vermis.
    c. Most common posterior fossa tumor in children.
    d. Seen more commonly in males than in females; usually presents in children 5 to 8 years old.
    e. Majority of medulloblastomas are found in cerebellar vermis (66%).
    f. Thirty percent invade brainstem; 40% have "drop" metastasis in spine. Leptomeningeal seeding of central nervous system (CNS) is also common.

> **Imaging** CT shows midline, dense lesion often with patchy but intense enhancement. On MRI, medulloblastoma ranges from isointense to hyperintense on $T_2$-weighted images and is hypointense on $T_1$-weighted images, again with patchy enhancement. This rapidly growing lesion can cause hydrocephalus via anterior displacement or obstruction of fourth ventricle. Medulloblastomas can be cystic (50%) and have calcifications (20%).

3. Ependymomas.
   a. Fifteen percent of posterior fossa tumors.
   b. Derived from undifferentiated ependymal cells that line floor and roof of fourth ventricle, lateral recesses, and foramina of Luschka.
   c. Most common location is fourth ventricle (95%).
   d. Solid, slow-growing, infiltrating tumor; difficult to remove surgically with poor prognosis (5-year survival rate is less than 25%).
   e. Invades surrounding cerebellar parenchyma and can have CNS seeding (30% to 40%).

**Imaging** CT or MRI reveals heterogeneous posterior fossa mass, often with calcifications. Mass is infiltrative, often extending out of foramina of Luschka.

4. Brainstem glioma.
   a. Can present with cranial nerve palsy and cerebellar dysfunction.
   b. Common locations.
      1. Pons (most common).
      2. Midbrain.
      3. Medulla less often.
   c. Hydrocephalus is uncommon, unless involving tectum.
   d. Vast majority are astrocytoma.
   e. Can be exophytic mass that can cause posterior displacement of fourth ventricle.
   f. Poor prognosis; 5-year survival rate is less than 30%.

**Imaging** Inhomogeneous mass within brainstem can be seen on CT or MRI. Enhancement is variable.

5. Hemangioblastoma.
   a. One or two percent of all cranial neoplasms of which only 20% occur in children; found more commonly in males than in females.
   b. Ten percent of cerebellar hemangioblastomas are associated with von Hippel-Lindau disease (see Chapter 37).

**Imaging** CT or MRI demonstrates predominantly cystic cerebellar mass with enhancing, well-circumscribed nodule. Adjacent hemorrhage is often present. Angiography may show hypervascular nidus.

6. Schwannomas.
   a. Derived from Schwann cells or myelin sheath of nerve root axons.
   b. In cerebellopontine (CP) angle, consider acoustic neuroma (VIII); also consider facial neuroma (less common).

c. Must consider neurofibromatosis (type II) and be aware of the presence of other intracranial lesions (meningiomas or gliomas).

> **Imaging** CT and MRI reveal solid tumors that strongly enhance and rarely calcify. Look for enlargement of internal auditory canal when considering acoustic or facial schwannomas.

7. Dermoid or epidermoid.
   a. Arise from congenital rests of tissue that remain in intracranial cavity, following incomplete separation of neuroectoderm from cutaneous ectoderm (at time of closure of neural tube).
   b. Any location is possible, but popular sites include:
      1. Midline.
      2. CP angle.
      3. Near pituitary.
      4. Middle cranial fossa.
   c. Reason for clinical presentation.
      1. Because of compression or obstruction of adjacent ventricular system.
      2. Chemical meningitis (spillage of cyst materials).
   d. May present with recurrent meningitis or *Staphlococcus aureus* meningitis.
      1. Caused by occult portal to outer skin.
      2. Known as dermal sinus tract.

> **Imaging** CT or MRI shows lobulated, usually cystic lesion with fat (low density on CT and high-signal intensity on $T_1$-weighted MR images). May see fat "spillage" rupture into extraaxial space.

B. Supratentorial.
   1. Astrocytomas.
      a. Thirty percent of supratentorial tumors are cerebral astrocytomas.
      b. Clinical presentation.
         1. Seizures.
         2. Increased intracranial pressure.
      c. Usually solid; less likely to be more benign juvenile pilocytic variety seen in posterior fossa.
      d. Common locations.
         1. Cerebral hemispshere.
         2. Optic chiasm or hypothalamic (20% to 50% have neurofibromatosis).
      e. Giant cell astrocytoma.

1. Characteristic tumor associated with tuberous sclerosis.
2. Located at foramen of Monro; can present with hydrocephalus.
3. Considered malignant transformation of tuber (hamartoma) that begins to grow and enhance.

> **Imaging** Imaging appearance is variable depending on grade of tumor; higher-grade, aggressive tumors are often larger, more infiltrative with extensive edema, and shift on CT and MRI (as compared with smaller, less edematous low-grade tumors). Enhancement of tumor also varies with grade.

2. Craniopharyngiomas.
   a. Arise from epithelial remnants of pouch of Rathke (embryonic tract between pharynx and pituitary).
   b. Location.
      1. Suprasellar (70%).
      2. Suprasellar and intrasellar (20%).
      3. Intrasellar (10%).
   c. Benign, slow-growing tumor; however, is difficult to remove.
      1. Significant risk of morbidity.
      2. Local recurrence is common and is often treated with radiation.
   d. Comprises 50% of pediatric suprasellar lesions; found in males more commonly than in females.
   e. Presentation peak is between 5 and 15 years of age (second peak is between 40 and 50 years of age).

> **Imaging** CT and MRI can demonstrate often large, suprasellar cystic lesion (90%) with contrast enhancement (90%) of solid portion of mass. Calcifications (90%) are usually present.

3. PNET.
   a. "Small blue cell" tumor; mostly undifferentiated cells.
   b. Rapidly growing, aggressive tumor with poor prognosis.
   c. Closely resembles medulloblastomas, neuroblastomas, pinealblastomas, retinoblastomas, and ependymoblastomas.
   d. Common site is deep white matter of parietal and frontal lobes with seeding of CNS.
   e. Often seen in infants and small children less than 5 years of age.

> **Imaging** CT and MRI show inhomogeneous, hyperdense or intense tumor, often with calcifications, cystic areas,

edema, and necrosis; tumor commonly hemorrhages. Contrast enhancement is present.

4. Choroid plexus tumors.
   a. Papillomas (much more common) or carcinomas.
   b. Rare; majority of papillomas are found in infants, versus carcinomas, which tend to be found in children less than 5 years of age.
   c. Arises from secretory cells of choroid plexus that produce CSF; therefore, hydrocephalus is often present from hypersecretion of tumor.
   d. Common location is lateral ventricle (trigone region).
   e. Because of hydrocephalus and propensity to occur in infants, presenting sign is usually increasing head circumference.
   f. Found in males more commonly than in females.

**Imaging** Ultrasound, CT, or MRI can show often quite large ventricular mass with lobulated cauliflower appearance. Calcifications are often present with homogeneous contrast enhancement. Look for resulting hydrocephalus.

5. Pineal tumors.
   a. Most common is germ cell tumor.
      *1.* Germinoma.
      *2.* Teratoma.
      *3.* Choriocarcinoma.
      *4.* Endodermal sinus.
   b. Less common is tumor of pineal origin.
      *1.* Pineoblastoma (highly malignant); associated with retinoblastoma.
      *2.* Pineocytoma (benign).
      *3.* Pineal cyst.
   c. Clinical presentation.
      *1.* Hydrocephalus (obstruction of aqueduct).
         *a.* Headache.
         *b.* Nausea or vomiting.
         *c.* Decreased level of consciousness.
      *2.* Parinaud syndrome (compression of tectum).
         *a.* Paralysis of upward gaze.
         *b.* Retraction nystagmus.
         *c.* Light-near dissociation (loss of pupil reflex with sparing of accommodation).
   d. Physiologic pineal calcifications are not seen in children under 8 years of age; therefore, any calcifications in this region in small children are highly suspicious for pineal tumor.

> **Imaging** CT or MRI can demonstrate commonly cystic pineal mass, often with calcifications (especially germ cell tumor, such as germinoma).

6. Oligodendroglioma.
   a. Arise from myelin-producing cells.
   b. Location: cerebral hemispheres, often parietal.
   c. Rare in children.

> **Imaging** Calcifications are common (70%) in this slow-growing tumor; may have small amount of peripheral edema. Commonly little or no enhancement is present.

7. Ganglioglioma and ganglioneuroma.
   a. Arise from neuronal elements (ganglion cells) and glial cells (neoplastic astrocytes).
   b. Uncommon, comprising only 3% of all pediatric brain tumors.
   c. Slow-growing.
   d. Common locations.
      1. Peripheral temporal.
      2. Occipital.

> **Imaging** Well-circumscribed, low-density lesion is seen on CT with variable edema and enhancement. Can present with calcifications (30%).

8. Ependymomas.
   a. Although usually posterior fossa tumor, 20% to 40% are supratentorial.
   b. Unlike posterior fossa, supratentorial ependymomas are usually parenchymal lesions (arising from ependymal rests).
   c. Common site is adjacent to frontal horns, lateral ventricles, or temporal and parietal lobes.
   d. Less likely to contain calcifications (unlike those of posterior fossa variety).

> **Imaging** CT or MRI demonstrates inhomogeneous appearance often with cystis areas; enhancement is variable.

## SUGGESTED READINGS

Altman N, Fitz CR, Chuang S, Harwood-Nash D, Cotter C, Armstrong D: Radiologic characteristics of primitive neuroectodermal tumors in children. *AJNR* 1985; 61:15-18.

Armington WG, Osborn AG, Cubberly DA, Harnsburger HR, Boyer R, Naidich TP, Sherry RG: Supratentorial ependymoma: CT appearance. *Radiology* 1985; 157:367-371.

Buetow PC, Smirniotopoulos JG, Done S: Congenital brain tumors: A review of 45 cases. *AJR* 1990; 155:587.

Eldevik OP, Blaivas M, Gabrielsen T, Hald JK, Chandler WF: Craniopharyngioma: Radiologic and histologic findings and recurrence. *AJNR* 1996; 17:1427-1440.

Kollias S, Barkovich AJ, Edwards MSB: Magnetic resonance analysis of suprasellar tumors of childhood. *Pediatr Neurosurg* 1991-2; 17:284-303.

Kriss TC, Kriss VM, Warf BC: Recurrent meningitis, the search for the dermoid or epidermoid tumor. *Pediatr Infect Dis* 1995; 14:697-700.

Jooma R, Kendall BE: Intracranial tumors in the first year of life. *Neuroradiology* 1982; 23:267-274.

Lee Y, van Tassel P, Bruner J, Moser R, Share J: Juvenile pilocystic astrocytomas: CT and MR characteristics. *AJR* 1989; 152:1263-1270.

Naidich TP, Zimmerman RA: Primary brain tumors in children. *Semin Roentgenol* 1984; 19:100-114.

Radkowski MA, Naidich TP, Tomita T, Byrd SE, McLone DG: Neonatal brain tumors: CT and MR findings. *J Comput Tomogr* 1988; 12:10-20.

Strong JA, Hatten HP, Brown MT, Debatin JF, Freidman HS, Oakes WJ, Tien R: Pilocytic astrocytoma: Correlation between the initial imaging features and clinical aggressiveness. *AJR* 1993; 161:369-372.

Swartz JD, Zimmerman RA, Bilaniuk LT: Computed tomography of intracranial ependymomas. *Radiology* 1982; 143:97-101.

Tien R, Barkovich AJ, Edwards MSB. MR imaging of pineal tumors. *AJNR* 1990; 11:557-565.

Tomita T, McLone DG, Flannery AM: Choroid plexus papillomas of neonates, infants and children. *Pediatr Neurosci* 1988; 14:23-30.

# 41
# Metabolic Brain Disorders

### Key Concepts

1. Metabolic brain abnormalities can be divided into groups based on the cellular organelle in which the abnormal biochemical process (often an enzymatic defect) takes place. Most of these disorders present early in life and are progressive, resulting in early death.
2. Traditionally, the three organelle groups are lysosomal, peroxisomal, and mitochondrial defects. When the white matter is preferentially involved (dysmyelinating process), the word "leukodystrophy" is used.
3. Mucopolysaccharidoses are caused by abnormal degradation of mucopolysaccharides due to faulty lysosomal enzymes, resulting in deposition of glycosaminoglycans in the central nervous system (CNS) and other organs. Common types include Hurler, Hunter, Sanfilipo, and Morquio syndromes.
4. Metachromatic leukodystrophy is a lysosomal leukodystrophy caused by a deficiency of arysulfatase A (enzyme needed for normal myelin sheath development).
5. Adrenoleukodystrophy is an X-linked metabolic peroxisomal disorder. The deficiency of acyl CoA synthetase leads to the accumulation of long-chain fatty acids with progressive multifocal dysmyelination of the CNS.

-A. Lysosomal.
   1. Lysosome function.
      a. Involved in "digestive" function of cell.
      b. Eliminates unwanted substances.
   2. Lysosomal storage disorders.
      a. Gaucher disease (see Chapter 36).
         1. Most common lysosomal storage abnormality.
         2. Usually does not involve CNS.
      b. Niemann-Pick disease.
         1. Deficiency of sphingomyelinase activity with resulting accumulation of sphingomyelin within reticuloendothelial system.
         2. Involved organs.
            *a.* Bone marrow ("Erlenmeyer flask" deformity, see Chapter 36).
            *b.* CNS.
               *1)* Lipid storage in neurons.
               *2)* Results in diffuse cerebral atrophy.
      c. Tay-Sachs disease.
         1. Deficiency of hexasaminidase enzymes, resulting in accumulation of ganglioside in neurons with eventual neuronal loss, demyelination, and early death.
         2. Strong association with Jewish descent.
      d. Mucopolysaccharidoses.
         1. Abnormal degradation of mucopolysaccharides, due to faulty lysosomal enzymes, resulting in deposition of glycosaminoglycans in CNS and other organs.
         2. Diagnosis can be made based on presence of urinary excretion of these incompletely degraded mucopolysaccharides (heparan sulfate, dermatan sulfate, and keratan sulfate).
         3. Most are autosomal recessive.
         4. Common types.
            *a.* Hurler syndrome.
            *b.* Hunter syndrome (X-linked recessive).
            *c.* Sanfilipo syndrome.
            *d.* Morquio syndrome.
         5. Clinical manifestations.
            *a.* Macrocephaly.
            *b.* Severe mental retardation (Hunter, Hurler, and Sanfillipo syndromes).
            *c.* Short stature (dwarf).
            *d.* Abnormal spine.
               *1)* Bullet-shaped vertebral bodies.
               *2)* Atlantoaxial subluxation.

  *6.* Recent treatment advances include bone marrow transplanation, which has shown promising results with reversal of some of systemic and CNS findings of disorder.

**Imaging** Prominent perivascular spaces, dural thickening, atrophy, and white-matter changes can be seen on both magnetic resonance imaging (MRI) and computed tomography (CT). White-matter lesions can be seen as diffuse, scattered, low-attenuation lesions on CT; MRI demonstrates low-signal lesions on $T_1$-weighted images and high-signal lesions on $T_2$-weighted lesions.

 3. Lysosomal leukodystrophy.
  a. Metachromatic leukodystrophy.
   *1.* Deficiency of arysulfatase A (enzyme needed for normal myelin sheath development).
   *2.* Results in accumulation of cerebroside sulfatide in macrophages and Schwann cells.
   *3.* Autosomal recessive.
   *4.* Clinical presentation.
    *a.* Usually presents early.
     *1)* Late infantile form.
     *2)* Gait disorders and spasticity.
    *b.* Can present later (more uncommon, milder, and slowly progressive juvenile and adult forms).
   *5.* Steady deterioration with infantile form; death occurs within 5 years.

**Imaging** MRI and CT can show diffuse cerebral atrophy with ex vacuo dilatation of ventricular system (seen late in course of disease). Abnormal white-matter signal can be detected on MRI (hypointense on $T_1$-weighted images and high signal on $T_2$-weighted images).

  b. Krabbe disease.
   *1.* Also known as globoid cell leukodystrophy.
   *2.* Deficiency of β-galactocerebrosidase that results in inability to break down cerebroside (constituent of myelin). The cerebroside collects in lysosomes forming globoid cells.
   *3.* Early onset (3 to 6 months) with irritability and spasticity. Death occurs within the first few years of life.

**Imaging** Abnormal high signal can be seen in thalami, caudate nuclei, and posterior limb of internal capsule on $T_1$-weighted images with abnormal white-matter high signal

($T_2$-weighted images). Late in disease, diffuse atrophy can be seen. Calcifications in basal ganglia may be detected on CT.

B. Peroxisomal.
  1. Peroxisomal function.
     a. Peroxisomes are required for synthesis of myelin components.
     b. Name is based on peroxide-based reaction that occurs within this organelle.
  2. Loss of general peroxisome function.
     a. Types.
        1. Zellweger (cerebrohepatorenal) syndrome.
           a. Most severe involvement with early death.
           b. Cystic renal disease.
           c. Poor liver function.
           d. Punctate calcifications of patella.
           e. CNS migration anomalies.
        2. Neonatal adrenoleukodystrophy.
        3. Infantile Refsum disease (mildest type).
     b. All are autosomal recessive.
     c. Demyelination and abnormal neuronal migration are present (especially in Zellweger syndrome).
     d. Associations.
        1. Dysmorphic features.
        2. Hypotonia.
        3. Seizures.
        4. Poor liver function.

**Imaging** All have white-matter abnormalities that may enhance (indicative of active inflammatory process in addition to diffuse demyelination). Decreased white-matter volume with particular thinning of corpus callosum noted.

  3. Loss of single peroxisome function.
     a. Adrenoleukodystrophy.
        1. X-linked disorder.
        2. Deficiency of acyl CoA synthetase leads to accumulation of long-chain fatty acids.
        3. Associated with adrenal insufficiency and progressive multifocal demyelination of CNS.
        4. Manifests in males, ages 3 to 7 years.
        5. Clinical presentation and course.
           a. Seizures.
           b. Blindness.

        c. Spasticity.
        d. Death ensues within few years of onset.

> **Imaging** Fairly symmetric demyelination of white matter can be seen on MRI and CT, predominantly near occipital trigone region with anterior spread over time. The presence of enhancement of anterior margin of diseased portion may be indicative of activity. Cerebellar white matter and tracts may also be involved. MRI spectroscopy has been helpful in early diagnosis of adrenoleukodystrophy (increased levels of lipid, choline, and inositol).

C. Mitochondrial.
  1. Mitochondrial function.
     a. Mitochondria supply energy to cell in form of adenosine triphosphate.
     b. Energy is provided via work of oxidative enzymes.
  2. Mitochondrial encephalomyopathies are caused by dysfunctional oxidative metabolism that can lead to elevated lactate and pyruvate blood levels.
  3. Involves gray matter and subcortical white matter.
  4. Types.
     a. Leigh disease (subacute necrotizing encephalomyopathy).
     b. MELAS.
        1. *M*itochondrial myopathy.
        2. *E*ncephalopathy.
        3. *L*actic *a*cidosis.
        4. *S*trokelike episodes.
     c. MERRF.
        1. *M*yoclonic *e*pilepsy.
        2. "*R*agged *r*ed *f*ibers" (pathologic description).
     d. Kearns-Sayre syndrome.
     e. Menkes' syndrome.
  5. Clinical presentation.
     a. Seizures (especially MELAS and MERFF).
     b. Short stature.
     c. Mental deterioration.

> **Imaging** Abnormal signal is seen primarily in gray matter (cortical and basal ganglia). Cortical atrophy is usually present as well.

D. Other leukodystrophies (often unknown etiology).
  1. Alexander disease.

a. Also known as fibrinoid leukodystrophy.
   b. No known enzymatic defect; no obvious heritable component.
   c. Clinical presentation.
      1. Macrocephaly.
      2. Seizures.
      3. Spasticity.
   d. Rosenthal fibers (dense glial filaments).
      1. Deposition near aqueduct can cause hydrocephalus.
      2. Accumulation near blood vessels can disrupt blood-brain barrier resulting in contrast enhancement.
   e. Early death (late infancy or early childhood).

**Imaging** CT and MRI can demonstrate preferential involvement of frontal white matter, which can develop cystic changes (late in disease). White-matter changes progress posteriorly as disease advances.

2. Canavan disease.
   a. Also known as spongiform leukodystrophy.
   b. Deficiency of aspartoacylase that results in increased *N*-acetyl aspartic acid in urine.
   c. Autosomal recessive; commonly seen in Ashkenazic Jewish population.
   d. Clinical course.
      1. Early infantile onset with hypotonia and seizures.
      2. Cortical blindness ensues because of preferential occipital involvement.
   e. Macrocephaly.
   f. Early death occurs (within first few years of life).

**Imaging** CT and MRI demonstrate symmetric white-matter abnormalities (low density of CT with high-signal lesions seen on $T_2$-weighted MRI images), preferentially in occipital lobes and then frontal lobes. Basal ganglia is relatively spared with exception of globus pallidus.

3. Cockayne syndrome.
   a. Autosomal recessive.
   b. Associated with dwarfism, mental retardation.
   c. No known enzymatic defect.

**Imaging** Calcifications (often extensive) are present in basal ganglia and cerebral and cerebellar cortexes. Diffuse atrophy with abnormal white-matter high signal is also present.

4. Pelizaeus-Merzbacher disease.
   a. Deficiency of proteolipid protein (lipophilin), important constituent of myelin.
   b. Rare; X-linked recessive.
   c. Clinical presentation.
      *1.* Choreoathetoid movements.
      *2.* Nystagmus.
      *3.* Ataxia.
   d. Sometimes classified with other sudanophilic leukodystrophies because of similar clinical presentation.
   e. Clinical course.
      *1.* Presents initially in infancy or early childhood.
      *2.* Slowly progressive; death occurs in adolescence or early adulthood.

> **Imaging** MRI shows diffuse high-signal intensity in white matter, consistent with lack of myelination (similar appearance to newborn brain). In severe cases, total lack of myelination is seen. Progressive white-matter atrophy also occurs.

**SUGGESTED READINGS**

Baram TZ, Goldman AM, Percy AK: Krabbes disease: MRI and CT findings, *Neurology* 1986; 36:111-115.

Becker LE: Lysosomes, peroxisomes and mitochondria: Function and disorder. *AJNR* 1992; 13:609-620.

Blaser SI, Clarke JTR, Becker LE: Neuroradiology of lysosomal disorders. *Neuroimaging Clin North Am* 1994; 4:283-298.

Brismar J, Brismar G, Gascon G, Ozand P: Canavan disease: CT and MR imaging of the brain. *AJNR* 1990; 11:809-810.

Engelbrecht V, Rassek M, Gartner J, Kahn T, Modder U: The value of new MRI techniques in adrenoleukodystrophy. *Pediatr Radiol* 1997; 27:207-215.

Jensen ME, Sawyer RW, Braun IF, Rizzo WB: MR imaging appearance of childhood adrenoleukodystrophy with auditory, visual and motor pathway involvement. *Radiographics* 1990; 10:53-66.

Kendall BE: Disorders of lysosomes, peroxisomes and mitochondria. *AJNR* 1992; 13:621-653.

Kimura M, Hasegawa Y, Yasuda K, Sejima H, Inoue M, Yamaguchi S, Ando Y, Ohno S: Magnetic resonance imaging with fluid-attentuated inversion recovery pulse sequences in MELAS syndrome. *Pediatr Radiol* 1997; 27:153-154.

Kumar AJ, Rosenbaum AE, Naidu S, Wener L, Citrin CM, Lindenberg R, Kim W, Zinreich SJ, Molliver ME, Mayberg HS: Adrenoleukodystrophy: Correlating MR imaging with CT. *Radiology* 1987; 165:497-504.

Lee C, Dineen TE, Brack M, Kirsch JE, Runge VM: The mucopolysaccharidoses: Characterization by cranial MR imaging. *AJNR* 1993; 14:1285-1292.

Murata R, Nakajima S, Tanaka A, Miyagi N, Matsuoka O, Kogame S, Inoue Y: MR imaging in patients with mucopolysaccharidoses. *AJNR* 1989; 10:1165-1170.

Pasco A, Kalifa G, Sarrazin JL, Adamsbaum C, Aubourg P: Contribution of MRI to the diagnosis of cerebral lesions in adrenoleukodystrophy. *Pediatr Radiol* 1991; 21:161-163.

Patel PJ, Kolawole TM, Malabarey TM, al-Hirbish AS, al-Jurrayan NA, Saleh M: Adrenoleukodystrophy: CT and MR findings. *Pediatr Radiol* 1995; 25;256-258.

Silverstein AM, Hirsh DK, Trobe JD, Gebarski SS: MR imaging of the brain in five members of a family with Pelizaeus-Merzbacher disease. *AJNR* 1990; 11:495-499.

Uchiyama M, Hata Y, Tada S: MR imaging of adrenoleukodystrophy. *Neuroradiology* 1991; 33:25-29.

# 42
## Head and Neck Lesions

---

### Key Concepts

1. The vast majority of head and neck lesions in children are benign.
2. Hemangioma is the most common "tumor" of the head and neck in infants; the two major types are capillary or "strawberry" (that usually involutes) and cavernous.
3. Inflammatory or infectious cervical adenopathy is quite common in the first 5 years of life. Retropharyngeal abscess can be an emergent condition because of the potential airway compromise.
4. Fibromatosis colli is a benign enlargement of the sternocleidomastoid muscle (SCM) that usually presents 10 to 14 days after birth with neonatal torticollis. No treatment is needed, since this disorder will resolve.
5. Rhabdomyosarcoma is the most common head and neck malignancy in children, usually presenting in the first decade of life. Common locations include orbit, nasopharynx, and sinuses.

A. Congenital.
   1. Lymphangioma or cystic hygroma.
      a. Sequestration of primitive embryonic lymph sacs.
         *1.* Capillary (tiny spaces).
         *2.* Cavernous (dilated lymphatics).
         *3.* Cystic hygroma (very large spaces or cysts).
      b. Often asymptomatic; 65% present at birth, 90% present by age 3.
      c. Common locations.
         *1.* Neck (75%).
         *2.* Axilla (20%).
         *3.* Can extend down into chest or mediastinum.
      d. May have sudden increase in size because of intralesional hemorrhage or infection.
      e. Associated with Turner, Noonan, and fetal alcohol syndromes.
      f. Treatment.
         *1.* Very difficult surgical removal ("like tissue paper") with frequent recurrence.
         *2.* Recent attempts have been at alcohol sclerosis of lesion prior to surgical approach.

   **Imaging** Ultrasound (US) can show septated, anechoic mass; can often be multilocular. Hemangiomatous components are common and can be seen with color Doppler. A lymphangioma can also hemorrhage and therefore, acutely enlarge. The lesion itself is very compressible and does not usually compress other structures or vessels; it just grows around and between them.

   2. Thyroglossal duct cyst (persistent thyroglossal duct, Fig. 42-1).
      a. Most common of congenital neck lesions.
      b. Embryology.
         *1.* Foramen cecum (base of tongue) goes through floor of mouth (mylohyoid).
         *2.* Loops around hyoid bone and goes through strap muscles of neck to reach thyroid bed.
      c. Remnant duct continues to secrete.
         *1.* Obstruction can result in palpable, mobile mass.
         *2.* Fistulous tract.
      d. Usually asymptomatic mass unless infected.
      e. Locations.
         *1.* Below level of hyoid bone (65%).
         *2.* Suprahyoid (20%).
         *3.* At level with hyoid (15%).
      f. Need to confirm thyroid position prior to surgical removal.

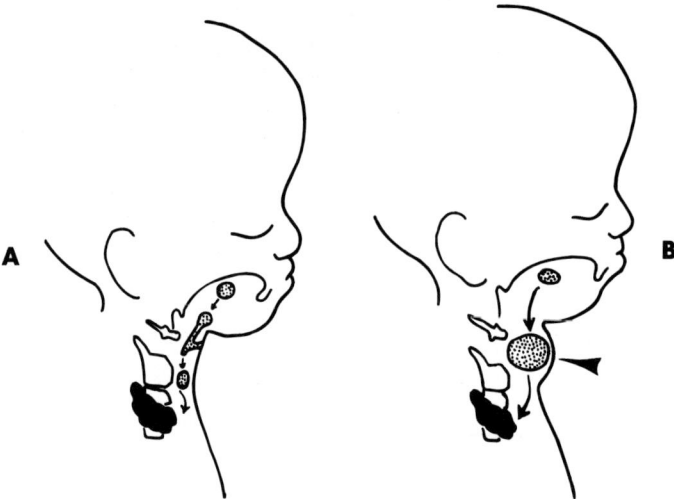

**Fig. 42-1** Thyroglossal duct cyst *(pathway).* **A,** Pathway of thyroglossal duct *(stippled area),* as it loops around hyoid bone on its path to normal thyroid location *(shaded structure).* **B,** Thyroglossal duct cyst *(arrowhead).*

    1. Ectopic or lingual thyroid can mimic thyroglossal duct cyst.
    2. Nuclear medicine scan or US can document thyroid position to prevent inadvertent removal of normal-functioning thyroid.

> **Imaging** US can reveal midline, anechoic cystlike mass on computed tomography (CT). Again, midline location, near hyoid bone is confirmatory.

3. Branchial arch (BA) anomalies.
    a. Embryology (Fig. 42-2).
        1. Six branchial arches form, separated by five clefts.
        2. Potential anomalies include cysts or sinus tract and fistula that arise from entrapped remnants of branchial clefts.
    b. Types.
        1. First BA.
            a. Forms external auditory canal, eustachian tubes, and mastoid air cells.
            b. Rare site for cyst or fistula.
            c. If anomaly occurs, site would be superficial and high (near ear or parotid).
        2. Second BA.
            a. Forms palatine tonsil.
            b. Most common; 95% of all BA abnormalities.

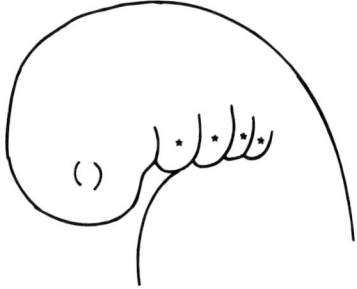

**Fig. 42-2** Branchial arches. Embryo (at 4 weeks) with appearance of branchial arches *(asterisk)* that go on to form structures of neck.

        c. Unilocular, cystic mass; anterior to sternocleidomastoid muscle.
          *1)* Can pass between internal and external carotid.
          *2)* Lateral to internal jugular at carotid bifurcation.
        d. Can acutely present with infection (look for rim enhancement).
        e. Can have sinus tract usually near mandibular angle.
     3. Third BA.
        a. Forms inferior parathyroid and thymus.
        b. Tract can occur that extends posteriorly to carotid (not medially as above for second arch).
        c. Thymic cyst may extend to neck.
     4. Fourth BA.
        a. Forms superior parathyroid and piriform sinus.
        b. Very rare; need to differentiate BA cyst at this level from laryngocele.
        c. Sinus tract may extend from piriform sinus to thyroid (causing recurrent thyroiditis).
  4. Hemangioma.
    a. Most common tumor of head and neck in infants.
    b. Usually superficial and variable in location.
    c. Types.
       *1.* Capillary ("strawberry") hemangioma of infancy (usually involutes).
       *2.* Cavernous (dilated, blood-filled spaces that tend to persist).

**Imaging** Usually multiseptated, hypoechoic lesion that can have intense color Doppler signal on US; overlying skin is often discolored (cavernous hemangiomas can have bluish tinge).

5. Juvenile nasopharyngeal angiofibroma.
   a. Benign but highly vascular lesion in posterior nasopharynx.
   b. Presents almost exclusively in adolescent males.
   c. Presents with epistaxis, nasal obstruction.
   d. Most common benign sinonasal tumor in children.
   e. Do not biopsy; these lesions are embolized via interventional angiography prior to surgical removal if necesssary.

   **Imaging** Facial radiograph may show soft-tissue nodule in posterior maxillary sinus or nasopharynx. Bowing of posterior wall of maxillary sinus is also commonly present. CT demonstrates intense enhancement of lesion. Serpentinous flow void within lesion can be seen on magnetic resonance imaging (MRI). Angiography shows increased vascularity of lesion, often with vessels from maxillary artery branch of external carotid artery.

6. Dermoid or epidermoid.
   a. Common congenital tumor of head and neck.
   b. Often pedunculated.
      1. Nasopharyngeal teratoma.
      2. "Hairy polyp" that can fill nasopharyngeal and/or oral cavities.

   **Imaging** US can show usual cystic quality of mass, while CT and MRI can demonstrate extent of lesion and other distinguishing characteristics like fat and calcifications.

7. Fibromatosis colli (neonatal torticollis).
   a. Benign enlargement of SCM; usually right sided.
   b. Unknown pathogenesis.
      1. Perhaps birth trauma causing pressure necrosis.
      2. Secondary fibrosis of SCM may then occur.
   c. Usually presents 10 to 14 days after birth; 20% have persistent torticollis.
   d. No treatment needed; usually resolves within 4 to 8 months.

   **Imaging** Diffuse enlargement of SCM with no adjacent adenopathy or enhancement seen on CT. Isoechoic or hypoechoic mass that moves synchronously with muscle can be seen within SCM; US is modality of choice.

B. Inflammatory or infectious.
   1. Cervical adenopathy.
      a. Quite common in first 5 years of life.
         1. Be aware of tuberculous adenitis.

2. Also known as scrofula.
   b. Retropharyngeal abscess.
      1. Well-circumscribed fluid collection.
      2. Anterior displacement of airway with widened retropharyngeal space (see Chapter 1).
      3. Often have adjacent cellulitis and myositis with increased density and stranding of subcutaneous fat (due to engorged vessels and lymphatics).
   c. Acquired immunodeficiency syndrome.
      1. Diffuse cervical adenopathy can be present.
      2. Parotid masses, usually cysts (lymphoepithelial).

> **Imaging** CT or US can show hypoechoic or low-density nodules that can become frank abscess (often multilocular), causing significant displacement of normal neck structures (especially airway).

2. Ranula.
   a. Mucus retention cyst from floor of mouth resulting from obstruction of salivary gland, often sublingual.
   b. Can be mistaken for epidermoid or dermoid cyst.
   c. Types.
      1. Simple (confined to floor of mouth).
      2. Diving or plunging ranula (dissection into submandibular or inferior parapharyngeal space).

> **Imaging** Fluid-density lesion is seen on CT or MRI confined to floor of mouth at expected location of sublingual duct or extending below mylohyoid (plunging ranula).

C. Vascular.
   1. Prominent internal jugular vein is normal variant.
      a. Usually on right.
      b. Can increase in size with valsalva maneuver.
   2. Jugular vein thrombosis.
      a. Associations.
         1. Adenitis or abscess.
         2. Tumor compression.
         3. Hypercoagulability.
      b. Can occur with long-term central venous lines.
         1. Clot can also propagate into superior vena cava (SVC).
         2. SVC syndrome: Swelling of head and neck due to occulsion of SVC.
   3. Cervical aortic arch (see Chapter 20).

D. Neoplastic masses.
   1. Rhabdomyosarcoma.
      a. Most common malignancy of pediatric head and neck; presents in first decade of life.
      b. Location.
         *1.* Orbit (38%).
         *2.* Nasopharynx (33%).
         *3.* Paranasal sinuses.
      c. Types.
         *1.* Embryonal.
         *2.* Alveolar.
         *3.* Botryoid.
         *4.* Undifferentiated.

   > **Imaging** CT and MRI demonstrate very aggressive tumor with bony destruction and inhomogenous soft-tissue mass that rapidly displaces and invades surrounding structures. High percentage have intracranial extension.

   2. Neuroblastoma.
      a. Less than 2% of head and neck lesions are primary neuroblastoma.
      b. Usually metastatic lesions; most commonly to dura mater or bony-skull metastases.
      c. Infiltrative, often with vascular invasion.

   > **Imaging** Inhomogenous, enhancing lesions (usually with bony destruction) can be seen on CT and MRI.

   3. Lymphoma.
      a. Painless neck mass.
      b. Types.
         *1.* Usually non-Hodgkin type (75%) in children.
         *2.* Hodgkin type in adolescents.
      c. Look for disease elsewhere.
         *1.* Especially in abdomen when head and neck Burkitt lymphoma lesions are present.
         *2.* Also look in chest and mediastinum.
         *3.* Orbit.

   > **Imaging** Homogenous adenopathy can be seen on CT, MRI, and US (often hypoechoic); rapid progession with bony involvement suggests Burkitt type.

   4. Salivary gland tumors.
      a. Rare in first two decades of life; usually involve parotid.

b. Types.
   *1.* Hemangioma or hemangioendothelioma.
      *a.* Most common parotid tumor in children.
      *b.* Usually seen in first 6 months of life. Occurs more frequently in girls than in boys.
   *2.* Pleomorphic adenoma (most common primary tumor of salivary glands in children).
   *3.* Mucoepidermoid carcinoma.
   *4.* Acinar cell.

**SUGGESTED READINGS**

Abramson SJ, Berdon WE, Ruzal-Shapiro C, Stolar C, Garvin J: Cervical neuroblastoma in eleven infants: A tumor with favorable prognosis. *Pediatr Radiol* 1993; 23:253-257.

Baker LL, Dillon WP, Hieshima GB, Dowd CF, Frieden IJ: Hemangiomas and vascular malformations of the head and neck: MR characteristics. *AJNR* 1993; 14:307-314.

Benson MT, Dalen K, Mancuso AA, Kerr HH, Cacciarelli AA, Mafee MF: Congenital anomalies of the branchial apparatus: Embryology and pathologic anatomy. *Radiographics* 1992; 12:943-960.

Bianchi A, Cudmore RE: Salivary gland tumors in children. *J Pediatr Surg* 1978; 13:519-521.

Crawford SC, Harnsberger HR, Johnson L, Aoki JR, Giley J: Fibromatosis colli of infancy: CT and sonographic findings. *AJR* 1988; 151:1183-1184.

Dunnick NR, Reaman GH, Head GL, Shawker TH, Ziegler JL: Radiographic manifestations of Burkitts lymphoma in American patients. *AJR* 1979; 132:1-6.

Friedman AP, Haller JO, Goodman JD, Nagar H: Sonographic evaluation of neck masses in children. *Radiology* 1983; 147:693-697.

Glasier CM, Siebert JJ, Williamson SL, Siebert RW, Corbitt SL, Rodgers AB, Lange TA: High resolution ultrasound of soft tissue masses in children. *Pediatr Radiol* 1987; 17:233-237.

Harnsberger HR, Mancuso AA, Muraki AS, Byrd SE, Dillon WP, Johnson LP, Hanafee WN: Branchial cleft anomalies and their mimics: Computed tomography evaluation. *Radiology* 1984; 152:739-748.

Kraus R, Han BK, Babcock DS, Oestriech AE: Sonography of neck masses in children. *AJR* 1986; 146:609-613.

Miller MB, Rao VM, Tom BM: Cystic masses of the head and neck: Pitfalls in CT and MRI interpretation. *AJR* 1992; 159:601-607.

Raney RB, Handler, SD: Management of neoplasms of the head and neck in children. *Head Neck Surg* 1981; 3:500-507.

Senac MO, Seagal HD: CT diagnosis of nasopharyngeal teratoma in a newborn. *AJNR* 1987; 8:710-712.

Sherman NH, Rosenberg HK, Heyman S, Templeton J: Ultrasound evaluation of neck masses in children. *J Ultrasound Med* 1985; 4:127-134.

Sheth S, Nussbaum AR, Hutchins GM, Sanders RC: Cystic hygromas in children: Sonographic pathologic correlation. *Radiology* 1987; 162:821-824.

Siebert RW, Seibert JJ: High resolution ultrasonography of the parotid gland in children. *Pediatr Radiol* 1986; 16:374-379.

Siegel MJ, Glaser HS, Amour TE, Rosenthal DD: Lymphangiomas in children: MR imaging. *Radiology* 1989; 170:467-470.

Wadsworth DT, Siegel MJ: Thyroglossal duct cysts: Variability of sonographic findings. *AJR* 1994; 163:1475-1477.

Wright GL, Smith RJH, Katz CD, Atkins JH: Benign parotid diseases of childhood. *Laryngoscope* 1985; 95:915-920.

# 43
# Spine

## Key Concepts

1. Spinal dysraphism is an abnormality in the separation of the infolding neural tube from the cutaneous ectoderm. Types include spina bifida aperta, spina bifida cystica, and occult spinal dysraphism.
2. Spina bifida aperta (also known as myelomeningocele) is an open neural tube defect with exposed neural tissue, most commonly located in the lumbosacral spine.
3. Occult spinal dysraphism (like tethered cord syndrome or diastematomyelia) can have a normal skin–covered back, yet 50% have a variety of lumbosacral cutaneous stigmata such as hemangiomas, sacral dimples or pits, hairy patches, or a skin tag or tail.
4. Dermoid or epidermoid are predominantly cystic lesions that can have dermal sinus tracts continuous with the thecal sac due to faulty neural tube closure. Recurrent meningitis is often the presenting symptom in children with this lesion.
5. Neoplasms of the pediatric spine include intramedullary tumors such as astrocytoma or ependymoma (usually cervical or upper thoracic) and extramedullary, intradural lesions such as "drop" metastases (often from posterior fossa tumors, such as medulloblastoma).

A. Development of human spine.
   1. Two distinct stages.
      a. Neurulation.
         *1.* Spinal cord forms following closure of neural tube (approximately third-to-fourth week of gestation).
         *2.* Closure begins centrally and extends cranially and caudally.
         *3.* Adjacent mesenchyme forms somites which become vertebral bodies, ribs, and paraspinal muscles.
      b. Canalization with retrogressive differentiation (Fig. 43-1).

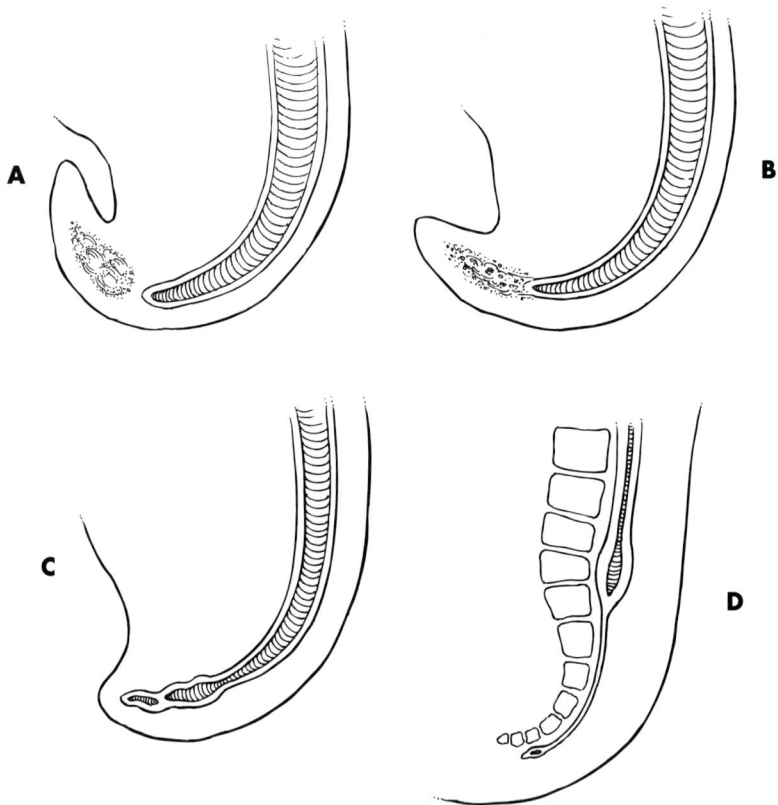

**Fig. 43-1** Canalization with retrogressive differentiation. **A,** Appearance of caudal cell mass distal to developing spinal cord. **B** and **C,** This mass of cells gradually develops internal lumen ("canalization") that connects to central canal of spinal cord above. **D,** Development of conus medullaris (distal spinal cord), filum terminale, and ventriculus terminalis. (Adapted from Barkovich, AJ: *Pediatric neuroimaging,* ed 1. Philadelphia, Lippincott-Raven, 1990; p. 230.)

1. Caudal portion or conus medullaris forms in this second separate process.
2. Undifferentiated cell aggregate called caudal cell mass forms inferior to neural tube. This mass of cells develops internal lumen (canalization) that connects to central canal of spinal cord above.
3. This cell mass decreases in size with decreasing central canal lumen as well ("retrogressive differentiation"), finally forming conus medullaris, filum terminale, and ventriculus terminalis (residual central canal of conus medullaris or so-called "fifth ventricle").
2. Abnormal spinal development.
   a. Abnormality in separation of infolding neural tube from cutaneous ectoderm can result in dysraphism of spine.
   b. Categorization of spinal dysraphism.
      1. Spina bifida aperta.
         a. Exposed neural tissue.
         b. 1:1000 births; higher in children of English or Irish descent.
         c. Meningoceles, myeloceles, meningomyeloceles.
         d. Open neural tube at skin surface because of posterior spinal defect; most commonly at lumbosacral spine.
         e. Associations.
            1) Chiari type II malformation of hindbrain.
            2) Syrinx.
            3) Diastematomyelia.
            4) Hydrocephalus.
            5) Neurogenic bladder.

**Imaging** Imaging is primarily needed for evaluation of previously noted complications associated with meningomyelocele. Computed tomography (CT) and magnetic resonance imaging (MRI) can determine presence and extent of hydrocephalus or syrinx. Renal ultrasound (US) and voiding cystourethrogram evaluate neurogenic bladder and/or associated vesicoureteral reflux.

      2. Spina bifida cystica.
         a. Skin-covered back mass.
         b. Types.
            1) Meningocele (herniated sac of meninges).
            2) Lipomeningomyelocele.
               a) Extension of lipomatous mass from subcutaneous fat into spinal canal via posterior spina bifida defect.

  *b)* Lipoma also tethers cord.

> **Imaging** US can show posterior orientation of low-lying spinal cord (lower than third lumbar vertebra [L3]) that terminates into echogenic mass (lipoma). MRI similarly demonstrates tethered cord within high-signal fat that often fills distal spinal canal in addition to posterior spinal defect.

  3) Myelocystocele.
   *a)* Localized cystic dilatation of distal end of spinal cord that is continuous with central canal (hydrosyringomyelia is present). This cystic dilatation herniates through posterior spinal defect.
   *b)* Uncommon form of spinal dysraphism.
3. Occult spinal dysraphism.
 *a.* Can have normal back; yet 50% have variety of lumbosacral cutaneous stigmata.
  *1)* Hemangiomas.
  *2)* Sacral clefts, pits.
  *3)* Hairy patch.
  *4)* Skin tag or tail.
 *b.* Because of lack of ossification of posterior spinal elements of lumbosacral area (which ossify at 3 months of age), screening US can be performed in infants less than 3 months of age with previously described high-risk lumbosacral cutaneous stigmata.
 *c.* Clinical symptoms of tethered cord syndrome are often not apparent until child becomes ambulatory.
  *1)* Bowel or bladder incontinence or dysfunction.
  *2)* Back and leg pain.
  *3)* Scoliosis.
  *4)* Limp or limb atrophy.
  *5)* Spasticity.
  *6)* Foot abnormalities (pes cavus).
 *d.* Tethered cord syndrome.
  *1)* Tight filum terminale with conus medularis that lies below L3 level in neonate.
  *2)* Spinal lipoma can also tether cord.
   *a)* Intradural lipoma (4%).
   *b)* Lipomyelomeningocele (84%).
   *c)* "Fatty" filum terminale (12%).

> **Imaging** Thickened, tight, or foreshortened filum terminale can be seen on US and MRI, causing abnormal traction on

> conus medullaris. Normal filum terminale should be less than 2 mm. Look for dorsal adherence of low-lying spinal cord in prone position and echogenic or high-signal material (lipomatous elements) within thecal sac.

    e. Meningocele (anterior or lateral).
    f. Dermal sinus tract.
        1) Extends from dural surface to skin surface.
        2) May end blindly in dura versus intradural extension to tether spinal cord or involve intradural lipoma.
        3) Midline defect due to abnormal neural tube folding.
            a) Higher incidence in cranial and lumbar areas.
            b) Last regions of neural tube to fuse.
        4) Can present with recurrent meningitis or *Staphylococcus aureus* meningitis.
        5) Associated with dermoid or epidermoid (50%).

**Imaging** US may show hypoechoic track extending from skin surface; however, dermal sinus tract can be missed on US. MRI is more sensitive for small, subcutaneous tract.

    g. Diastematomyelia.
        1) Splitting or partial duplication of spinal cord.
        2) Often associated with bony or fibrous spur that divides cord and may cause tethering.
        3) Often seen with vertebral segmentation abnormalities or hydromyelia (50%).
        4) Usually occurs between ninth thoracic vertebrae (T9) and first sacral vertebrae (S1).
        5) Five percent of nonidiopathic scoliosis cases are due to diastematomyelia.
        6) Majority of cases occur in females (80%), up to 50% have foot abnormalities, such as clubfoot.

**Imaging** Radiographs may show bony vertebral defect. On MRI and US, look for splitting of spinal cord into two hemicords.

  c. Caudal regression.
    1. Insult to caudal mesoderm (fourth week of gestation).
    2. Result is spectrum ranging from absent portions of sacrum to sirenomelia ("mermaid" or fusion of lower extremities with hypoplastic caudal spine and pelvis).
    3. Strong association with diabetic mothers.

4. More severe cases usually involve anal atresia and distal genitourinary abnormalities.

**Imaging** Absent or hypoplastic bony sacrum and lower lumbar vertebral bodies can be seen on radiographs. MRI may show squared-off conus medullaris (distal spinal cord).

   d. Neurenteric cysts (see Chapter 7).
      1. "Splitting" of notochord that results in abnormal, persistent communication between endoderm and ectoderm (gut and dorsal skin).
      2. Found in lower cervical or upper thoracic region, often as posterior mediastinal mass or cyst.
      3. Because of disruption of adjacent somites or mesoderm, associated vertebral body anomalies are present.
   e. Teratoma.
      1. Sacrococcygeal.
         a. Solid and cystic lesion.
         b. Location.
            1) Visible, palpable, posterior external mass.
            2) Presacral with mass extending within abdomen or pelvis.
         c. Can be highly vascular and difficult to remove surgically because of problems with hemostasis (may require preoperative embolization of large feeding vessels to tumor).

**Imaging** US, CT, and MRI can demonstrate often large, predominantly cystic lesion. Look for intraabdominal extension of tumor along retroperitoneum.

      2. Dermoid or epidermoid.
         a. Cystic lesions.
         b. Form from dermal or epidermal rests; can have dermal sinus tract because of faulty neural tube closure (see previous discussion).
         c. Formation has also been associated with lumbar puncture.
         d. Dermoids are predominantly in lumbosacral area; epidermoids can be anywhere along spine.

**Imaging** Small cystic lesion can be seen on US or MRI, although MRI better demonstrates any associated sinus tract to thecal sac.

   f. "Hydrosyringomyelia."
      1. Hydromyelia is dilated central canal of spinal cord.

2. Syringomyelia (syrinx) is fluid connection lateral to and independent of central canal.
3. Causes of syringomyelia.
   a. Chiari malformation (especially Chiari type II with meningomyelocele).
   b. Tumor.
   c. Scarring from arachnoiditis.
   d. Trauma.

> **Imaging** MRI is best imaging choice for evaluation of hydromyelia or syringomyelia (although two can be indistinguishable). Sagittal and axial views of spine can delineate extent of fluid collection and demonstrate possible cause (imaging of posterior fossa). In absence of clear Chiari malformation, contrast material should be given to rule out neoplasm as cause of syringomyelia.

B. Neoplasms of spine.
  1. Intramedullary.
     a. Location (usually cervical or upper thoracic).
     b. Types.
        *1.* Astrocytoma (60%).
        *2.* Ependymoma (30%).
     c. Presentation.
        *1.* Extremity weakness.
        *2.* Pain.

> **Imaging** MRI with gadolinium enhancement best delineates spinal cord tumor. These lesions are often inhomogenous, with cystic or necrotic areas. Adjacent syringomyelia is common. Intraoperative US (following removal of posterior bony elements) is helpful in distinguishing tumor margins for surgical resection.

  2. Extramedullary or intradural.
     a. Metastasis.
        *1.* "Drop mets" (seeding of tumor into spinal canal from intracranial sources).
           a. Medulloblastomas.
           b. Ependymomas.
           c. Pineal tumors.

> **Imaging** Focal nodules, thickened nerve roots, and thecal sac can be seen on CT, myelography, and MRI (with
> *Continued*

> *Continued from previous page*
> gadolinium contrast). These lesions are commonly seen in lumbosacral region.

    2. Neuroblastoma.
       *a.* Metastatic lesions more commonly involve bony vertebrae but can have intrathecal metastases.
       *b.* Direct extension of tumor into spinal canal via neural foramen can occur with both abdominal and posterior mediastinal primary neuroblastoma.
    3. Leukemia or lymphoma.
       *a.* Vertebral bony involvement is more common than actual meningeal leukemic infiltration.
       *b.* Once in central nervous system, leukemia is difficult to eradicate because of blood-brain barrier.
  b. Meningiomas (uncommon in children).
  c. Neurofibroma (schwannoma).
    *1.* Strong association with neurofibromatosis.
    *2.* Focal scoliosis and vertebral erosions can occur.

> **Imaging** Classic "dumb-bell shaped" lesion can be seen on CT and MRI with neural foraminal widenening.

## SUGGESTED READINGS

Barnes PD, Lester PD, Yamanashi WS, Prince. JR: Magnetic resonance imaging in infants and young children with spinal dysraphism. *AJNR* 1986; 7:465-472.

Byrd SE: Imaging of the spine in infants and children. *Curr Opin Radiol* 1990; 2:885-894.

Byrd SE, Darling CF, McLone DG: Developmental disorders of pediatric spine. *Radiol Clin North Am* 1991; 29:711-752.

Davis PC, Hoffman JC, Ball TI, Wyley JB, Braun IF, Fry SM, Drvaric DM: Spinal abnormalities in pediatric patients: MR imaging findings compared with clinical, myelographic, and surgical findings. *Radiology* 1988; 166:679-685.

Korsvik HE, Keller MS: Sonography of occult dysraphism in neonates and infants with MR correlation. *Radiographics* 1992; 12:297-306.

Kriss TC, Kriss VM, Warf BC: Recurrent meningitis: The search for the dermoid or epidermoid tumor. *Pediatr Infect Dis J* 1995;14:697-700.

Kriss VM, Kriss TC, Babcock DS: The ventriculus terminalis of the spinal cord in the neonate: A normal variant on sonography. *AJR* 1995; 165:1491-1493.

Kriss VM, Kriss TC, Desai NS, Warf BC: Occult spinal dysraphism in the infant: Clinical and sonographic review. *Clin Pediatr* 1995; 34(12):650-654.

Naidich TP, Fernbach SK, McLone DG, Shkolnick A: Sonography of the caudal spine and back: Congenital anomalies in children. *AJR* 1984; 142:1229-1242.

Prenger EC: Magnetic resonance imaging of the pediatric spine. *Semin Ultrasound CT MR* 1991; 12:410-428.

Raghavendra BN, Epstein FJ: Sonography of the spine and spinal cord. *Radiol Clin North Am* 1985; 23:91-104.

Reimer R, Onofrio BM: Astrocytomas of the spinal cord in children and adolescents. *J Neurosurg* 1985; 63:669-675.

Scatliff JH, Kendall BE, Kingsley DPE, Britton J, Grant DN, Hayward RD: Closed spinal dysraphism: Analysis of clinical, radiological, and surgical findings in 104 consecutive patients. *AJR* 1989; 152:1049-1057.

Sherman JL, Barkovich AJ, Citrin CM: MR appearance of syringomyelia: New observations. *AJNR* 1986; 7:985-995.

Stanley PO, Senac MO, Segall HD: Intraspinal seeding from intracranial tumors in children. *AJR* 1984; 144:157-161.

Sze G, Krol G, Zimmerman RD, Deck MDF: Intramedullary disease of the spine: Diagnosis using Gd-enhanced MRI. *AJNR* 1988; 9:847-858.

Zieger M, Dorr U: Pediatric spinal sonography. Part I: Anatomy and examination technique. *Pediatr Radiol* 1988; 18:9-13.

# 44
# Orbital Lesions

---

### Key Concepts

1. Pediatric orbital lesions can be divided into three compartments:
   a. Globe.
   b. Intraconal (posterior to the globe, inside the space bounded by the extraocular muscles).
   c. Extraconal (posterior to the globe, outside the space bounded by the extraocular muscles).
2. Retinopathy of prematurity (ROP) or retrolental fibrodysplasia is caused by oxygen toxicity with the increased oxygen content causing neovascularity of the retina.
3. Retinoblastoma is the most common intraocular neoplasm of childhood. This lesion presents early in life (90% by age 3), is commonly bilateral, and has a strong association with pineal lesions ("third eye").
4. Optic nerve glioma most commonly presents in children less than 15 years of age, and has a strong association with neurofibromatosis.
5. Orbital infection can be divided into two types: preseptal versus postseptal. Postseptal infection is a more ominous condition than preseptal infection because of the potential for intracranial spread.

A. Globe lesions.
   1. Anophthalmos.
      a. Congenital absence of eye.
      b. Very rare.
      c. Etiology.
         *1.* Isolated failure of optic pit formation versus forebrain and neural tube malformation.
   2. Microphthalmos.
      a. Unilateral (70%); often associated with orbital cyst (usually retrobulbar).
      b. Lens formation may or may not occur; if lens is present, cataracts are common.
      c. Detachment of retina can be present.

   **Imaging** Small, malformed globe can be seen on computed tomography (CT) or magnetic resonance imaging (MRI).

   3. Buphthalmos.
      a. Congenital glaucoma.
      b. Increased intraocular pressure with optic nerve damage.
      c. Bilateral (80%); may be heritable.

   **Imaging** Enlarged, yet often deformed globe is present.

   4. Coloboma.
      a. Congenital defect in globe; often posterior, near optic nerve insertion.
      b. Associated with retinal detachment.
      c. Differentiate from staphyloma.
         *1.* Acquired defect of globe.
         *2.* Can be related to persistent increased intraocular pressure, possibly from infection or injury.

   **Imaging** Outpouching of globe, near optic nerve insertion; can be seen posteriorly on CT or MRI.

   5. Persistent hyperplastic primary vitreous.
      a. Primitive hyaloid artery.
         *1.* Embryologic vessel.
         *2.* Runs from ophthalmic artery to posterior aspect of lens.
         *3.* Primary vitreous (highly vascular) should give way to more gelatinous secondary or adult vitreous by eighth month of gestation.
      b. Persistence of these embryologic structures is almost always unilateral (90%) and is associated with retinal detachment, glaucoma, and cataracts.

**Imaging** CT or MRI can show small globe with vitreous demonstrating increased density on CT or hypointensity on $T_2$-weighted images. Linear density may be present between posterior lens and retina (persistent hyaloid artery). Echogenic vitreous can be seen on ultrasound (US).

6. Coats disease.
    a. Vascular abnormality of retina with aneurysmal and telangiectatic changes and exudative ophthalmopathy.
    b. No systemic abnormality, but 60% have retinal detachment.

**Imaging** CT and MRI demonstrate normal-sized orbit with increased density in vitreous chamber. Look for associated retinal detachment.

7. ROP.
    a. Used to be known as retrolental fibrodysplasia.
    b. Etiology.
        *1.* Caused by oxygen toxicity in premature infant.
        *2.* Increased oxygen content causes neovascularity of retina.

**Imaging** Small globe with increased signal on $T_1$-weighted MRI images; history of oxygen therapy or prematurity is obviously helpful in diagnosis.

8. Drusen.
    a. Caused by hyaline bodies of optic nerve; often bilateral.
    b. Heritable.

**Imaging** Single, smooth, round calcification may be seen at optic nerve insertion on CT.

9. Retinoblastoma.
    a. Most common intraocular neoplasm of childhood.
    b. Arises from retinal photreceptor cells; primitive neuroectodermal tumor type.
    c. Rare; 1:20,000.
    d. Presents early in life (90% by age 3).
    e. Presents with leukocoria (lack of red reflex).
    f. Bilateral lesions (30%); familial (chromosome 13).
    g. Strong association with pineal lesions (third eye or trilateral retinoblastoma).
    h. Treament.
        *1.* Enucleation and radiation.

2. Be aware that radiation-induced malignancies such as osteosarcoma of maxilla or bony orbit may occur 8 to 15 years after treatment.

> **Imaging** Characteristic calcified lesion of posterior orbit (90%) is seen on CT. Little tumor enhancement is present. Remember to evaluate pineal region for associated lesions.

   10. Other lesions of globe (rare in children).
      a. Melanoma.
      b. Metastases.

B. Intraconal lesions.
   1. Optic nerve glioma.
      a. Can involve optic nerve, chiasm, optic tracts, or all three.
      b. Majority present in children less than 15 years of age (85%); peak incidence is 4 to 6 years of age.
      c. Strong association with neurofibromatosis; majority will have intracranial lesions (70%).

> **Imaging** Fusiform enlargement of optic nerve can be seen on CT and MR images. Some enhancement may be present, but certainly not as much as is seen in meningioma (see following discussion).

   2. Meningioma.
      a. Primary optic nerve sheath tumor.
      b. Unusual lesion in children.
      c. More commonly seen in neurofibromatosis (type II).

> **Imaging** CT and MRI demonstrate thickening of sheath with encircling of optic nerve. Intense enhancement occurs.

   3. Hemangioma.
      a. Can be either intraconal or extraconal lesions.
      b. Capillary hemangiomas.
          1. Also known as hemangioma of infancy.
          2. Capillary (strawberry) hemangiomas; often have associated facial hemangiomas.
          3. These lesions usually spontaneously involute with time (although may initially increase in size over first 2 to 3 years of life).
      c. Cavernous hemangiomas.
          1. Dilated vascular spaces that can hemorrhage.
          2. Usually present with mass effect and/or blurred vision.
          3. Do not spontaneously regress.

> **Imaging** Smooth, well-defined soft-tissue density is seen posterior to globe in intraconal space with extensive enhancement on CT.

4. Grave disease.
   a. Rare; less than 3% of cases are seen in children.
   b. Clinical presentation.
      *1.* Proptosis (80% are bilateral).
      *2.* Hyperthyroidism.

> **Imaging** Diffuse extraocular muscle swelling and proptosis can be seen on CT or MRI.

5. Lymphoma (see following discussion).
6. Vascular lesions.
   a. Venous varix.
      *1.* Intermittant exophthalmos is present; associated with valsalva maneuver, coughing, crying, or bending over at waist.
      *2.* Varix usually has more superior location within orbit.

> **Imaging** Well-defined, yet often tortuous vessel is seen within orbit on CT that demonstrates intense enhancement. In order to actually see varix, imaging during maneuver that induces finding is often required.

   b. Carotid-cavernous fistula.
      *1.* Traumatic injury to intracavernous carotid artery, resulting in communication with cavernous sinus.
      *2.* Systemic arterial flow is shunted into venous system (superior orbital vein), resulting in pulsatile exophthalmos and venous engorgement.
      *3.* Treatment.
         *a.* Balloon embolization of fistula.

> **Imaging** Enlarged superior orbital vein with multiple, engorged, collateral vessels emanating from cavernous sinus can be seen on CT or MRI. Angiography can also demonstrate abnormal cavernous sinus and collateral vessels with subsequent treatment (embolization).

7. Pseudotumor.
   a. Idiopathic; painful inflammatory process.
   b. Unilateral (80%).
   c. Diagnosis of exclusion.
   d. Responds well to steroids.

> **Imaging** Variable appearance that includes swelling of extraocular muscles (yet sparing of muscle insertion at sclera), well-defined mass (can mimic hemangiomas although usually not as enhancing), or increased density of orbital fat on CT.

C. Extraconal lesions.
   1. Lymphangioma.
      a. Sequestration of lymph sacs often with hemangiomatous elements.
      b. Hemorrhage or infection can occur with subsequent sudden increase in size of lesion.
      c. Common location is medial aspect of orbit.

   > **Imaging** CT or MRI can demonstrate lobulated fluid-filled mass with variable enhancement (especially if infected or contains hemangiomatous component).

   2. Lymphoma.
      a. Non-Hodgkin variety (often Burkitt type).
      b. Can involve lacrimal gland.
      c. Majority of orbital lymphomas either develop or simultaneously have systemic lymphoma (75%).

   > **Imaging** Variable appearance on CT from well-defined lesion to diffuse infiltration of orbital tissues. Involvement of extraocular muscles often occurs. Contrast enhancement is also variable. Adjacent osseous erosion may be present.

   3. Dermoid or epidermoid.
      a. Arises from embryonic rests (usually dermoids) following neural tube closure.
      b. Presentation.
         *1.* Painless proptosis.
         *2.* Palpable lump.
      c. Common location is lateral or superior orbit.

   > **Imaging** Well-defined lesions on CT with low-density-fat (or usually cystic) components.

   4. Infection.
      a. Preseptal versus postseptal (separated by thin membrane, orbital septum, which is reflection of periosteum upon tarsal plates).

b. Preseptal.
   1. Usually arises from adjacent cellulitis.
   2. May have superficial abscess.
c. Postseptal.
   1. Usually related to adjacent spread of infection from sinuses.
   2. More ominous condition than preseptal infection because of potential for intracranial spread.

> **Imaging** Soft-tissue swelling with stranding of adjacent subcutaneous tissues can be seen in preseptal infections on CT with little contrast enhancement. Postseptal infections are similar; stranding of orbital fat and extraocular muscle swelling can be seen. Enhancement may be present, particularly with adjacent sinus disease and/or bony involvement. Fluid collections with rim enhancement are concern for abscess and should be surgically drained.

5. Rhabdomyosarcoma.
   a. Etiology is presumed congenital mesenchymal rests with malignant potential within orbit.
   b. Most common primary orbital tumor in children.
   c. Presentation is usually rapidly progressive proptosis.

> **Imaging** CT and MRI reveal aggressive tumor often with sinus and bony extension and destruction. Intracranial extension also can occur. Mild homogeneous enhancement is usually present.

6. Metastases.
   a. Commonly involves bony orbit.
   b. Often bilateral.
   c. Common types.
      1. Neuroblastoma.
         a. Periorbital ecchymosis.
         b. "Raccoon eyes."
      2. Ewing sarcoma.
      3. Leukemia or lymphoma.

> **Imaging** Bone destruction often with associated soft-tissue mass can be seen on CT and MRI orbital images.

7. Langerhans cell histiocytosis (see Chapter 35).
   a. Bony lesion of skull or orbit.
   b. Often has soft-tissue extension (histiocytic mass) that can enter orbit.

> **Imaging** Deformed bony orbit with irregular margins (occasionally sclerotic) can be seen on CT. Soft-tissue component (centered on bone) is often present.

## SUGGESTED READINGS

Abramson DH, Servodidio CA: Retinblastoma in the first year of life. *Ophthalmic Paediatr Genet* 1992; 13:191-203.

Albert A, Lee BC, Saint-Louis L, Deck MD: MRI of optic chiasm and optic pathways. *AJNR* 1986; 7:255-258.

Armington WG, Bilaniuk LT: Radiologic evaluation of the orbit: Conal and intraconal lesions. *Semin Ultrasound CT MR* 1988; 9:455-473.

Azar-Kia B, Naheedy MH, Elias DA, Mafee MF, Fine M: Optic nerve tumors: Role of CT and MR imaging. *Radiol Clin North Am* 1987; 25:561-581.

Berrocal T, Orbe A, Prieto C, Al-Assir I, Izquierdo C, Paster I, Abelairos J: US of color Doppler imaging of ocular and orbital disease in the pediatric age group. *Radiographics* 1996; 16:251-272.

Bilaniuk LT, Atlas SW, Zimmerman RA: Magnetic resonance imaging of the orbit. *Radiol Clin North Am* 1987; 25:509-528.

Enzmann D, Donaldson SS, Marshall WH, Kriss JP: Computed tomography in orbital pseudotumor. *Radiology* 1976; 120:597-601.

Flanders AE, Espinosa GA, Markiewicz DA, Howell DD: Orbital lymphoma. Role of CT and MR. *Radiol Clin North Am* 1987; 25:601-613.

Hopper KD, Haas DK, Sherman JL: Radiologic evaluation of congenital and pediatric lesions of the orbit. *Semin Ultrasound CT MR.* 1988; 9:413-427.

Mafee MF, Goldberg MF, Greenwald MJ, Schulman J, Malmed A, Flanders AE: Retinoblastoma and simulating lesions: Role of CT and MR imaging. *Radiol Clin North Am* 1987; 25:667-682.

Mafee MF, Goldberg MF, Valvassori GE, Capek V: CT in the evaluation of patients with persistent hyperplastic primary vitreous (PHPV). *Radiology* 1982; 145:713-717.

Price HI, Batnitzky S, Danzinger A, Karlin CA, Goldberg L: The neuroradiology of retinoblastoma. *Radiographics* 1982; 2:7-23.

Ramji FG, Slovis TL, Baker JD: Orbital sonography in children. *Pediatr Radiol* 1996; 26:245-258.

Sobel DF, Kelly W, Kjos BO, Char D, Brant-Zawadzki M, Norman D: MR imaging of orbital and ocular disease. *AJNR* 1985; 5:259-264.

Vade A, Armstrong D: Orbital rhabdomyosarcoma in childhood. *Radiol Clin North Am* 1987; 25:701-704.

# Index

**A**
Abdomen
  acute, 117-125
  anterior wall defects, 85
  manifestations of child abuse, 263-264
  neonatal bowel obstruction, 72-86
  neonatal masses, 72, 84-85
    differential diagnosis, 84*b*
  trauma to, 266-272
    key concepts, 266
Abdominal radiography
  with annular pancreas, 139
  with appendicitis, 120
  with bezoar, 95
  with bowel trauma, 268
  with choledochal cysts, 130
  with colonic duplications, 111
  of duodenal atresia or stenosis, 75
  duodenal hematoma, 263
  of esophageal atresia and tracheoesophageal fistula, 90
  with functional megacolon, 114
  with gallstones, 134
  with graft-*versus*-host-disease, 115
  with hemolytic uremia, 115, 225
  of Hirschsprung disease, 80
  with hypertrophic pyloric stenosis, 73
  of ileal atresia, 81-82
  with infectious gastroenteritis, 104
  with inguinal hernia, 123
  with intussusception, 122
  of jejunal atresia, 81-82
  with meconium ileus, 81
  of meconium peritonitis, 83
  of mesenteric, 104
  of midgut volvulus, 76
  with necrotizing enterocolitis, 119
  of omental cysts, 104
  with pancreatic trauma, 268
  of pancreatitis, 141
  with pneumatosis intestinalis, 112
  with pneumoperitoneum, 118
  of proximal small bowel obstruction, 77
  with pseudomembranous colitis, 114

Abscess, retropharyngeal, 7-8
  cervical adenopathy with, 391
Abuse, child, 258-265
Acetabula, Graf US classification of, 306, 307*f*
Achalasia, 93-94
Achondrogenesis, 333
Achondroplasia, 332, 333
Achondroplastic dwarfism, 362
Acinar cell tumors, 393
Acquired immunodeficiency syndrome, 36-37
  bony abnormalities in, 329
  cervical adenopathy in, 391
  esophagitis in, 93
  pneumonia in, 29
Actinomycosis, 36
Acute abdomen, 117-125
Acute disseminated encephalomyelitis, 364, 368
Acute renal failure, 224-225
  neonatal, 223
Acute tubular necrosis, neonatal, 223
Acyanotic heart disease, 154, 156-164
Acyanotic pulmonary artery abnormalities, 163
Adamantinoma, 283, 288-289
ADEM; *see* Acute disseminated encephalomyelitis
Adenocarcinoma
  clear cell, 240
  cystadenocarcinoma, 239
  pancreatic, 142
Adenoma
  hepatic, 131
  pleomorphic, 393
Adenomatoid malformation, cystic, 44, 45-46
Adenopathy
  cervical, 390-391
  with middle mediastinal masses, 64
Adhesions, bowel, 123-124
Adolescent idiopathic scoliosis, 296
Adrenal hyperplasia, congenital, 243
Adrenocortical tumor or hyperplasia, 228
Adrenoleukodystrophy, 378, 381-382
  neonatal, 381
Adult respiratory distress syndrome, 40
African Burkitt lymphoma, 34
Agyria, 349
AIDS; *see* Acquired immunodeficiency syndrome
Air leak problems
  neonatal, 16, 19-20
  with surfactant deficiency disorder, 17

---

Page numbers followed by *f* indicate figures; those followed by *t* indicate tables; and those followed by *b* indicate boxes.

Index    **413**

Air-contrast enema studies
  for juvenile polyps, 113
  for polyposis syndromes, 113
Airway, 2-15
  anatomy, 3
    normal, 3, 4f
    normal variants, 3, 5f, 6f
  anteroposterior film of, 3, 4f
  "buckling" of, 3, 5f
  imaging, 5, 6f
  key concepts, 2
  lateral film of, 3, 4f
  malignant primary lesions of, 10
  masses, 2, 8-10
  obstruction by foreign body, 9-10
  pathology, 3-14
    congenital or developmental, 10-14
    infectious or inflammatory, 3-8
  physiology, 3
  reactive disease, 50, 51
  "steepling" of, 2
  viral disease, 30
Airway fluoroscopy
  with airway obstruction by foreign body, 10
  with tracheomalacia, 14
Airway radiography, for Epstein-Barr virus, 34
Alagille syndrome, 133
Albers-Schönberg disease, 324
Alexander disease, 382-383
  imaging findings, 383
  macrocephaly in, 362
Allergic alveolar granulomatosis, 55
Allergic bronchopulmonary aspergillosis, 35-36
  chest radiographic findings, 36
Allergic conditions
  differential diagnosis, 33
  reaction to contrast material, pulmonary edema with, 39
Alveolar edema, 40
Alveolar granulomatosis, allergic, 55
Alveolar proteinosis, 55-56
Amenorrhea
  key concepts, 235
  primary, 236-237
Anemia
  congenital, with bony abnormalities, 327-328
  hemolytic, splenomegaly with, 144
  sickle cell
    bony abnormalities in, 327-328
    bony manifestations, 321
    differential diagnosis, 279
    early radiographic signs, 328
Anencephaly, 342, 344
Aneurysm
  pulmonary artery, 41
  renal, 228
  vein of Galen, 359
Angiofibroma, juvenile, 10
Angiography; *see also* Magnetic resonance angiography
  with carotid-cavernous fistula, 408
  with cervical aortic arch, 187
  with coarctation of aorta, 161
  with cor triatriatum, 162
  with juvenile nasopharyngeal angiofibroma, 390

  with pancreatic neoplasms, 142
  for pulmonary arteriovenous malformations, 48
  for renal artery stenosis, 227
  with vascular rings, 186
Angiomatosis, encephalotrigeminal, 348
Angiomyolipoma, 230, 233
Ankylosing spondylitis, 54
Annular pancreas, 138-139
  imaging findings, 77, 139
  neonatal, 77
Anophthalmos, 405
Anorectal malformations, 111
"Anteater nose," 319
Anterior abdominal wall defects, 85
Antral atresia, 73
Antral webs, congenital, 74
Anus, imperforate, 78, 109
Aortic arch
  cervical, 187
  congenital abnormalities of, 187-191
    key concepts, 181
  double, 185f, 185-186
    with tracheomalacia, 13
  embryology of, 182, 182f
  interrupted, 161, 189
    surgical repair for, 174
  left, 182-183, 183f
  patterns, 182-185
  radiographic approach to, 150-151
  right, 183-185, 184f
    with tracheomalacia, 13
Aortic dissection, with middle mediastinal masses, 64
Aortic masses, 64-65
Aortic shunts to pulmonary artery, 174
Aortic stenosis, 160-161
  categorization of, 153-154
  imaging findings, 160-161
  statistics, 154
  subvalvular, 160
  supravalvular, 160
  valvular, 160
Aortic valve, bicuspid, 155
Aortopulmonary graft, 174
Aortopulmonary window, 159
AP window; *see* Aortopulmonary window
Apert syndrome, 298
Appendicitis, 117, 119-120
"Apple-peel" atresia, 81
Aqueductal stenosis, 362
Arachnoid cyst, 362
Arch abnormalities, 318, 319f
Arteriohepatic dysplasia, 133
Arteriovenous malformations
  pulmonary, 42, 47-48
  renal, 228
Arthritis
  juvenile rheumatoid, 54, 301, 311
  septic, 274, 277-278
Arthrogryposis multiplex congenita, 338
ASD; *see* Atrial septal defect
Askin tumor, 56
Aspergillosis
  allergic bronchopulmonary, 35-36
  saprophytic to mycetoma, 35

*Aspergillus*, 35-36
  invasive, 36
Asphyxia, perinatal, 360
Aspiration, neonatal, 21
Aspiration pneumonia, 31-32
Aspirin overdose, 39
Asplenia, 177, 178, 178f, 179
Asthma, 51; *see also* Reactive airway disease
  differential diagnosis, 33
Astrocytoma
  giant cell, 373-374
    foramen of Monro, 362, 373
  imaging findings, 371
  juvenile pilocytic, 370
  macrocephaly with, 361
  pilocytic, 371
  posterior fossa, 371
    macrocephaly with, 361
  spinal, 395
  supratentorial, 373-374
Atelectasis, 26
  in surfactant deficiency disorder, 18b
Atlantoaxial subluxation, 294-295
ATN; *see* Acute tubular necrosis
Atresia
  choanal, 10-11
  tracheal, 11
Atrial septal defects, 156, 158
  categorization of, 153
  sinus venosus or "high," 42
  statistics, 154, 155
  surgical repair for, 172, 173
Atrioventricular canal, 158-159
  categorization of, 153
  statistics, 154
Avascular necrosis
  of hip, 301, 308
  with sickle cell anemia, 321, 328
AVC; *see* Atrioventricular canal
AVMs; *see* Arteriovenous malformations
Axial skeleton, 293-300

**B**
Back pain, 279
  nontraumatic, 274, 278
Backwash ileitis, 114
Bacterial encephalitis, 367
Bacterial pneumonia, 30-31
Bacterial tracheitis, 5-6
"Ballooning" of hypopharynx, 5, 6f
Barium studies
  with achalasia, 94
  enema, with appendicitis, 120
  fluoroscopy during, with gastroesophageal
    reflux disease, 92
  with malabsorption, 106
  swallow
    with esophageal masses, 94
    with esophagitis, 93
    for foreign bodies, 93
    with vascular rings, 186
Barlow maneuver, 302
Bartter syndrome, 225
Battered babies, *see* Abuse, child
  CNS manifestations, 261

Beckwith-Wiedemann syndrome
  hepatoblastoma in, 132
  macroglossia in, 14
  Wilms tumor in, 231-232
Bell-clapper deformity, 241, 242f
Bent limb dwarfism, 333-334
Bezoar, 95
Biliary atresia
  neonatal jaundice with, 127-128
  types of, 127, 128f
Biliary disease, acquired, 134-135
Biliary tree dilatation, 135
Bladder
  abnormalities, 209-213
  development and disorders, 206-215
  exstrophy, 209
  formation, 209
  injury, 270
  innervation, 209-210
  lazy, 213
  neurogenic, 206, 211
  unstable, 212
Blalock-Hanlon operation, 174
Blalock-Taussig procedure, 172
Blalock-Taussig shunt, 173
Blastoma
  chondroblastoma, 287
  hepatoblastoma, 131-132
  pulmonary, 56
Blastomycosis, 36
Blood flow; *see* Pulmonary blood flow
Blount disease, 310
"Blue-baby operation," 173
Bochdalek hernia, 25
Bone age evaluation, 325-326
Bone density, dysplasias and, 336-337
Bone infarctions, 321, 327-328
Bone lesions, 282-292
  benign, 278, 283
  categorization of, 283-284
  characteristics of, 283-284
  cystic, 289-291
  cysts
    aneurysmal, 283, 290
    unicameral, 282, 283, 289-290
  fibrous, 288-289
  key concepts, 282
  malignant, infiltrative, or progressive, 283-284
  skull, 293, 298
Bone marrow; *see* Marrow
Bone metastases, 278
Bone scans
  for avascular necrosis of hip, 308
  for back pain, 279
  child abuse screening, 259
  for discitis, 278
  fracture findings, 247
  for osteomyelitis, 274, 276
  stress fractures, 248
Bone shortening, 332
Bone tumors, 280
Bone-in-bone finding, 324, 327
Bony abnormalities, 321-331
  congenital anemias with, 327-328
  with congenital heart disease, 152-153

Index **415**

key concepts, 321
metabolic disease, 322-323
"Boot-shaped" heart, 150, 166
Bourneville disease, 348
Bowel
  adhesions, 123-124
  canalization of, 75, 76f
  dysgenesis, 80
  edema, with thumbprinting, 115
  large; see also Colon
    abnormalities, 109-116
    development, 110, 110f
    neonatal obstruction, 77-82
  neonatal masses, 72-86
  sausage, 115
  "saw-tooth" contractions of, 80
  "shock bowel," 268
  small bowel
    abnormalities, 97-108
    atresia, 81, 83f
    obstruction, 77-82
    stenosis, 83f
    trauma, 268
Bowel disease, inflammatory, 93, 97, 105, 114
Bowel duplication cyst, 103
Bowel loops, 25
  bulbous, 80
  dilated, 73
  neonatal distended, 72
Bowel obstruction
  causes of, 123-124
  distal small bowel, 77-82
  double bubble pattern of, 73, 75-77, 139
  neonatal, 73-82
  patterns of, 72, 73
  proximal small bowel, 77
  pseudoobstruction, 80
Bowing fractures, 247, 248f
"Box-shaped" heart, 150, 169
BPD; see Bronchopulmonary dysplasia
Brain development, 343-344
Brain disorders
  lysosomal, 379-381
  metabolic, 378-385
  peroxisomal, 381-382
Brain malformations, congenital, 342-353
  Chiari, 345
    neonatal, 359
    type I, 345
    type II, 342, 345
    type III, 345
  destructive lesions, 351-352
  key concepts, 342
  with macrocephaly, 362
Brain stem glioma, 372
Brain tumors, 361, 370-377
Branchial arches
  anomalies, 388-389
  embryology, 388, 389f
Brodie abscess, 277
Bronchiectasis, 52, 53
Bronchiolitis, 30
Bronchiolitis obliterans, 33
  hypoplastic pulmonary arteries with, 41

Bronchogenic cysts, 87
  intrapulmonary, 46
  mediastinal, 46, 65
  parenchymal, 91
Bronchopulmonary aspergillosis, allergic, 35-36
Bronchopulmonary dysplasia, 18b, 20-21
Bronchopulmonary sequestration, 46-47
  extralobar, 47
  intralobar, 46-47
Bronchoscopy, with tracheomalacia, 14
Bronchus
  esophageal, 12-13, 90-91
  tracheal ("pig bronchus"), 12
"Brown tumors," 325
"Bubbly" findings
  with adamantinoma, 288
  with cystic masses, 46
  double bubble pattern
    with bowel obstruction, 73, 75-77, 139
    with duodenal atresia or stenosis, 102
  with ossifying fibroma, 288
  "soap-bubble," 81
"Bucket-handle" fractures, 258, 260
Buckle fractures, 248, 248f
"Buckling" of airway, 3, 5f
Budd-Chiari syndrome, 133
Bullet-shaped vertebral bodies, 337, 379
Buphthalmos, 405
Burkitt lymphoma, 63, 392
  African, 34

**C**

"Café-au-lait" spots, 338, 347
Caffey syndrome, 261, 280
Calcaneal line, 314, 315
Calcaneal-talar angle, 315, 315f, 316
  normal, 314
Calcifications, intracranial gyral, 348
CAM; see Cystic adenomatoid malformation
Camurati-Englemann disease, 324
Canalization with retrogressive differentiation, 396f, 396-397
Canavan disease, 362, 383
Cancer; see also specific carcinomas
  differential diagnosis, 280
Candidiasis, 35, 93
Capillary (strawberry) hemangioma, 386, 389
  orbital, 407
Captopril scans, with renal artery stenosis, 227
Carcinoid
  colonic, 116
  small bowel, 107
Carcinoma
  choriocarcinoma, 61, 239, 375
  choroid plexus, 361, 375
  clear cell adenocarcinoma, 240
  colonic, 116
  cystadenocarcinoma, 239
  hepatocellular, 132
  mucoepidermoid, 393
  pancreatic adenocarcinoma, 142
  renal cell, 230, 233
  teratocarcinoma, 61
Cardiac masses, 66

Cardiac vessels
    great vessels, 147-192
    situs, 152
    situs indeterminus, 152
Cardiomegaly, 149-150
    differential diagnosis, 154
Cardiomyopathy, left heart, 162
"Cardiothymic notch," 61
Caroli disease, 129f, 130
Carotid-cavernous fistula, 408
Carpet of polyps, 113
Cartilaginous dysplasias, 338
Cartilaginous lesions, 286-288
Castleman disease, 64
Caudal regression, 399-400
Cecal colitis, 115
Cecum, development of, 98, 98f
Celiac disease, 106
Central nervous system
    child abuse manifestations, 261-263
    infections, 364-369
        congenital, 365
        key concepts, 364
    "shaken-baby" injury, 262-263
        key concepts, 258
Central nervous system tubers, hamartomas on, 348
Cerebellum
    disorders of, 350-351
    hypoplasia or agenesis of, 351
Cerebral edema or infarction, 263
Cerebral hemispheres, abnormal thickness,
        folding, and organization of, 349-350
Cerebrohepatorenal syndrome, 381
Cervical adenopathy, 390-391
    inflammatory or infectious, 386
Cervical aortic arch, 187
Cervical spine, normal variants, 293
"Champagne glass" iliac bones, 332
CHD; see Congenital heart disease
Chediak-Higashi syndrome, 33
Chemotherapy-induced osteosarcoma, 285-286
Chest, 1-70
    neonatal, 16-28
Chest radiography
    with aberrant left coronary artery, 162
    with achalasia, 94
    for air leak, 20
    for allergic bronchopulmonary aspergillosis, 36
    of alveolar proteinosis, 56
    with anomalous innominate artery, 187
    of anterior mediastinal masses, 62
    of aortic leak, 64-65
    with aortic stenosis, 160-161
    with AP window, 159
    of Askin tumor, 56
    for aspergillosis, 35
    of aspiration pneumonia, 32
    asthma findings, 51
    with atrial septal defect, 158
    for bronchiolitis obliterans, 33
    of bronchogenic cysts, 46, 65, 91
    of bronchopulmonary dysplasia, 20-21
    of bronchopulmonary sequestrations, 47
    of cardiac masses, 66
    with cervical aortic arch, 187
    with chronic lung disease, 163
    for chylothorax, 23
    with coarctation of aorta, 161, 189
    for collagen vascular, 54
    congenital heart disease evaluation, 149
    for congenital lobar emphysema, 27, 45
    for congenital lung cysts, 27
    with cor triatriatum, 162
    with corrected transposition of great vessels, 191
    for cystic adenomatoid malformation, 26, 46
    cystic fibrosis findings, 53
    for diaphragmatic hernia, 25
    of duplication (enteric) cysts, 92
    with Ebstein malformation, 169
    with endocardial cushion defect, 159
    with endocardial fibroelastosis, 162
    for esophageal bronchus, 13
    of extramedullary hematopoiesis, 69
    of ganglioneuroma, 69
    of hamartoma, 56
    of hiatal hernia, 66
    of Hodgkin lymphoma, 63
    for hypogenetic lung, 48
    with hypoplastic left heart, 160
    for invasive *aspergillus*, 36
    for Langerhans cell histiocytosis, 54
    with left heart lesions, 163
    for lymphangiectasia, 24
    of lymphangioma-hemangioma, 66
    of middle mediastinal masses, 64
    for neonatal aspiration, 21
    for neonatal pneumonia, 22
    of neurenteric cyst, 91
    of neuroblastoma, 68
    of neurofibroma, 67
    of obstructive airway disease, 30
    with patent ductus arteriosus, 158
    for persistent pulmonary hypertension of the
        newborn, 23
    for pertussis, 35
    postoperative findings, 175
    for pulmonary arteriovenous malformations, 48
    with pulmonary artery stenosis, 163
    with pulmonary atresia, 168-169
    of pulmonary blastoma, 56
    for pulmonary edema, 23
    for pulmonary embolus, 43
    for pulmonary hemorrhage, 22
    for pulmonary hemosiderosis, 55
    for pulmonary hypertension, 41
    for pulmonary hypoplasia, 24
    for pulmonary interstitial emphysema, 19
    of pulmonary metastatic disease, 56
    for pulmonary sequestration, 27
    with pulmonary sling, 186
    for restrictive lung, 24-25
    of round pneumonia, 31
    of *S. aureus*, 34
    for surfactant deficiency disorder, 19
    with Tetralogy of Fallot, 166
    of thymus, 61
    for tracheal agenesis or atresia, 11
    for tracheal bronchus, 12
    for tracheomalacia, 14
    for transient tachypnea of the newborn, 17
    with transposition of great vessels, 168, 190
    with tricuspid atresia, 168

pulmonary, 44
renal, 194-205
of spleen, 142-143
tumors, 361
urologic, 196-204
vertical talus, 317-318, 318f
Congenital dysplasia of hip; see Developmental dysplasia of the hip
Congenital heart disease, 148-155, 172-176
   acyanotic, 156-164
   categories of, 148, 153
   cyanotic, 165-171
   diagnosis, 149
   differential diagnosis, 153-155
   key concepts, 148
   left-to-right shunts, 157-159
   radiographic approach to, 149-153
   situs, 152
   situs abnormalities with, 177
   soft tissues and bones with, 152-153
   surgical repair of, 173-174
      radiographic findings of, 174-175
Congenital lobar emphysema, 27, 44, 45
Congenital malformations; see Congenital abnormalities
Contrast material, allergic reaction to, 39
Contrast studies
   barium
      with achalasia, 94
      with appendicitis, 120
      fluoroscopy during, with GERD, 92
      with malabsorption, 106
   barium swallow
      with esophageal masses, 94
      with esophagitis, 93
      for foreign bodies, 93
      with vascular rings, 186
   with bezoar, 95
   with bowel dysgenesis, 80
   with chronic granulomatous disease of childhood, 95
   computed tomography
      of aortic injury, 65
      with pancreatic neoplasms, 142
   contraindications, 114, 115
   cystography, for bladder injury, 270
   enema
      with appendicitis, 120
      with colonic atresia, 82
      with Hirschsprung disease, 80
      with inflammatory bowel disease, 114
      for juvenile polyps, 113
      with malrotation, 101
      with microcolon, 82
      for polyposis syndromes, 113
   with esophageal atresia and tracheoesophageal fistula, 90
   of esophageal bronchus, 91
   gadolinium MRI, with drop mets, 401-402
   with gastric duplications, 94
   with gastric volvulus, 96
   with graft-versus-host-disease, 115
   of inflammatory bowel disease, 105
   of laryngotracheoesophageal cleft, 90
   with malabsorption, 106

with malignant colonic tumors, 116
with peptic ulcer disease, 95
of SMA syndrome, 106
upper gastrointestinal examination; see Upper gastrointestinal examination
water-soluble
   of patent omphalomesenteric duct, 103
   of patent urachus, 210
Cooley operation, 174
Copper deficiency, 261
Copper storage abnormality, 133
Cor triatriatum, 154, 162
Coronary heart disease
   with congenital lobar emphysema, 45
   with lymphangiectasia, 24
Corpus callosum
   agenesis of, 346, 347f, 359
   anomalies of, 342, 345-346
Cortical desmoid, 311
Cortical hyperostosis, infantile, 261
Cough
   depressed, 32
   whooping, 34
Craniometaphyseal dysplasia, 337
Craniopharyngioma, 361, 370, 374
Craniosynostosis, 293, 298-299
   universal, 299
"Crescent sign," 308
Cretinism, 326
CRITOE mnemonic for elbow epiphyses, 252-253, 254f
   example how to use, 253
Crohn's disease; see Inflammatory bowel disease
Croup, 2
   membranous, 5-6
   viral, 3-5
Crouzon disease, 298
Cryptococcus, 36
Cryptorchidism, 240-241
C-T angle; see Calcaneal-talar angle
Cushing syndrome, 322
Cyanotic heart disease, 165-171
   with decreased pulmonary flow, 153, 154, 166-169
   with increased pulmonary flow, 153, 154, 169-170
Cystadenocarcinoma, 239
Cystadenoma, 239
Cystic adenomatoid malformation, 25-26, 44, 45-46
   types, 25-26, 26f, 45
Cystic astrocytoma, 361
Cystic bronchopulmonary dysplasia, 20
Cystic fibrosis, 50, 51-53
   differential diagnosis, 32
   pancreatic malformations with, 141
   peptic ulcer disease with, 94
Cystic hygroma, 387
Cystic lesions, 289-291
Cystic masses
   "bubbly," 46
   neonatal
      differential diagnosis, 84b, 130
      key concepts, 126
Cystic nephroma, multilocular, 232

# 420  Index

Cysticercosis, 367, 368
Cysts
   arachnoid, 362
   bronchogenic, 46, 65
   choledochal, 128-130
   dermoid or epidermoid
      brain, 373
      of head and neck, 390
      orbital, 409
      spinal, 400
   developmental, 65-66
   duplication, etiology of, 75, 76f
   epidermoid, 290-291
      brain, 373
      categorization of, 283
   medullary disease, 204
   midgut, 103-104
   neurenteric, 400
   pericardial, 66
   pineal, 375
   splenic, 143
   thymic, 60
   thyroglossal duct, 387-388, 388f
   urachal, 211
   with von Hippel-Lindau disease, 348
Cytomegalo virus infection, 93

## D

Dactylitis, 321
   with sickle cell anemia, 327
Dandy-Walker malformation, 359, 362
Dandy-Walker syndrome, 350-351
Dandy-Walker variant, 351
Daytime frequency, 212
DDH; see Developmental dysplasia of the hip
De Morsier syndrome, 347
"Delta sign," 366
Deposition dysplasia, 337-338
Dermal sinus tract, 399
Dermoid cysts
   in brain, 361, 373
   of head and neck, 390
   orbital, 409
   ovarian, 239
   spinal, 395, 400
   splenic, 143
Desmoid tumor, cortical, 311
Developmental cysts, 65-66
   in foregut, 87, 91-92
Developmental disorders, congenital, with macrocephaly, 362
Developmental dysplasia of the hip, 302-305
   clinical examination for, 304
   clinical screening for, 302
   Graf classification of, 306, 307f
   imaging findings, 303-304
   indications for imaging, 302
   lines and angles of, 303, 305f
   radiographic examination, 303
   ultrasound examination for, 301, 303-304, 304
      at 4 to 6 weeks, advantages, 304
      timing of, 303-304
   undetected (missed), 304-305
Dextrocardia, 179
Diaphragmatic hernia, 25

Diaphragms, congenital, 74
Diaphyseal dysplasia, 324
Diastematomyelia, 395, 399
Diastrophic dwarfism, 338-339
Diethylenetriaminepentacetic acid, renal scans
   of multicystic dysplastic kidney, 203
   for uretero-pelvic junction obstruction, 202
   with uretero-vesical junction obstruction, 201
DiGeorge syndrome, 32, 60
Dimercaptosuccinic acid scans
   with reflux nephropathy, 226
   renal, 219
Discitis, 274, 278-279
Dislocating dysplasias, 338-339
Distal jejunal atresia, 81-82
Distal small bowel obstruction, 77-82
Diverticulation, 343
   disorders of, 346-347
Doppler ultrasound
   with chronic renal failure, 227
   color
      with hemangioma, 389
      with lymphangioma, 387
   of hemangioendothelioma, 131
   with ovarian torsion, 237
   with renal vein thrombosis, 224
Dorsal induction, 344-345
Double aortic arch, 185f, 185-186
   with tracheomalacia, 13
"Double bubble" pattern
   with bowel obstruction, 139
   in neonates, 73, 75-77
   with duodenal atresia or stenosis, 102
Double outlet right ventricle, 167
Down syndrome
   atlantoaxial subluxation in, 294-295
   duodenal atresia or stenosis in, 101
   endocardial cushion defect in, 158
   heart disease in, 155
   imaging for Special Olympics participants, 295
   lymphangioma-hemangioma in, 65
   macroglossia in, 14
Drooping lily sign, 200, 200f
"Drop mets" or drop metastases, 395, 401-402
   differential diagnosis, 278
Drug overdose, 39
Drusen, 406
DTPA; see Diethylenetriaminepentacetic acid
"Dumb-bell shaped" lesions, 402
Duodenal atresia, 75, 101-102
   etiology of, 75, 76f
Duodenal hematoma, 97, 104
   child abuse, 258, 263
   traumatic, 266
Duodenal injury, 268
Duodenal lesions, 139
Duodenal stenosis, 75, 101-102
Duodenum
   coiled-spring appearance of, 263
   "stack of coins" appearance, 105, 263
Duplication cysts
   enteric, 91-92
      etiology, 88f, 92
   etiology of, 75, 76f
   neonatal, 126

Dwarfism, 333-335
  achondroplastic, 332, 362
  acromelic, 334-335
  bent limb, 333-334
  campomelic, 333-334
  diastrophic, 338-339
  mesomelic, 333-334
  rhizomelic, 333
  short-limb, 338
  skeletal dysplasia with, 332
Dyschondroesteosis, 334
Dysgerminoma, 239
Dysmyelinating disorders, 362
Dysplasia epiphyseal hemimelica, 335
Dysraphism, 395
Dyssegmental dysgenesis, 339
Dyssynergia, 212-213

## E

Eagle-Barrett syndrome; *see* Prune-belly syndrome
Ebstein malformation, 153, 169
Ecchymosis, periorbital, 410
ECD; *see* Endocardial cushion defect
"Egg-on-string" heart configuration, 150, 168, 190
Eisenmenger complex, 41, 163
Elbow
  epiphyses, 252-253, 254*f*
  fractures, 246
  humeral or capitellar line imaging, 252, 254*f*
  Little Leaguer's elbow, 253, 254*f*
  nursemaid's elbow, 253, 255*f*
  trauma, 251-253
Elfin faces, 160
Ellis–van Creveld syndrome, 334
Embryonal cell tumors, 239
Embryonal sarcoma
  rhabdomyosarcoma, 214
  undifferentiated, 132
Embryonal tumors, 206
Emphysema
  congenital lobar, 27, 44, 45
  pulmonary interstitial, 18*b*
Encephalitis, 366-368
  bacterial, 367
  herpes simplex, 364, 366
  human immunodeficiency virus, 367
  parasitic, 367-368
  subacute sclerosing panencephalitis, 367
  viral, 366-367
Encephalocele, 344-345
Encephalomyelitis, acute disseminated, 364, 368
Encephalomyopathy, 382
Encephalopathy, 382
Encephalotrigeminal angiomatosis, 348
Enchondroma, 283, 286
Enchondromatosis, 338
Endocardial cushion defect, 158-159
Endocardial fibroelastosis, 154, 161-162
Endocrine disorders, bony abnormalities in, 321, 324-326
Endocrine hypertension, 228
Endodermal sinus, 61, 62, 375
Endodermal sinus tumors, 240

Endoscopic retrograde cholangiography, with pancreas divisum, 139
Endoscopy, for peptic ulcer disease, 95
Endotracheal tube, aberrant placement of, 26
End-stage lung disease, 163
Enema studies
  with appendicitis, 120
  with colonic atresia, 82
  with Hirschsprung disease, 80
  with inflammatory bowel disease, 114
  with malrotation, 101
  with microcolon, 82
  single-contrast
    for juvenile polyps, 113
    for polyposis syndromes, 113
Enemas
  for reduction of intussusception, 122-123
    air technique, 122-123
  water-soluble, 78-79
    for distal obstruction in neonate, 72
    for meconium ileus, 81
Enuresis, nocturnal, 212
Eosinophilic granuloma, 53, 278; *see also* Langerhans cell histiocytosis
  bony abnormalities in, 330
Ependymoma
  "drop mets," 401
  imaging findings, 372, 376
  posterior fossa, 370, 372
    macrocephaly with, 361
  spinal, 395
  supratentorial, 376
Epidermoid cysts, 290-291
  in brain, 361, 373
  categorization of, 283
  of head and neck, 390
  orbital, 409
  skull, 298
  spinal, 395, 400
  splenic, 143
Epidermolysis bullosa, 93
Epididymitis, 241
Epiglottitis, 2, 6-7, 7*f*
Epilepsy, myoclonic, 382
Epiphyseal dysplasias, 335-336
Epiphyseal injuries, 240*b*, 249-251
  classification of, 250*b*-251*b*, 252*f*
  imaging findings, 250*b*, 251*b*
  Salter-Harris classification of, 250*b*-251*b*, 252*f*
Epiphyseal osteomyelitis, primary, 277
Epiphyses
  elbow, 252-253, 254*f*
  slipped capital femoral, 308-309
  stippled, 333
Epispadias, 207
Epithelial tumors, 239
Epstein-Barr virus, 34
Equinovarus, 314, 317, 317*f*
Erlenmeyer flask deformity, 308, 337
Esophageal atresia, 87, 90
  with fistula, 87, 88-90, 89*f*
  without fistula, 88-89, 89*f*
Esophageal bronchus, 12-13, 90-91
Esophageal cysts, 87

Esophageal filling defects, 93, 94
Esophageal masses, 66, 94
Esophagitis, 93
Esophagus
    abnormalities, 87-96
    foreign body in, 93
    pathology, 92-94
Ewing sarcoma, 280, 283, 291
    metastasis, 56, 410
Exostosis; see Osteochondroma
External genitalia, ambiguous, 243
Extramedullary hematopoiesis, 69, 327

**F**

Facial radiography
    for juvenile angiofibroma, 10
    for juvenile nasopharyngeal angiofibroma, 390
"Fallen fragment" sign, 282
Familial polyposis coli, 113
Fanconi syndrome, 328
Fatigue fracture, 247
Fatty liver, 53
FCD; see Fibrous cortical defect
Female genitals, 236-240
    acquired disorders, 237-239
    congenital disorders, 236-237
    neoplasms, 239-240
    normal anatomy, 236
    prepubescent, 236
    pubertal, 236
Female hypospadias, 207-209
Females
    cloacal malformations, 208, 208f
    urinary tract infection, 217
Feminization, testicular, 243
Femur
    proximal femoral focal deficiency, 333
    slipped capital epiphysis, 308-309
Fetal circulation, persistent, 23
Fetal renal hamartoma, 230, 232
Fibrinoid leukodystrophy, 383
Fibrocortical defects, 283
    in knee, 309
Fibrodysplasia, retrolental, 404, 406
Fibroma
    cardiac, 66
    chondromyxoid, 287
    nonossifying, 288
        in knee, 309
    ossifying, 283, 288
    ovarian, 239
    small bowel, 107
Fibromatosis colli, 386, 390
Fibrous cortical defect, 282, 288
Fibrous dysplasia, 282, 283, 289, 338
Fibrous histiocytoma, malignant, 283
Fibrous lesions, 288-289
Filling defects, esophageal, 93, 94
"Finger-in-glove" finding, 36, 51
Flat foot, 318, 319f
Fluid, neonatal lung, 26
Fluid overload, 39
Fluoroscopy
    airway
        with airway obstruction by foreign body, 10
        with tracheomalacia, 14

of gastroesophageal reflux, 32, 92
    for urinary tract infection, 217-218
Fontan procedure, 172, 173
Foot, 314-320
    congenital abnormalities of, 316-319
    normal alignment of, 315, 315f
    radiographic evaluation of, 315-316
        components, 314
        weight-bearing films, 315-316
"Football" sign, 118
Foramen of Monro giant cell astrocytoma, 362, 373
Forearm, Madelung deformity of, 334
Forefoot, 314, 315, 316
Foregut abnormalities, 87-96
    congenital malformations, 88-92
    developmental cysts, 87, 91-92
    foreign bodies, 93
    key concepts, 87
Foregut development, 88, 89f
Foreign bodies
    airway obstruction by, 9-10
    "ball-valve," 10
    chronic, 32
    in foregut, 93
Fracture foolers, 249
Fractures
    bowing, 247, 248f
    bucket-handle, 258, 260
    child abuse and, 258
    corner, in child abuse, 260
    of elbow, 246
    fatigue, 247
    greenstick, 247, 248f
    growing, 298
    incomplete, 247-249
    insufficiency, 247
    Jefferson fractures, 295
    key concepts, 246
    long-bone, in child abuse, 259-260
    multiple, differential diagnosis, 261
    plastic, 247, 248f
    posterior rib, 260
    pseudo-Jefferson, 295
    skull, 298
        in child abuse, 260-261
    stress, 247-248, 248f
    Toddler's fracture, 246, 248-249
    torus or buckle, 248f
    types of, 246, 247-249, 248f
Free air, 118
Functional megacolon, 113-114
Fungal infections, 36
Fungal pneumonia, 35-36

**G**

Gadolinium contrast magnetic resonance imaging, with drop mets, 401-402
Gag, depressed, 32
Gallbladder
    acute noncalculous distension of, 134
    enlarged, 134
Gallbladder hydrops, 134
Gallbladder polyps, 135
Gallbladder sludge, 53
Gallstones, 134
Ganglioglioma, 376

Ganglion, intraosseous, 283, 290
Ganglioneuroblastoma, 68
Ganglioneuroma, 68-69, 376
Gardner syndrome, 95, 113, 284
Gastric atresia, 94
Gastric duplications, 87, 94
Gastric lesions, 139
Gastric masses, 95-96
Gastric outlet abnormalities, 73-74
Gastric volvulus, 96
  neonatal, 74
Gastritis, 95
Gastroenteritis
  eosinophilic, 106
  infectious, 97, 104
Gastroesophageal reflux, 32, 87
Gastroesophageal reflux disease, 92-93
Gastrointestinal system, 71-146
  atresias, 73
  duplication cyst, 65
  neonatal masses, 84b
Gastroschisis, 85
Gaucher disease, 337-338, 379
  categorization of, 283
  splenomegaly with, 144
Genitals
  ambiguous external, 243
  development and disorders, 235-244
  female, 236-240
  male, 240-242
  malformations, 197
  neonatal masses, 84b
Genitourinary system, 193-244
  fistula, 78
GERD; see Gastroesophageal reflux disease
Germ cell tumors, 61-62
  ovarian, 239
  pineal, 375
Germinal matrix hemorrhage, 356, 357b
Germinoma, 375
Giant cell astrocytoma, 373-374
  foramen of Monro, 362, 373
Giant lymph node hyperplasia, 64
Giant osteoid osteoma, 285
Glenn operation, 173
Glioma
  brain stem, 372
  optic nerve, 404, 407
  slow-growing, 361
Globe lesions, 405-407
Globoid cell leukodystrophy, 380
Glomerulonephritis, 224-225
  chronic, 226
Gonads, 236
Goodpasture's syndrome, 55
Graf classification of acetabula, 306, 307f
Graft-versus-host-disease, 115
Granuloma, chronic granulomatous disease of childhood, 33
Granulomatosis
  allergic alveolar, 55
  Wegener, 55
Granulosa cell tumors, 239
Grave disease, 407-408
Great vessels, 147-192
  anomalies with cervical aortic arch, 187
  transposition of, 165, 166-168, 170
    corrected, 167, 191
    D loop, 190
    L loop, 191
    surgical repair for, 174
Greenstick fractures, 247, 248f
"Ground glass" finding, 282
Growing fracture, 298
Growth arrest lines, 311
Growth plate dysfunction, 251
Growth plate injuries, 240b, 249-251
  classification of, 250b-251b, 252f
  imaging findings, 250b, 251b
  Salter-Harris classification of, 250b-251b, 252f
Growth recovery lines, 311
Gyrus
  agyria, 349
  intracranial calcifications, 348
  pachygyria, 349
  polymicrogyria, 349

**H**
"Hair-on-end" skull, 327
Hairy polyps, 390
Hamartomas, 56
  CNS tuber, 348
  fetal renal, 230, 232
  mesenchymal, 131
  splenic, 143
Hand-foot syndrome, 279, 321, 327
Hand-Schüller-Christian disease or syndrome, 53-54, 330
Harcke views (hip), 304, 307f
"Harlequin eye," 298, 299
"Hazy lungs of prematurity," 18b
Head
  neonatal, 354-363
    congenital anomalies, 359-360
    large, 360-361
    ultrasound of, 355
Head and neck lesions, 386-394
  congenital, 387-390
  inflammatory or infectious, 390-391
  neoplastic masses, 392-393
  vascular, 391
Heart, 147-192
  "boot-shaped" appearance, 150, 166
  "box-shaped" appearance, 150, 169
  oval or "egg-on-a-string" appearance, 150, 168, 190
  pathognomonic configurations, 150, 151f
  "shaggy heart," 35
  size, 149-150
  snowman appearance of, 170
Heart disease, congenital
  acyanotic, 156-164
  cyanotic, 165-171
  radiographic approach to, 149-153
  surgical repair of, 173-174
Hemangioblastoma, 348, 372
Hemangioendothelioma, 130-131
  bone lesions, 283
  salivary gland, 393
Hemangioma
  airway, 2, 9
  bone lesions, 283

Hemangioma—cont'd
  capillary (strawberry), 386, 389, 407
  cavernous, 389, 390, 407
  colonic, 115
  esophageal, 94
  facial, 407
  head and neck, 386, 389
  hepatic, 126, 130
  of infancy, 407
  intraconal, 407
  lower urinary, 214
  lymphangioma-hemangioma, 65, 66
  salivary gland, 393
  skull, 298
  small bowel, 107
  splenic, 143
Hematoma
  duodenal, 97, 104
    in child abuse, 258, 263
    traumatic, 266
  in hip, 306
  jejunal or ileal, 104-105
  mediastinal, 172
  midgut, 104-105
  muscular or soft tissue, 256
Hematopoiesis, extramedullary, 69, 327
Hematopoietic disorders, 321, 327-330
Hemolytic anemias, 144
Hemolytic uremia, 114-115, 223, 225
Hemophilia, 328-329
Hemorrhage
  germinal matrix, 356, 357b
  intracranial, 354, 355-359
    grading of, 356, 357b
  intraparenchymal, 357b
  intraventricular, 356, 357b
  parenchymal lesions, 263
  pulmonary, 22, 55
  subdural, 262-263
  subperiosteal, 260
Henoch-Schönlein purpura, 104-105
Hepatic adenoma, 131
Hepatic cirrhosis, 132-134
Hepatic masses
  benign, 130-131
  malignant, 131-132
Hepatic trauma, 267
Hepatic venooclusive disease, 133
Hepatitis, 127
Hepatobiliary system, 126-136
Hepatoblastoma, 126, 131-132
Hepatocellular carcinoma, 132
Hepatosplenobiliary masses, 84b
Hermaphrodites, 243
Hernia
  diaphragmatic, 25
  hiatal, 66
  inguinal, 123, 240f, 241
  internal, 100
  Morgagni, 25
  paraduodenal, 100
Heroin overdose, 39
Herpes simplex virus infection
  encephalitis, 364, 366-367
  esophagitis, 93

Heterotaxy syndrome, 177, 179
Heterotopias, 349-350
Hiatal hernia, 66
High arch (foot), 318, 319f
Hilar enlargement, 53
Hilgenreiner's line, 303, 305f
Hindfoot, 314, 315, 316
Hindfoot valgus, 316
Hindfoot varus, 316
Hindgut abnormalities, 109-116
  acquired, 112-116
  congenital, 110-112
Hindgut development, 110, 110f
Hinman syndrome, 212-213
Hip, 301, 302-309
  avascular necrosis of, 301, 308
  developmental dysplasia of, 301, 302-305, 307f
  effusion, 301, 305-308
  instability, Harcke views, 304, 307f
Hirschsprung disease, 109, 111-112
  neonatal, 79-80
  total colonic, 79-80
Histiocytosis X; see Langerhans cell histiocytosis
Histogenesis disorders, 347-349
*Histoplasmosis*, 35
HIV; see Human immunodeficiency virus
Hodgkin lymphoma, 63, 392
Holoprosencephaly, 346-347, 362
Honeycomb lung, 54, 55, 163
Horseshoe kidney, 197-199, 198f
HPS; see Hypertrophic pyloric stenosis
Human immunodeficiency virus
  encephalitis with, 367
  pneumonia with, 29
Hunter syndrome, 337, 378, 379
  macrocephaly in, 362
Hurler syndrome, 337, 378, 379
  macrocephaly in, 362
  macroglossia in, 14
Hutch diverticulum, 211
Hyaline membrane disease; see Surfactant
  deficiency disorder
Hyaloid artery
  persistent, 406
  primitive, 405
Hydranencephaly, 342, 351-352, 362
Hydrocele, 235, 240f, 241
Hydrocephalus, 354, 362
  communicating, 365
  with macrocephaly, 361
  with meningitis, 365-366
  with pineal tumors, 375
Hydrometrocolpos, 236-237
Hydronephrosis, 194, 201-203
Hydrostatic enema, 122
Hydrosyringomyelia, 400-401
Hygroma
  cystic, 387
  with meningitis, 366
Hypercalcuria, 225
Hyperparathyroidism
  primary, 324-325
  secondary, 321, 325
Hypertension, 227-228
  adrenal, 228

endocrine, 228
pulmonary, 41
  persistent, of the newborn, 23, 41
  renovascular, 227-228
Hyperthyroidism, 326
Hypertrophic pyloric stenosis, 73
Hypervitaminosis, 326
Hypervitaminosis A, 279
Hypochondroplasia, 333
Hypogammaglobulinemia, 33
Hypogenetic lung, 48
Hypoparathyroidism, 325
Hypopharynx, "ballooning" of, 5, 6f
Hypophosphatasia, 336
Hypoplastic left heart, 159-160
  categorization of, 153-154
  statistics, 154
Hypoplastic left ventricle, 174
Hypoplastic lung, 41
  secondary, 48
Hypoplastic pancreas, 140
Hypoproteinemia, 40
Hypospadias, 207-209
Hypothyroidism, 326
Hypoxia, vasodilatory, 360

## I

Ileal atresia, 81-82
Ileal dilatation, segmental, 80
Ileal hematoma, 104-105
Ileal-cecal intussusception, 120, 121f
Ileitis, backwash, 114
Ileus, neonatal, 73
Iliac bones, "champagne glass," 332
Immunodeficiency, 32-33; *see also* Acquired immunodeficiency syndrome
Imperforate anus, 78
Infants; *see also* Neonates
  brain tumors in, 361
  cortical hyperostosis, 261
  idiopathic scoliosis, 296
  inspiratory stridor, 2
  osteomyelitis, 275, 276
  osteopetrosis, 323
  polycystic kidney disease, 204
  premature
    "hazy lungs," 18b
    head ultrasound screening, 355
    intracranial hemorrhage in, 354
    pulmonary insufficiency, 18b
Infections
  airway, 3-8
  central nervous system, 364-369
  fungal, 36
  head and neck lesions, 390-391
  musculoskeletal, 274-281
  orbital, 404, 409-410
  urinary tract, 216-222
Infectious gastroenteritis, 97, 104
Infectious mononucleosis, 144
Infectious splenomegaly, 144
Inflammation
  airway, 3-8
  head and neck lesions, 390-391
Inflammatory bowel disease, 93, 97, 105, 114

Inguinal hernia, 123
  and hydrocele, 240f, 241
Inhalational injury, 39
Injuries; *see also* Trauma
  duodenal, 268
  growth plate or epiphyseal, 240b, 249-251
  mesenteric, 268
  seat-belt, 268
  straddle-type, 270
  visceral organ, in child abuse, 263-264
Innominate artery
  anomalous, 186-187, 187f
  anomalous compression of, 13
Inspiratory stridor, 2
Insufficiency fracture, 247
Insulinoma, 142
Internal jugular vein, prominent, 391
Interstitial edema, 40
Intestinal lymphangiectasia, 106
Intracranial gyral calcifications, 348
Intracranial hemorrhage
  grading of, 356, 357b
  in premature infants, 354, 355-359
Intradural tumors, 401-402
Intramedullary neoplasms, 401
Intraoperative ultrasound
  with pancreatic neoplasms, 142
  with spinal cord tumors, 401
Intraosseous ganglion, 283, 290
Intraparenchymal hemorrhage, 357b
Intrauterine growth retardation, 362
Intravenous pyelography
  for bladder injury, 270
  for ectopic ureter, 200f, 201
  with horseshoe kidney, 199
  with medullary sponge disease, 204
  with polycystic kidney disease, 204
  with renal agenesis, 197
  with renal duplex, 199
  with ureterocele, 200
  with uretero-vesical junction obstruction, 201
Intraventricular hemorrhage, 356, 357b
Intraventricular tumors, 361
Intussusception, 117, 120-123
  air reduction of, 122-123
  hydrostatic reduction of, 122
  ileal-cecal, 120, 121f
Ischemia, perinatal, 360
Islet cell hyperplasia, 141
Ivemark syndrome, 179
"Ivory" vertebra, 329

## J

Jatene procedure, 167, 173
Jaundice, neonatal, 127-130
  persistent, 126
Jefferson fractures, 295
Jejunal atresia, distal, 81-82
Jejunal hematoma, 104-105
Jeune syndrome, 334
Joubert syndrome, 351
JRA; *see* Juvenile rheumatoid arthritis
Jugular vein
  prominent internal, 391
  thrombosis of, 391

Juvenile angiofibroma, 10
Juvenile idiopathic scoliosis, 296
Juvenile nasopharyngeal angiofibroma, 390
Juvenile nephronophthisis, 204
Juvenile pilocytic astrocytoma, 370
Juvenile polycystic kidney disease, 204
Juvenile polyps, 109, 112-113
Juvenile rheumatoid arthritis, 54, 301, 311

## K

Kasabach-Merritt syndrome, 143
Kasai procedure, 127
Kawasaki syndrome, 134, 162
Kearns-Sayre syndrome, 382
Kidney; *see also under* Renal
　acquired disease, 223-229
　agenesis, 196-197
　congenital abnormalities, 194-205
　development of, 196
　dysfunction, pulmonary edema with, 39
　embryology, 195*f*, 195-196
　horseshoe, 197-199, 198*f*
　leukemia or lymphoma infiltration, 232-233, 233
　masses, 230-234
　　in neonate, 84*b*, 84-85
　multicystic dysplastic, 194, 203
　page, 228
　polycystic disease, 194, 203-204
　pseudokidney, 122
　trauma to, 268-270, 269*f*
Kinky hair syndrome; *see* Menkes' syndrome
Kleeblattschädel syndrome, 298
Klinefelter syndrome, 243
Knee, 301, 309-311
　growth recovery lines, 311
　internal derangement of, 254
　trauma to, 253-255
Knee radiography
　with Blount disease, 310
　with chondromalacia, 255, 309
　with cortical desmoid, 311
　with dorsal defect of patella, 310
　with Osgood-Schlatter disease, 255, 310
　with tibia vara, 311
Kniest syndrome, 335-336
"Knock knees," 310
Krabbe disease, 362, 380-381

## L

Lactic acidosis, 382
Lactobezoar, 74-75, 95
"Lacy" lesions or granulomas, 54
Ladds bands, 75-76, 100, 101
Langerhans cell histiocytosis, 53-54, 278, 283
　bony abnormalities in, 321, 330
　in lung, 50
　orbital, 410
　splenomegaly with, 144
Large bowel; *see also* Colon
　abnormalities, 109-116
　development, 110, 110*f*
　obstruction, neonatal, 77-82
Larsen syndrome, 338
Laryngomalacia, 2, 13
Laryngotracheoesophageal cleft, 90
Lazy bladder, 213

LCH; *see* Langerhans cell histiocytosis
Lead lines, 326-327
Lead poisoning, 326-327
Leaky lung syndrome, 18*b*, 22
Left aortic arch, 182-183, 183*f*
Left coronary artery
　aberrant, 162
　anomalous, 153-154
Left heart
　cardiomegaly, 149-150
　cardiomyopathy, 162
　hypoplastic, 159-160
　　categorization of, 153-154
　lesions, 156, 163
　　categorization of, 153-154
　　obstructive, 159-163
　myocarditis, 162
Left subclavian artery, aberrant, right aortic arch with, 13, 183-184, 184*f*, 185
Left ventricle
　cardiomegaly, 150
　hypoplastic, 174
Left-to-right shunts, 157-159
Legg-Calvé-Perthes syndrome, 306, 308
Leigh disease, 382
Leiomyomas
　esophageal, 94
　gastric, 95
　small bowel, 107
Leiomyosarcoma, 107
Leptomeningeal cyst, 298
Lesch-Nyhan syndrome, 225
Lesions; *see also* Masses; Neoplasms; Tumors
　benign splenic, 143
　bone, 282-292
　　benign, 278
　bony skull, 293, 298
　brain, destructive, 351-352
　cartilaginous, 286-288
　congenital lung, 45-48
　cystic, 289-291
　"dumb-bell shaped," 402
　duodenal, 139
　fibrous, 288-289
　gastric, 139
　head and neck, 386-394
　marrow, 291
　orbital, 404-411
　osseous, 284-286
　splenic, benign, 143
Letterer-Siwe disease, 54
　bony abnormalities in, 330
　splenomegaly with, 144
Leukemia
　bony abnormalities in, 329
　categorization of, 283
　differential diagnosis, 278, 280
　kidney infiltration, 230, 232-233
　metastasis to orbit, 410
　spinal, 402
　splenomegaly with, 144
　testicular involvement, 242
Leukodystrophy, 378
　adrenoleukodystrophy, 378, 381-382
　fibrinoid, 383
　globoid cell, 380

Index    427

lysosomal, 380-381
metachromatic, 378, 380
spongiform, 383
of unknown etiology, 382-384
Levocardia
situs inversus and, 179
situs solitus and, 178-179
Ligament of Treitz, 98
LIP; *see* Lymphocytic interstitial pneumonitis
Lipomas
colonic, 115
of corpus callosum, 346
interhemispheric, 346
small bowel, 107
Lipomeningomyelocele, 397-398
Lissencephaly, 349
Little Leaguer's elbow, 250*b*, 253, 254*f*
Liver; *see also under* Hepatic
fatty, 53
metastasis in, 132
starry-sky appearance of, 127
LLS; *see* Leaky lung syndrome
Lobar emphysema, congenital, 27, 44, 45
Long-bone fractures, 259-260
Lower urinary tract
development and disorders, 206-215
embryology, 207, 208*f*
masses, 206, 214-215
Lung; *see also under* Pulmonary
abscesses, 52
bilateral atelectasis of, 11
congenital abnormalities, 44
congenital cysts, 27
congenital lesions, 45-48
types of, 44
"granular," 19
"hazy," of prematurity, 18*b*
honeycomb, 54, 163
hypogenetic, 48
Langerhans cell histiocytosis in, 50
restrictive, 24-25
tumors, 56-57
vascular branching patterns, 169
Lung disease
chronic, 163
end-stage, 163
Lung disorders, chronic, 50-57
Lye ingestion, 93
Lymphangiectasis, 24
intestinal, 106
Lymphangioma, 387
orbital, 409
splenic, 143
Lymphangioma-hemangioma, 65, 66
Lymphocytic interstitial pneumonitis, 29, 37
in AIDS, 36
Lymphoid hyperplasia, 109, 113
Lymphoma, 95, 278, 283
anterior mediastinal masses with, 62-63
bony abnormalities in, 329
bowel, 97
Burkitt, 63, 392
African, 34
colonic, 116
head and neck, 392
Hodgkin, 63

kidney infiltration, 230, 232-233
metastasis to orbit, 410
middle mediastinal masses with, 64
non-Hodgkin's, 62-63
orbital, 409
pancreatic, 142
small bowel, 106-107
spinal, 402
splenomegaly with, 144
Lysosomal brain disorders, 379-381
Lysosomal leukodystrophy, 380-381
Lysosomal storage disorders, 379-380
Lysosome function, 379

**M**
Macrocephaly, 354, 360-362
Macrocrania, benign, 361
Macroglossia, 14
Madelung deformity of forearm, 334
Magnetic resonance angiography
of aortic injury, 65
of bronchopulmonary sequestrations, 47
of pulmonary sequestration, 27
Magnetic resonance imaging
with acute disseminated encephalomyelitis, 368
with adrenoleukodystrophy, 382
with Alexander disease, 383
with aneurysmal bone cysts, 290
with anomalous innominate artery, 187
of aortic injury, 65
with astrocytoma, 371
avascular necrosis findings, 308, 328
for back pain, 279
with bacterial encephalitis, 367
brain stem glioma on, 372
of bronchopulmonary sequestrations, 47
with Canavan disease, 383
with carotid-cavernous fistula, 408
with caudal regression, 400
with Chiari malformations, 345
with choroid plexus tumors, 375
of coarctation of aorta, 161
with Coats disease, 406
with coloboma, 405
with congenital CNS infections, 365
with corpus callosum agenesis, 346
craniopharyngiomas on, 374
with cryptorchidism, 241
with cysticercosis, 368
with Dandy-Walker syndrome, 350-351
with Dandy-Walker variant, 351
of dermal sinus tract, 399
with dermoid or epidermoid cysts, 373, 390
of diastematomyelia, 399
with discitis, 278
with encephalocele, 345
with ependymomas, 372, 376
gadolinium contrast, with drop mets, 401-402
of ganglioneuroma, 69
giant cell astrocytoma on, 374
with Grave disease, 408
growth plate or epiphyseal trauma, 251*b*
of hemangioblastoma, 372
of hepatic metastasis, 132
with herpes simplex encephalitis, 367
with heterotopias, 350

**428** Index

Magnetic resonance imaging—cont'd
  with hydranencephaly, 352
  with hydrometrocolpos, 237
  for hydrosyringomyelia or syringomyelia evaluation, 401
  with juvenile nasopharyngeal angiofibroma, 390
  large head imaging, 361
  with lipomeningomyelocele, 398
  with lissencephaly, 349
  with lymphoma, 392
  medulloblastoma, 371
  of meningocele, 69
  of mesenchymal hamartoma, 131
  with metachromatic leukodystrophy, 380
  of microphthalmos, 405
  with mucopolysaccharidosis, 380
  of neuroblastoma, 68
  of neurofibroma, 67
  with optic nerve glioma, 407
  with optic nerve meningioma, 407
  with orbital lymphangioma, 409
  with orbital metastases, 410
  with orbital rhabdomyosarcoma, 410
  of osteochondritis dissecans, 310
  with osteoid osteoma, 284
  for osteomyelitis, 276
  with osteosarcoma, 286
  with peliosis hepatis, 131
  with Pelizaeus-Merzbacher disease, 384
  periventricular leukomalacia findings, 359
  with persistent hyperplastic primary vitreous, 406
  with pineal tumors, 376
  with precocious puberty, 239
  with primitive neuroectodermal tumors, 374-375
  of pulmonary sequestration, 27
  with pulmonary sling, 186
  ranula on, 391
  with retinopathy of prematurity, 406
  with rhabdomyosarcoma, 392
  with schizencephaly, 350
  with schwannomas, 373
  for SCIWORA, 295
  spina bifida aperta evaluation, 397
  with spinal cord tumors, 401
  of spinal dermoid or epidermoid, 400
  with spinal neurofibroma, 402
  with subacute sclerosing panencephalitis, 367
  of subdural hemorrhage, 263
  with tethered cord syndrome, 398-399
  of tracheomalacia, 14
  with vein of Galen aneurysm, 360
Majewski syndrome, 334
Malabsorption, 53, 105-106
Male genitals, 240-242
Males
  hypospadias, 207
  urinary tract infection in, 217
Malignant fibrous histiocytoma, 283
Malignant tumors
  of bone, 283-284
  colonic, 116
  hepatic, 131-132
  lower urinary, 214-215
  pancreatic, 142
  of small bowel, 107

Malrotation
  of bowel, 75
  of small bowel, 99f, 99-101, 102f
Marfan syndrome, 332, 339
  middle mediastinal masses in, 64
Marrow hyperplasia, 327
Marrow lesions, 291
Marrow tumors, 283
Masses; *see also* Neoplasms; Tumors
  airway, 8-10
  cardiac, 66
  esophageal, 66, 94
  gastric, 95-96
  head and neck, 392-393
  lower urinary, 214-215
  malignant, lower urinary, 214-215
  mediastinal, 58-70
  middle mediastinal, 63-66
  neonatal bowel, 72-86
  neonatal lung, 16
  posterior mediastinal, 66-69
  renal, 230-234
Mayer-Rokitansky-Küster-Hauser syndrome, 197, 236
McCune-Albright disease, 338
McCune-Albright syndrome, 289
MCDK; *see* Multicystic dysplastic kidney
Meckel diverticulum, 102-103, 103f
Meconium, 21
Meconium ileus, 52, 81
Meconium ileus equivalent, 53
Meconium peritonitis, 82-83
Meconium plug syndrome, 79
Mediastinal masses, 58-70
  anterior mediastinum, 59-63
  differential diagnosis, 58, 59f
  key concepts, 58
  middle mediastinum, 63-66
  mnemonic for, 58
  posterior mediastinum, 66-69
Medullary cystic disease, 204
Medullary pyramids, 226
Medullary sponge disease, 204
Medulloblastoma, 361, 370, 371
  "drop mets," 395, 401
Megacalyces, congenital, 201
Megacolon, functional, 113-114
Megacystis, 213
Megacystis-microcolon syndrome, 213
Melanoma
  of globe, 407
  metastasis to small bowel, 107
MELAS, 382
Melorheostosis, 324
Membranous croup, 5-6
Meningioma
  optic nerve, 407
  spinal, 402
Meningitis, 364, 365-366
Meningocele, 69
Menkes' (kinky hair) syndrome, 261, 336, 382
"Mermaid," 399
MERRF, 382
Mesenchymal hamartoma, 131
Mesenchymal tumors, 239

Mesenteric cysts, 103, 104
  neonatal, 126
Mesenteric injury, 268
Mesoblastic nephroma, 230, 232
Mesonephros embryology, 195-196
Metabolic bone disease, 321, 322-323
Metabolic brain disorders, 378-385
Metachromatic leukodystrophy, 378, 380
Metaiodobenzylguanidine scans, for pheochromocytoma, 228
Metanephros embryology, 196
Metaphyseal dysplasias, 335
Metastases
  to bone, 278, 280
  "drop mets," 278, 395, 401-402
  of globe, 407
  hepatic, 132
  orbital, 410
  pulmonary, 56-57
  to skull, 298
  small bowel, 107
  to spine, 401-402
Metatarsus adductus, 314, 316$f$, 316-317
Microcolon, 81, 82
  megacystis-microcolon syndrome, 213
  neonatal, 72
Microileum, 82
Microphthalmos, 405
Middle cerebral artery, resistive index of, 357, 358$f$
  with hypoxia, 360
Midfoot, 314, 315
Midgut
  abnormalities of, 97-108
  acquired pathology of, 104-107
  congenital pathology, 99-104
  cysts, 103-104
  development of, 98$f$, 98-99
Midgut volvulus, 97, 100, 101
  bowel obstruction with, 124
  neonatal, 75-76
Mineralization, abnormal, 336-337
"Missing tracheal segment" sign, 33
Mitochondrial brain disorders, 382
Mitochondrial encephalomyopathies, 382
Mitochondrial function, 382
Mitochondrial myopathy, 382
Mixed germ cell tumors, 61
Mononucleosis, 8
Morgagni hernia, 25
Morphine overdose, 39
Morquio syndrome, 337, 378, 379
MRI; *see* Magnetic resonance imaging
Mucocutaneous lymph node syndrome, 134
Mucoepidermoid carcinoma, 393
Mucopolysaccharidoses, 337, 378, 379-380
  macrocephaly with, 362
  macroglossia with, 14
Mucormycosis, 36
Mucoviscidosis, 51-53
Mucus plugs, 26
Multicystic dysplastic kidney, 194, 203
Multilocular cystic nephroma, 232
Multiple pneumonia, 32-33
  in AIDS, 36-37
  differential diagnosis, 29

Muscular trauma, 256-257
Musculoskeletal system, 273-340
  infection, 274-281
  trauma, 246-257
Mustard procedure, 167
Mustard-Senning technique, 174
Mycetoma, 35
Myelination, 344
Myelocystocele, 398
Myelography, with drop mets, 401-402
Myelomeningocele; *see* Spina bifida aperta
Myocardial infarction, 392
Myocarditis, left heart, 162
Myopathy, mitochondrial, 382
Myositis ossificans, 256-257
Myositis ossificans progressiva, 256-257
Myositis ossificans traumatica, 256
Myxoma, cardiac, 66

**N**

Nasopharyngeal angiofibroma, juvenile, 390
Nasopharyngeal teratoma, 390
Naumoff syndrome, 334
Near-drowning, 39
Neck; *see* Head and neck
Neck radiography
  for hemangiomas, 9
  for macroglossia, 14
  for papilloma, 9
  for tracheomalacia, 14
Necrotizing encephalomyopathy, subacute, 382
Necrotizing enterocolitis, 118-119
Neimann-Pick disease, 283
Neonates
  abdomen, 72-86
  acute renal failure, 223, 224
  adrenoleukodystrophy, 381
  aspiration, 21
  bowel masses, 72-86
  bowel obstruction, 73-82
  chest, 16-28
    medically treated conditions, 17-25
    surgically treated conditions, 25-27
  distended bowel loops, 72
  head, 354-363
    congenital anomalies, 359-360
    large, evaluation of, 360-361
    ultrasound of, 354, 355, 355$f$
  hepatitis, 127
  jaundice, 127-130
    persistent, 126
  normal radiography of, 72
  osteomyelitis, 276
  pneumonia, 21-22
  polycystic kidney disease, 204
  respiratory distress in, 16
  torticollis, 390
  transient tachypnea of the newborn, 17
Neoplasms; *see also* Masses; Tumors
  brain, 370-377
  female gonads, 239-240
  head and neck masses, 392-393
  male genitalia, 242
  ovarian, 239-240
  pancreatic, 142

Neoplasms—cont'd
  of spine, 395, 401-402
  supratentorial, 373-376
Neoplastic adenopathy, 64
Nephroblastomatosis, 231
Nephrocalcinosis, 225-226
Nephroma
  mesoblastic, 230, 232
  multilocular cystic, 232
Nephronophthisis, juvenile, 204
Nephropathy, reflux, 217, 226
Nephrotoxic agents, 225
Nesidioblastosis, 141-142
Neural tube closure, 343
  disorders of, 344-345
Neurenteric cysts, 65, 87, 91, 400
Neuroblastoma, 67-68, 361
  bone lesions, 283
  head and neck, 392
  malignant, 68
  metastasis to bone, 278, 280
  metastasis to lung, 56
  metastasis to orbit, 410
  metastasis to skull, 298
  spinal, 402
  staging, 68
Neuroectodermal tumors, primitive, 361, 374
Neurofibroma, 67
  lower urinary, 214
  spinal, 402
Neurofibromatosis, 347-348
  hallmark findings, 342
Neurogenic bladder, 206, 211
Neurologic system, 341-411
Neuronal differentiation, disorders of, 347-349
Neuronal migration, 343-344
  disorders of, 349-350
Neuronal proliferation, 343
  disorders of, 347-349
Neurulation, 396
Neutropenic colitis, 115
Newborn; *see* Neonates
NF; *see* Neurofibromatosis
NHL; *see* Non-Hodgkin's lymphoma
Niemann-Pick disease, 379
Nocturnal enuresis, 212
NOF; *see* Nonossifying fibroma
Non-Hodgkin's lymphoma, 62-63
  head and neck, 392
Nonossifying fibroma, 288
  in knee, 309
Nonrenal retroperitoneal masses, 84*b*
Noonan syndrome
  intestinal lymphangiectasia in, 106
  lymphangiectasia in, 24
  lymphangioma-hemangioma in, 65
  middle mediastinal masses in, 64
Norwood procedure, 174
Nuclear medicine; *see also specific radiopharmaceuticals*
  bone scans
    for avascular necrosis of hip, 308
    for back pain, 279
    child abuse screening, 259
    for discitis, 278
    fracture findings, 247
    for osteomyelitis, 274, 276
    stress fractures, 248
  for choledochal cysts, 130
  cystography, 219
  for gastroesophageal reflux disease, 92
  for hemangioendothelioma, 131
  liver scans
    with biliary atresia, 128
    for neonatal hepatitis, 127
  for multicystic dysplastic kidney, 203
  for patent omphalomesenteric duct, 103
  for pheochromocytoma, 228
  for pulmonary embolus, 43
  for reflux nephropathy, 226
  reflux studies, 32, 219
  for renal artery stenosis, 227
  for testicular torsion, 235, 242
  for uretero-pelvic junction obstruction, 202
  for uretero-vesical junction obstruction, 201
Nursemaid's elbow, 253, 255*f*

O

Obstruction
  airway, by foreign body, 9-10
  choanal, 10
  neonatal bowel, 72-86
  posterior urethral valves, 213-214
Obstructive airway disease, 30
Oligodendroglioma, 376
Oligohydramnios, 196
Ollier disease, 286, 338
Omental cysts, 103, 104, 126
Omphalocele, 85
Omphalomesenteric (vitelline) duct
  patent, 102-103, 103*f*
  types of, 102, 103*f*
Optic nerve glioma, 404, 407
Orbital infection, 409-410
Orbital lesions, 404-411
Ortolani maneuver, 302
Osgood-Schlatter disease, 255, 310
Osseous lesions, 284-286
Ossifying fibroma, 283, 288
Osteoblastoma, 278, 283, 284-285
Osteochondritis dissecans, 310
Osteochondroma, 283, 286-287
Osteochondromatoses, 338
Osteodystrophy, renal, 321, 325
Osteogenesis imperfecta, 261, 332
Osteogenic sarcoma, 280
  metastatic to lung, 56
Osteoid osteoma, 278, 283, 284
  giant, 285
Osteoma, 283, 284
  osteoid, 278, 283, 284
  giant, 285
Osteomalacia, 321, 323
Osteomyelitis, 274, 275-277, 278, 279
  in knee, 309
  with sickle cell anemia, 321, 327
Osteopathia striata, 324
Osteopenia, 321, 322, 336
Osteopetrosis, 261, 323-324, 336
Osteophytes, talar, 319
Osteopoikilosis, 324
Osteoporosis, 322-323

Osteosarcoma, 282, 283, 285-286
  in knee, 309
Osteosclerosis, 321, 323-324
  dysplasias with, 336-337
Ostium primum, 158
Ostium secundum, 158
Ovarian cysts, 126
Ovarian neoplasms, 235, 239-240
Ovarian torsion, 235, 237

**P**

Pachygyria, 349
Page kidney, 228
Pain, back, 279
  nontraumatic, 274, 278
Paintbrush finding, 204
Pancreas, 137-145
  acquired malformations of, 140-142
  annular, 77, 138-139
  congenital malformations of, 138-140
  development of, 138, 138$f$
  ectopic, 95-96, 139
  hypoplastic, 140
  neoplasms of, 142
  trauma to, 267-268
Pancreas divisum, 139
Pancreatic ducts, mucus inspissation of, 141
Pancreatitis, 137, 140-141
  traumatic, 266, 267
Pancreatoblastoma, 142
Papillomas, 8-9
  choroid plexus, 361, 375
PAPVR; see Partial anomalous pulmonary venous return
Paraduodenal hernia, 100
Parasitic encephalitis, 367-368
Parathyroid disorders, 324-325
Parenchymal bronchogenic cysts, 91
Parenchymal hemorrhagic lesions, 263
Parinaud syndrome, 375
Parosteal osteosarcoma, 285
Partial anomalous pulmonary venous return, 24
Patella, 309-310
Patent ductus arteriosus, 153, 156, 157-158
  surgical corrections and palliative procedures for, 173
  therapy for, 172
Patent urachus, 210, 210$f$
PDA; see Patent ductus arteriosus
Peliosis hepatis, 131
Pelizaeus-Merzbacher disease, 384
Pelkan sign, 322
Pelvis
  radiography of, 303, 305$f$
    with hip effusion, 307-308
    with septic arthritis, 277-278
  ultrasound of
    with ambiguous external genitalia, 243
    with precocious puberty, 238-239
Peptic ulcer disease, 87, 94-95
Peribronchial cuffing or edema, 30
Pericardial cysts, 66
Pericardial effusion, 162
Perihilar infiltrates, 30
Perinatal asphyxia, 360
Perinatal polycystic kidney disease, 203-204

Periosteal osteosarcoma, 285
Periosteal reaction, 260, 274, 279-280
  differential diagnosis, 261
  physiologic, 260
Periostitis
  diffuse symmetric, 279
  "sunburst," 286
Periventricular leukomalacia, 354, 358-359
Perkin's line, 303, 305$f$
Peroxisomal brain disorders, 381-382
Peroxisomal function, 381
  general loss, 381
  single loss, 381-382
Persistent fetal circulation, 23
Persistent hyperplastic primary vitreous, 405-406
Persistent pulmonary hypertension of the newborn, 23, 41
Pertussis, 34-35
Pes cavus, 318, 319$f$
Pes planus, 318, 319$f$
Peutz-Jeghers syndrome, 95, 113
pH probe evaluation of gastroesophageal reflux disease, 93
Pheochromocytoma, 223, 228
Phytobezoar, 95
PIE; see Pulmonary interstitial emphysema
Pierre Robin syndrome, 14
"Pig bronchus," 12
Pilocytic astrocytoma, 371
  juvenile, 370
Pineal cysts, 375
Pineal tumors, 375-376
  "drop mets," 401
Pineoblastoma, 375
Pineocytoma, 375
"Pink Tet," 166
Pituitary disorders, 326
"Plastic" fractures, 247, 248$f$
Pleomorphic adenoma, 393
Plicae colicularis, 213
Pneumatosis, 80
Pneumatosis intestinalis, 112
Pneumococcal pneumonia, 29
*Pneumocystis carinii* pneumonia, 29, 36
Pneumomediastinum, neonatal, 16, 19, 20
Pneumonia, 29-37
  neonatal, 21-22, 26
  "round," 29, 31
Pneumoperitoneum, 118
Pneumothorax
  with diaphragmatic hernia, 25
  neonatal, 16, 19-20
Polycystic kidney disease, 194, 203-204
  autosomal dominant, 194, 204
  autosomal recessive, 203-204
  infantile, 204
  juvenile, 204
  neonatal, 204
  perinatal, 203-204
Polyhydramnios, 101
Polymicrogyria, 349
Polyposis syndromes, 113
Polyps
  colonic, 115
  gastric, 95
  hairy, 390

Polyps—cont'd
    juvenile, 109, 112-113
    lower urinary, 214
    small bowel, 107
Polysplenia, 152, 177, 178, 178f, 179, 180
Pompe disorder, 162
Porencephaly, 351, 352
Portal hypertension, 144
Portal vein, preduodenal, 77
Portal venous gas, 118-119
Posterior fossa
    disorders, 350-351
    lesions, 370, 371-373
    tumors, 361
Posterior laminar line, 294, 294f
Posterior rib fractures, 260
Potter's syndrome, 196
Pott's disease, 33, 297
Potts operation, 174
PPHN; see Persistent pulmonary hypertension of the newborn
Preduodenal portal vein, 77
Premature infants; see also Infants; Neonates
    "hazy lungs," 18b
    head ultrasound screening, 355
    intracranial hemorrhage in, 354, 355-359
    pulmonary insufficiency of, 18b
Prenatal ultrasound
    for anencephaly, 344
    with cystic adenomatoid malformation, 46
    of duodenal atresia or stenosis, 75
Primitive neuroectodermal tumors, 361, 374-375
Pronephros, 195
Prostaglandin administration
    bone toxicity, 327
    differential diagnosis, 279
    gastric distension with, 75
Proximal femoral focal deficiency, 333
Proximal small bowel obstruction, 77
Prune-belly (Eagle-Barrett) syndrome, 206, 211-212
    megacystis in, 213
Pseudocoarctation of aorta, 161, 189
Pseudohermaphrodites, 243
Pseudohypoparathyroidism, 325
Pseudo-Jefferson fracture, 295
Pseudokidney, 122
Pseudomembranous colitis, 114
Pseudoobstruction, bowel, 80
Pseudoprune, 212
Pseudosubluxation, 293, 294, 294f
Pseudotruncus, 168, 170
Pseudotumors
    bony, 329
    orbital, 408
    thymic, 60
Puberty, precocious, 237-239
Pulmonary arteriovenous malformations, 42, 47-48
Pulmonary artery
    abnormalities of, 40-41
        acyanotic, 163
    aortic shunts to, 174
    hypoplastic, 41
    "pruned-tree," 41
    stenosis, 163

Pulmonary atresia, 153, 168-169
Pulmonary blastoma, 56
Pulmonary blood flow, 38-43
    decreased, 152
        cyanotic heart disease with, 153, 154, 166-169
    increased, 152
        cyanotic heart disease with, 153, 154, 169-170
    radiographic approach to, 151-152
    redistribution of, 40
    symmetry of, 152
Pulmonary edema, 39-40
    mechanisms for, 38, 39
    neonatal, 22-23
Pulmonary emboli, 38, 42-43
Pulmonary hemorrhage
    idiopathic, 55
    neonatal, 22
Pulmonary hemosiderosis, 55
Pulmonary hypertension, 41
    idiopathic primary, 163
    persistent, of the newborn, 23, 41
Pulmonary hypoplasia, 23-24, 41
    bilateral renal agenesis with, 196
    secondary, 48
Pulmonary insufficiency of the premature, 18b
Pulmonary interstitial emphysema, 18b, 19
Pulmonary sequestration, 26-27
Pulmonary sling, 186, 186f
    with tracheomalacia, 13
Pulmonary stenosis
    critical, 153
Pulmonary thromboembolic disease, 42-43
Pulmonary varix, 42
Pulmonary vasculitis, 55
Pulmonary veins
    abnormalities, 41-42
    "meandering," 42
    pruning appearance, 163
Pulmonary venous return
    cardiac, 41
    infradiaphragmatic, 41
    partial anomalous, 42
    supracardiac, 41
    total anomalous, 41
Pulsus tardus and parvis, 227
Purified protein derivative (PPD) test, 33
PVL; see Periventricular leukomalacia
Pyknodysostosis, 324, 334-335
Pyle dysplasia, 337
Pyloric atresia, 73
Pyloric muscle, 73, 74f

R
"Raccoon eyes," 410
"Rachitic rosary," 323
RAD; see Reactive airway disease
Radiation-induced osteosarcoma, 285-286
Radiography
    abdominal; see Abdominal radiography
    of abdominal trauma, 266
    of adamantinoma, 289
    airway, for Epstein-Barr virus, 34
    of aneurysmal bone cysts, 290
    approach to congenital heart disease, 149-153
        repair findings, 174-175

for avascular necrosis of hip, 308
with back pain, 279
bony findings
　with eosinophilic granuloma, 330
　in hypothyroidism, 326
　in lead poisoning, 326-327
　osteomyelitic, 276
　of thalassemia, 327
chest; *see* Chest radiography
with childhood osteomyelitis, 276
of chondroblastoma, 287
of chondromyxoid fibroma, 287
with chondrosarcoma, 288
DDH examination, 303
of diastematomyelia, 399
with discitis, 278
of enchondroma, 286
with epiphyseal osteomyelitis, 277
with Ewing sarcoma, 291
facial
　for juvenile angiofibroma, 10
　for juvenile nasopharyngeal angiofibroma, 390
of fibrous cortical defect, 288
of fibrous dysplasia, 289
of foot, 315, 315*f*, 316
fracture findings, 247
with gastric volvulus, 96
greenstick fractures, 247
growth plate or epiphyseal trauma, 250*b*, 251*b*
for hip effusion, 307-308
of imperforate anus, 78
of intraosseous ganglion, 290
with juvenile rheumatoid arthritis, 311
knee; *see* Knee radiography
leukemia findings, 329
Little Leaguer's elbow, 253
myositis ossificans traumatica, 256
neck; *see* Neck radiography
with neonatal or infantile osteomyelitis, 276
with neurogenic bladder, 211
normal neonatal, 72
nursemaid's elbow, 253
of ossifying fibroma, 288
with osteoblastoma, 285
of osteochondroma, 287
with osteoma, 284
with osteomalacia, 323
of osteomyelitis, 274
with osteosarcoma, 286
of pelvis, 303, 305*f*
　with hip effusion, 307-308
　with septic arthritis, 277-278
of periosteal reaction, 280
with renal osteodystrophy, 325
scoliosis evaluation, 296
skull
　with craniosynostosis, 299
　with epidermoid cyst, 291
spinal, with Schmorl node, 298
stress fractures, 248
for surfactant deficiency disorder, 26
Toddler's fracture, 249
torus fractures, 248
with unicameral bone cysts, 290
for Wilson-Mikity syndrome, 21

"Ragged red fibers," 382
Ranula, 391
Rashkind procedure, 174
Rastelli operation, 174
Reactive airway disease, 50, 51
Rectosigmoid ratio, 80
Reflux
　gastroesophageal, 32, 87, 92-93
　vesicoureteral, 217, 219-221
Reflux esophagitis, 87
Reflux nephropathy, 217, 221, 226
Refsum disease, 381
Renal arteriovenous malformation or aneurysm, 228
Renal artery stenosis, 223, 227
Renal blastema, 231
Renal cell carcinoma, 230, 233
Renal cysts, 126
Renal duplex, 199-201
　with ectopic ureter, 200-201, 201*f*
　with ureterocele, 199-200, 200*f*
Renal ectopia, 197
　crossed-fused, 197, 198*f*
Renal failure
　acute, 224-225
　neonatal, 223
　chronic, 226-227
Renal hamartoma, fetal, 230, 232
Renal medical disease, 225
Renal osteodystrophy, 321, 325
Renal scans, with dimercaptosuccinic acid, 219
Renal ultrasound
　with chronic glomerulonephritis, 226
　with chronic renal failure, 227
　with glomerulonephritis, 224-225
　with hemolytic uremia, 225
　with renal artery stenosis, 227
　with renal vein thrombosis, 224
　spina bifida aperta evaluation, 397
　with Tamm-Horsfall proteinuria, 224
　for UTI imaging, 218-219
Renal vein thrombosis, 224
Rendu-Osler-Weber syndrome, 42, 47
Renovascular hypertension, 227-228
Resistive index of middle cerebral artery, 357, 358*f*
　with hypoxia, 360
Respiratory distress, in newborn, 16
Respiratory distress syndrome; *see* Surfactant deficiency disorder
Respiratory syncytial virus, 29, 30
Restrictive lung, 24-25
Reticulum cell sarcoma, 283
Retinitis, 54
Retinoblastoma, 404, 406-407
Retinopathy of prematurity, 404, 406
Retrograde urethrography
　for urethral injury, 271
　for urethral strictures, 214
Retrolental fibrodysplasia, 404, 406
Retropharyngeal abscess, 7-8, 8
　cervical adenopathy with, 391
Rhabdomyoma, 66
Rhabdomyosarcoma
　bone, 283
　head and neck, 386, 392

Rhabdomyosarcoma—cont'd
  lower urinary, 214
  male genital, 242
  metastatic to lung, 56
  orbital, 410
  vaginal, 240
Rheumatic fever, 162
Rheumatoid arthritis, 54
  juvenile, 301, 311
RI; *see* Resistive index
Ribs
  deformities with congenital heart disease, 153
  paddle-shaped, 337
Rickets, 261, 321, 323
Right aortic arch, 183-185, 184*f*
  with aberrant left subclavian artery, 183-184, 184*f*
    with tracheomalacia, 13
  with isolated left subclavian artery, 185
  with mirror-image branching, 184*f*, 184-185
Right subclavian artery, aberrant or isolated, left aortic arch with, 183, 183*f*
Right ventricle
  cardiomegaly, 149
  double outlet, 167
Rolland-Desbuquois dyssegmental dysgenesis, 339
ROP; *see* Retinopathy of prematurity
Rosenthal fibers, 383
Round cell tumors, 283
Round pneumonia, 29, 31
"Rugger-jersey" spine, 325

## S

Sacrococcygeal teratoma, 400
"Sail sign," 61
Saldino-Noonan syndrome, 334
Salivary gland tumors, 392-393
Salter-Harris classification of growth plate injuries, 250*b*-251*b*, 252*f*
Sanfilipo syndrome, 337, 378, 379
Sarcoid, 54-55
Sarcoma; *see also* Rhabdomyosarcoma
  chondrosarcoma, 287-288
  Ewing sarcoma, 280, 283, 291
  metastasis to lung, 56
  metastasis to orbit, 410
  osteogenic, 280
  osteosarcoma, 285-286
  reticulum cell, 283
  undifferentiated embryonal, 132
Sarcoma botryoides, 206, 214
"Saw-tooth" contractions of bowel, 80
SCFE; *see* Slipped capital femoral epiphysis
Scheuermann kyphosis, 297
Schizencephaly, 350
Schmorl node, 297-298
Schwachman syndrome, 140, 335
Schwachman-Diamond syndrome, 140, 335
Schwannomas, 372-373
  spinal, 402
Scimitar syndrome, 48
  hypoplastic pulmonary arteries in, 41
  partial anomalous pulmonary venous return in, 42
  pulmonary hypoplasia in, 23-24
SCIWORA; *see* Significant cord injury without radiographic abnormality
Scleroderma, 54

Sclerosing cholangitis, 135
Sclerosing panencephalitis, subacute, 367
SCM; *see* Sternocleidomastoid muscle
Scoliosis, 293, 295-297
  Cobb measurement, 296, 297*f*
Scrofula, 391
Scurvy, 261, 279
Seat-belt injury, 266, 268
Seminoma, 61-62
Sentinel loop finding, 141
Septic arthritis, 274, 277-278
Septic hip, 305
Septooptic dysplasia, 347
Sertoli-Leydig cell tumors, 239
Sesamoids, 249
Sex differentiation, 242-243
"Shaggy heart," 35
"Shaggy mucosa," 93
Shaken-baby injury, 258, 262*f*, 262-263
Shenton's line, 303
"Shock bowel," 268
Short rib–polydactyly syndromes, 334
Short stature, 332
"Shouldering"
  duodenal bulb, "string sign" with, 73
  subglottic region, 2
Sickle cell anemia, 279
  bony abnormalities in, 321, 327-328
Significant cord injury without radiographic abnormality, 293, 295
Silverman-Handmaker (dyssegmental dysgenesis), 339
Single photon emission computed tomography, for back pain, 279
Single ventricle, 168
  surgical repair for, 173
Sinus venosus, 158
Situs abnormalities, 177-180
Situs ambiguous or indeterminus, 152, 179-180
  branching patterns of, 178, 178*f*
Skeletal dysplasias, 332-340
  with abnormal mineralization or bony density, 336-337
  with macrocephaly, 362
Skeleton
  axial, 293-300
  surveys for child abuse, 258, 259
Skull, 298-299
  bony lesions, 293, 298
  cloverleaf, 299
  "hair-on-end," 327
  metastases, 298
  radiography of
    with craniosynostosis, 299
    with epidermoid cyst, 291
Skull fractures, 298
  in child abuse, 260-261
Slipped capital femoral epiphysis, 308-309
Sludge, 134
SMA syndrome, 106
Small blue cell tumors, 242, 374
Small bowel abnormalities, 97-108
  acquired pathology, 104-107
  atresia
    "apple-peel," 81
    types of, 81, 83*f*

congenital pathology, 99-104
cysts, 103-104
malrotation, 99f, 99-101
obstruction
 distal, 77-82
 proximal, 77
tumors, 106-107
Snowman finding, 170
"Soap-bubble" finding, 81
Soft tissues
with congenital heart disease, 152-153
trauma to, 256-257
Sonography; *see* Ultrasound
Special Olympics, imaging for Down syndrome participants, 295
SPECT; *see* Single photon emission computed tomography
Spherocytosis, 144
Spina bifida aperta, 395, 397
Spina bifida cystica, 395, 397-398
Spinal dysraphism, 395
categorization of, 397-399
occult, 395, 398-399
Spinal radiography, with Schmorl node, 298
Spine, 294-298, 395-403
canalization with retrogressive differentiation, 396f, 396-397
development of, 396-401
 abnormal, 397-401
key concepts, 395
metastasis to, 401-402
 drop mets, 401-402
neoplasms of, 395, 401-402
 extramedullary or intradural, 401-402
 intramedullary, 401
normal variants, 293, 294-295
"rugger-jersey," 325
significant cord injury without radiographic abnormality, 293, 295
Spleen, 137-145
accessory, 142
acquired malformations of, 143-144
ambiguous situs, 142
asplenia, 177, 178, 178f, 179
benign lesions of, 143
congenital malformations of, 142-143
ectopic, 143
injury to, 266, 267
polysplenia, 177, 178, 178f, 179, 180
size guidelines, 143-144
wandering, 143
Splenomegaly, 137, 144
Splenules, accessory, 142
Spondyloepiphyseal dysplasia, 335
Spondylolysis, 278, 279
Spondylometaphyseal dysplasia, 335
Spongiform leukodystrophy, 383
"Stack of coins" finding, 105, 263
*Staphylococcus aureus*, 34
"Starry-sky" finding, 127
"Steepling" or steeple sign, 2, 3, 5, 6f
Sternocleidomastoid muscle, benign enlargement of, 386, 390
Sternotomy, 174-175
Still disease, 311

Stomach; *see also under* Gastric
abnormalities, 87-96
congenital malformations, 87
development, 89, 89f, 98, 98f
neonatal distension, 73-75
pathology, 94-96
Storage diseases; *see also specific diseases*
splenomegaly with, 144
Straddle-type injuries, 270
Strawberry hemangioma, 386, 389
orbital, 407
Stress fractures, 247-248, 248f
differential diagnosis, 279
"Stress" images, for hip instability, 304, 307f
String sign, 105
with "shouldering," 73
Sturge-Weber syndrome, 348
Subacute sclerosing panencephalitis, 367
Subclavian artery
aberrant left, right aortic arch with, 13, 183-184, 184f, 185
aberrant or isolated right, left aortic arch with, 183, 183f
Subclavian artery patch, 174
Subdural effusions, 366
Subdural hemorrhage, 262-263
Subglottic narrowing, 3, 6f
Subglottic region, "shouldering" of, 2
Subluxation, atlantoaxial, 294-295
Subperiosteal hemorrhage, 260
Sulcation, disorders of, 349-350
"Sunburst" periostitis, 286
Superior mesenteric artery; *see* SMA
Suprasellar craniopharyngiomas, 374
Supratentorial lesions, 370, 373-376
Surfactant B deficiency, 17-19
Surfactant deficiency disorder, 16, 17-19
classification of, 18b
evolving, 18b
hallmark radiographic findings, 26
Surgery; *see also specific procedures*
congenital heart disease repair, 173-174
intraoperative ultrasound
 with pancreatic neoplasms, 142
 with spinal cord tumors, 401
Swallowing dysfunction, 32
Sweat test, 52
Swyer-James syndrome, 33, 41
Synostosis
coronal, 298
lambdoid, 298-299
metopic, 298
sagittal, 298
Synovitis, toxic, 305-306
Syphilis, 279
Syringomyelia, 401
Systemic lupus erythematosus, 54

**T**

Tachypnea, transient, of the newborn, 17
*Taenia solium*, 367
Talar breaks, 319
Talar line, 314, 315
Talar osteophytes, 319

Talus
  congenital vertical, 317-318, 318f
  oblique, 318
Tamm-Horsfall proteinuria, 223, 224
TAPVR; see Total anomalous pulmonary venous
    return
Tarsal coalition, 314, 318-319
Taussig-Bing syndrome, 167
Tay-Sachs disease, 362, 379
"Teardrop" distance, 277-278
Technetium-99m scans
  disopropyl iminodiacetic acid, of liver, 127
  with hemangioendothelioma, 131
  for osteomyelitis, 274, 276
  pertechnetate, of patent omphalomesenteric
    duct, 103
  sulfur
    for gastroesophageal reflux disease, 93
    with hepatic adenoma, 131
    with testicular torsion, 242
Telangiectatic osteosarcoma, 285
Teratocarcinoma, 61
Teratoma, 61, 361, 400
  gastric, 95
  nasopharyngeal, 390
  ovarian, 239
  pineal, 375
  sacrococcygeal, 400
Testicular feminization, 243
Testicular torsion, 235, 241-242, 242f
Tethered cord syndrome, 395, 398-399
Tetralogy of Fallot, 153, 166
  cardiomegaly with, 149
  components of, 165
  statistics, 154
"Texas longhorn" finding, 346
Thalassemia, bony abnormalities in, 327
Thanatophoric dwarfism, 333
"Third eye," 404
Thoracic bony cage abnormalities, 48
Thoracotomy, 175
Thorax, bell-shaped, 24
Thromboembolic disease, pulmonary, 42-43
Thrombosis, with meningitis, 366
Thumbprint sign
  with bowel edema, 2, 115
  with epiglottitis, 7, 7f
"Thymic wave," 61
Thymolipoma, 60
Thymoma, 60
Thymus, 60-61
  absent, 32
Thyroglossal duct
  cyst, 387-388, 388f
  persistent, 387-388
Thyroid disorders, 325-326
Tibia, Toddler's fracture, 248-249
Tibia vara, 310, 311
Toddler's fracture, 246, 248-249
TOF; see Tetralogy of Fallot
TORCH infections, 364, 365
  neonatal, 359
Torticollis, 390
Torus or buckle fractures, 248, 248f

Total anomalous pulmonary venous return, 153,
    165, 169-170
Toxic synovitis, 305-306
Toxicity, 326
Tracheal agenesis or atresia, 11, 12f
Tracheal bronchus, 12
Tracheitis, bacterial, 5-6
Tracheobronchitis, 2
Tracheoesophageal cleft, 32
Tracheoesophageal fistula, 14, 32, 90
  esophageal atresia with, 88-90, 89f
  esophageal atresia without, 88-89, 89f
  H-type, 87, 89f, 90
  types of, 88-89, 89f
Trachcoesophageal septum, 11, 11f
Tracheolaryngobronchitis, acute, 3-5
Tracheomalacia, 13-14
"Tram tracks"
  with bronchiectasis, 53
  in Sturge-Weber syndrome, 348
Transfusion reaction, 39
Transient tachypnea of the newborn, 17
Transposition of great vessels, 165, 166-168,
    170, 190
  corrected, 167, 191
  D loop, 190
  L loop, 191
  large shunt, 153
  small shunt, 153
  surgical repair for, 173, 174
Trauma, 245-272
  abdominal, 266-272
  bladder, 270
  bowel, 268
  elbow, 251-253
  hepatic, 267
  knee, 253-255
  muscular, 256-257
  musculoskeletal, 246-257
  nonaccidental, 258-265
  pancreatic, 267-268
  renal, 268-270, 269f
  soft tissue, 256-257
  splenic, 267
  ureters, 270
  urethral, 270-271
  urinary tract, 268-271
Treacher Collins syndrome, 10
Treitz, ligament of, 98
Trevor disease, 335
Trichobezoar, 95
Trichorhinophalangeal dysplasia, 334
Tricuspid atresia, 153, 168, 173
Truncus arteriosus, 153, 170, 189-190
TTN; see Transient tachypnea of the newborn
Tuberculosis, 33
Tuberculous adenitis, 390
Tuberous sclerosis, 348, 362
Tumors; see also Masses; Neoplasms
  adrenocortical, 228
  brain
    in children, 361
    in infants, 361
  "brown tumors," 325

choroid plexus, 375
colonic, 115-116
germ cell, 61-62
 ovarian, 239
 pineal, 375
lower genitourinary tract, 206
macrocephaly and, 361
marrow, 283
pineal, 375-376
posterior fossa, 361
pulmonary, 56-57
round cell, 283
salivary gland, 392-393
small blue cell, 242, 374
small bowel, 106-107
thymic, 60
vaginal, 240
Wilms tumor, 231-232
Turner syndrome, 242-243
 horseshoe kidney in, 199
 lymphangioma-hemangioma in, 65
 middle mediastinal masses in, 64
Typhlitis, 115

**U**
Ulcerative colitis, 109, 114
Ulcers
 "cobble-stone ulcerations," 105
 peptic ulcer disease, 94-95
Ultrasound; *see also* Doppler ultrasound
 for abdominal trauma, 266
 angiomyolipoma on, 233
 of annular pancreas, 139
 of appendicitis, 120
 with benign macrocrania, 361
 of benign splenic lesions, 143
 of biliary atresia, 127-128
 biliary tree dilatation, 135
 with cervical adenopathy, 391
 of choledochal cysts, 130
 with choroid plexus tumors, 375
 of coarctation of aorta, 161
 of colonic duplications, 111
 with congenital CNS infections, 365
 with corpus callosum agenesis, 346
 with cryptorchidism, 241
 DDH examination, 301, 303-304
 of dermal sinus tract, 399
 dermoid or epidermoid, 390, 400
 dynamic "stress" images for hip instability (Harcke views), 304, 307*f*
 with dyssynergia, 213
 with ectopic spleen, 143
 with fibromatosis colli, 390
 of gallstones, 134
 with gastric duplications, 94
 Graf classification of acetabula, 306, 307*f*
 head
 in neonates, 354
 of perinatal asphyxia, 360
 screening for premature infants, 355
 with vein of Galen aneurysm, 360
 of hemangioendothelioma, 130-131
 of hemangioma, 130, 389

 of hematoma, 105
 of hemolytic uremia, 115
 with hepatic cirrhosis, 133
 with hepatoblastoma, 132
 with hepatocellular carcinoma, 132
 for hip effusion, 301, 306-307
 with horseshoe kidney, 199
 with hydranencephaly, 352
 with hydrocele, 241
 with hydrocephalus, 361
 with hydrometrocolpos, 237
 with hypertrophic pyloric stenosis, 73
 of hypoplastic pancreas, 140
 of imperforate anus, 78
 with infectious gastroenteritis, 104
 of inguinal hernia, 123
 intracranial hemorrhage on, 358
 intraoperative
 with pancreatic neoplasms, 142
 with spinal cord tumors, 401
 of intussusception, 122
 large head imaging, 360-361
 of leukemia or lymphoma infiltration in kidneys, 233
 with lipomeningomyelocele, 398
 with lissencephaly, 349
 with lymphangioma, 387
 with lymphoma, 107, 392
 of malignant pancreatic masses, 142
 of malrotation, 101
 of medullary cystic disease, 204
 with medullary sponge disease, 204
 with meningitis complications, 366
 of mesenchymal hamartoma, 131
 of mesenteric, 104
 with mesoblastic nephroma, 232
 of midgut volvulus, 76
 of multicystic dysplastic kidney, 203
 with multilocular cystic nephroma, 232
 neonatal head, 355, 355*f*
 of neonatal hepatitis, 127
 with nephroblastomatosis, 231
 with nesidioblastosis, 142
 with neurogenic bladder, 211
 of neutropenic colitis, 115
 of omental cysts, 104
 for osteomyelitis, 276
 with ovarian torsion, 237
 for pancreatic trauma, 268
 with pancreatitis, 141
 with peliosis hepatis, 131
 pelvic
 with ambiguous external genitalia, 243
 with precocious puberty, 238-239
 periventricular leukomalacia findings, 358-359
 with persistent hyperplastic primary vitreous, 406
 with pheochromocytoma, 228
 of polycystic kidney disease, 204
 with posterior urethral valves, 214
 prenatal
 for anencephaly, 344
 with cystic adenomatoid malformation, 46
 of duodenal atresia or stenosis, 75
 with Prune-belly syndrome, 212

Ultrasound—cont'd
  of pyloric muscle, 73, 74f
  with reflux nephropathy, 226
  renal, spina bifida aperta evaluation, 397
  with renal agenesis, 197
  with renal cell carcinoma, 233
  with renal duplex, 199
  with renal ectopia, 197
  with schizencephaly, 350
  of splenic lymphangioma, 143
  for testicular torsion, 235
  with testicular torsion, 242
  with tethered cord syndrome, 398-399
  with thyroglossal duct cyst, 388
  of undifferentiated embryonal sarcoma, 132
  with unstable bladder, 212
  with urachal cyst, 211
  with ureterocele, 200
  with uretero-vesical junction obstruction, 201
  vaginal tumors on, 240
  with von Hippel-Lindau disease, 140
  Wilms tumor findings, 232
Upper gastrointestinal examination
  of annular pancreas, 77
  of congenital antral webs or diaphragms, 74
  of duodenal stenosis, 102
  with gastric and duodenal lesions, 139
  with hematoma, 105
  with hypertrophic pyloric stenosis, 73
  of malrotation, 101, 102f
  for reflux, 32
  of volvulus, 74, 76, 101, 102f
Urachal anomalies, 206, 210f, 210-211
Urachal cyst, 211
Urachal remnant or diverticulum, 210-211, 210f
Urachus, patent, 210, 210f
*Ureaplasma urealyticum*, 22
Ureterocele, 199-200, 200f
Uretero-pelvic junction obstruction, 201-202
Uretero-vesical junction obstruction, 201, 202
Ureters
  development and disorders, 206-215
  ectopic, 194, 200f, 200-201, 201f
  trauma to, 270
Urethra, 213-214
  development and disorders, 206-215
  injuries to, 270-271
  posterior valves, 213-214
Urethral strictures, 214
Urethrography; *see also* Voiding cystourethrography
  retrograde
    for urethral injury, 271
    for urethral strictures, 214
Urinary tract
  lower
    development and disorders, 206-215
    embryology, 207, 208f
    trauma to, 268-271
Urinary tract infection, 216-222, 217-219
  fluoroscopic examination, 217-218
  imaging modalities, 217-218
  indications for imaging, 217
  nuclear medicine, 219
  renal ultrasound, 218-219
  voiding cystourethrography, 217-218

Urogenital sinus defect, 207
Urologic abnormalities, congenital, 196-204
US; *see* Ultrasound
Uterine malformations, 237, 238f
UTI; *see* Urinary tract infection
Uveitis, 54

**V**
VACTERL, 78
Vaginal tumors, 240
Varicella, 34
Varices, 96
Vascular lesions
  head and neck, 391
  orbital, 408
Vascular rings, 33, 181, 185-187
  with tracheomalacia, 13
VCUG; *see* Voiding cystourethrography
Vein of Galen aneurysm, 359, 360
Venolobar syndrome, 42, 48
Venous varix, 408
Ventilation-perfusion scans, with pulmonary embolus, 43
Ventricular septal defect, 153, 156, 157
  statistics, 154, 155
  surgical repair for, 172, 173
Ventriculitis
  with intracranial hemorrhage, 356
  with meningitis, 365, 366
Ventriculomegaly, 356-357
Vertebra, "ivory," 329
Vertebra plana, 278
Vertebral bodies
  beaked or bullet-shaped, 337, 379
  collapsed, 278
  H-type, 321, 328
Vertical talus, congenital, 317-318, 318f
Vesicoureteral reflux, 216, 217, 219-221
  grading of, 219, 220f
VIPoma, 142
Viral airways disease, 30
Viral croup, 3-5
Visceral organ injury, 263-264
Vitamin A bone toxicity, 326
Vitamin D bone toxicity, 326
Vitelline cyst, 102, 103f
Vitelline duct, patent, 102-103, 103f
Vitelline sinus tract, 102
Vitreous, persistent hyperplastic primary, 405-406
Voiding
  child, 210
  infant, 209
Voiding cystourethrography
  with dyssynergia, 213
  for genitourinary fistula, 78
  with neurogenic bladder, 211
  with posterior urethral valves, 214
  with Prune-belly syndrome, 212
  spina bifida aperta evaluation, 397
  with urachal cyst, 211
  with urachal remnant or diverticulum, 211
  with ureterocele, 200
  with uretero-vesical junction obstruction, 201
  with urethral strictures, 214
  for urinary tract infection, 217-218
    timing of, 218

Volvulus
    gastric, 74, 96
    midgut, 97, 100, 101
        bowel obstruction with, 124
        neonatal, 75-76
Von Hippel-Lindau disease, 140, 348-349
Von Recklinghausen disease, 347-348
VSD; *see* Ventricular septal defect

**W**

Walker-Warburg syndrome, 349
Wandering spleen, 143
Water-soluble contrast studies; *see also* Contrast studies
    of patent omphalomesenteric duct, 103
    of patent urachus, 210
Water-soluble enema, 78-79
    for distal obstruction in neonate, 72
    for meconium ileus, 81
Waterston operation, 174
Wegener granulomatosis, 55

Weigert-Meyer rule, 199
Whitaker test, 202
"White" lung, 26
Whooping cough, 34
Williams syndrome, 225
Wilms tumor, 230, 231-232
    metastatic to lung, 56
Wilson disease, 133
Wilson-Mikity syndrome, 21
Wimberger sign, 322
"Windsock" finding, 102
Wiskott-Aldrich syndrome, 33
Wormian bones, 336

**Y**

Yolk sac, 61, 62
Yolk sac tumors, 239

**Z**

Zellweger (cerebrohepatorenal) syndrome, 381
Zollinger-Ellison syndrome, 94